PHARMACOLOGY - RESEARCH, SAFETY TESTING AND REGULATION

ZOLEDRONIC ACID

CLINICAL USES, THERAPEUTIC EFFECTS AND PHARMACOKINETICS

PHARMACOLOGY - RESEARCH, SAFETY TESTING AND REGULATION

Additional books in this series can be found on Nova's website under the Series tab.

Additional e-books in this series can be found on Nova's website under the e-book tab.

PHARMACOLOGY - RESEARCH, SAFETY TESTING AND REGULATION

ZOLEDRONIC ACID

CLINICAL USES, THERAPEUTIC EFFECTS AND PHARMACOKINETICS

RONALD CARMAN
EDITOR

nova publishers
New York

For permission to use material from this book please contact us:
Telephone 631-231-7269; Fax 631-231-8175
Web Site: http://www.novapublishers.com

Library of Congress Cataloging-in-Publication Data

Library of Congress Control Number: 2014944855

ISBN: 978-1-63321-525-2

Published by Nova Science Publishers, Inc. † New York

CONTENTS

PREFACE

Zoledronic acid is a third generation bisphosphonate which is administered intravenously once yearly at a dose of 5mg for multiple reasons including the treatment of post-menopausal women with osteoporosis to reduce the incidence of vertebral, hip and non-vertebral fractures and to increase bone mineral density (BMD), the prevention of clinical fractures after hip fracture in women and men, treatment of osteoporosis in men, prevention and treatment of glucocorticoid-induced osteoporosis (GIO), the prevention of post-menopausal osteoporosis (in the US) and the treatment of Paget's disease of the bone. This book discusses the clinical uses, therapeutic effects and pharmacokinetics of zoledronic acid.

Chapter 1 - Zoledronic acid is a bisphosphonate that was approved for the treatment of hypercalcemia of malignancy in 2001. Bisphosphonates are hydrolysis-resistant pyrophosphate derivatives that have a high affinity for bone and inhibit osteoclastic bone resorption. A once yearly infusion of zoledronic acid was approved for the treatment of post-menopausal osteoporosis in 2007; this therapy provides an alternative to oral bisphosphonate treatment of post-menopausal osteoporosis which is associated with an inconvenient mode of administration resulting in poor adherence and compliance. Since that time it has also been approved for the prevention of osteoporosis in post-menopausal women, to increase bone mass in men with osteoporosis, to decrease the incidence of new clinical fractures in patients at high risk of fracture (those with a recent low trauma hip fracture) and to treat and prevent glucocorticoid-induced osteoporosis in women and men who are expected to be on glucocorticoids for twelve months or longer. The data concerning combination use of zoledronic acid with other non-bisphosphonate therapy will be reviewed as will data concerning the long-term safety and head-to-head comparisons with other bone active drugs. The use of zoledronic acid in treating special populations will be discussed and suggestions for future research will be presented.

Chapter 2 - The biphosphonate zoledronic acid is indicated for the treatment of patients with osteolytic lesions from multiple myeloma for the prevention of skeletal related events. In patients with multiple myeloma the clonal expansion of plasma cells in the bone marrow results in the disruption of the homeostasis within the bone marrow microenvironment. Interactions between myeloma cells and bone marrow stromal cells directly increase growth and survival of myeloma cells through the dysregulation of growth factors and cytokines and accelerate the destruction of the bone.

Thus, most of multiple myeloma patients develop osteolytic bone lesions, which are often associated with bone pain and skeletal-related events which include spinal cord compression, pathologic fractures, or the need for surgery or radiation to the bone. Bisphosphonates are effective inhibitors of osteoclastic bone resorption. *In-vitro* evidences suggest that bisphosphonates may also have an antimyeloma activity.

Furthermore, they may synergize with anticancer agents used in the treatment of myeloma. Recent clinical data show a survival advantage for high-risk patients receiving zoledronic acid concurrently with antimyeloma therapies. This review summerizes the antimyeloma benefits of zoledronic acid combined with new drugs for the treatment of multiple myeloma patients.

Chapter 3 - Zoledronic acid is a bisphosphonate drug administered as an intravenous infusion which is licensed internationally for the treatment of osteoporosis. Pharmacologically, it can slow down bone resorption, potentiates an anabolic effect on bone-forming cells and promotes bone remodelling. Bone and cartilage turnover are affected in other musculoskeletal conditions including osteoarthritis (OA) and rheumatoid arthritis (RA). OA is the most common arthritic disease worldwide, with an increasing prevalence due to a rising ageing population and the epidemic of obesity worldwide. The most common joints affected in OA include the larger weight-bearing hip and knee joints, the hands and spine. Radiographic examination of affected joints often reveals joint space narrowing, cartilage degradation and bone marrow lesions observed by magnetic resonance imaging (MRI) scans.

Recent interest has focused on evaluating the therapeutic effects of bisphosphonate drugs to target OA pain and structural damage. This chapter presents the results of a systematic review assessing the currently available evidence on zoledronic acid in human and animal studies. In this chapter, the authors report the rationale for using zoledronic acid for OA from animal model data in the studies so far reported, discussing the effects of this drug on bone remodelling and inhibition of cartilage degradation.

The authors discuss how zoledronic acid could target lesions observed in the pathophysiology of OA, which include damage to the components of cartilage extracellular matrix (ECM) and peri-articular bone. The authors then report the effect of zoledronic acid in the clinical studies published so far for people with OA, including data on the use of this bisphosphonate as an adjunct to high tibial osteotomy surgery. The authors also discuss the impact of the use of zoledronic acid on improving knee pain in clinical trials and its effect on reducing the size of bone marrow lesions detected by magnetic resonance imaging (MRI) scans in the same studies.

In summary, this chapter outlines emerging data on the use of the bisphosphonate drug zoledronic acid in OA. Clinical trials published to date have shown an improvement in OA pain in the short term, coupled with an effect on the size of bone marrow lesions following infusion of zoledronic acid. It is possible that treatment with bisphosphonate drugs at earlier stages of the condition, as suggested by animal models of OA, may have a greater impact on modulating disease activity in this chronic, common arthritic disease.

Chapter 4 - Paget's disease of bone (PDB) is characterized by an increase in bone turnover located at one or more foci of the skeleton. The initial pathophysiological mechanism is the increase in osteoclastic bone resorption and bisphosphonates are the most commonly used treatments for PDB. The new bisphosphonates with greater potency and binding affinity to hydroxyapatite, like zoledronic acid, are very useful for short and long-term control of disease activity. Zoledronic acid is indicated for PDB in Europe and America at dose of 5 mg given intravenously. In 2005, a risedronate-controlled trial, showed that zoledronic acid, administered as a single 15 minute infusion is highly effective in controlling metabolic activity in PDB after 6 months of administration. Therapeutic response occurred in 96% of patients (normalization of alkaline phosphatase in 89% and a 75% reduction in 7% of patients), which is significantly superior to the results obtained by the other bisphosphonates, including risedronate, and also improved physical function and overall evaluation (measured by the SF-36 questionnaire). Other studies have demostrated similar results in terms of effectiveness of bone turnover control with a single 5 mg infusion of zoledronic acid. This drug has also proven effective in patients with active PDB that had not responded to other bisphosphonates in the previous 6 months. Regarding duration of response, zoledronic acid was still effective 75 months after a single infusion in most of the patients during the follow-up, with loss of therapeutic response in only 12.5 % of patients. Recently it has been reported that patients who had a relapse after a first dose of zoledronic acid may respond to a new 5 mg intravenous infusion. All these results make zoledronic acid the most effective therapy for the treatment of PDB to date, and the treatment of choice due to its efficiency, adherence and duration of response. The accepted indications for treatment of PDB include bone pain and neurological compression syndromes. Treatment before bone surgery is also recommended to prevent excess bleeding or hypercalcemia. Patients with high metabolic activity (alkaline phosphatase level more than twice the upper limit of normal) should also be treated. A controversial indication is treatment with bisphosphonates in asymptomatic PDB patients to prevent progression or complications. Zoledronic acid has changed the management of PDB. Currently, a 15-minute intravenous zoledronic acid infusion is able to maintain biochemical control of the disease for at least 6.5 years. This has important practical implications in the clinical management of PDB patients. Long-term control of metabolic activity will probably reduce the risk of complications such as deformity, fracture, deafness and degenerative joint disease.

Chapter 5 - Since their introduction to clinical practice more than 3 decades ago, bisphosphonates have been increasingly used for a wide range of skeletal disorders and other conditions including heritable skeletal disorders in children, postmenopausal and glucocorticoid-induced osteoporosis (GIO), and bone metastases in patients with malignancies. Bisphosphonates of first generation have side chains minimally modified (clodronate or etidronate) or a chlorophenyl group (tiludronate). Bisphosphonates of second generation (alendronate or pamidronate) have a nitrogen group in the side chain and their power is 10 to 100 times greater than the first generation compounds. Finally, among third-generation of bisphosphonates (ibandronate, risedronate and zoledronate), the two last with the N atom included in a heterocyclic ring, are 10,000 times more potent than first generation agents. Their main therapeutic use is as antiosteolitic agent in patients with pathologies with increased bone resorption including Paget disease, osteoporosis and tumoral osteolysis and as inhibitors of ectopic calcifications and ossifications. Although bisphosphonates are generally well tolerated, the adverse effects are not rare, and they often produce the interruption of treatment. The adverse effects on the upper gastrointestinal tract are common with oral bisphosphonates, especially if taken incorrectly, so benefits and risk should be weighed. Oral absorption of bisphosphonates is very poor, as they are only absorbed between 1-3%, being higher when administered fasting. Between 20-80% of the absorbed dose is taken up by the bone tissue, and the remaining dose is eliminated unchanged by the kidney. Protein plasma binding is variable between bisphosphonates (50-90%). This chapter describes and discusses the most important therapeutic effects together with the most relevant side-effects associated to the use of bisphosphonates.

Chapter 6 - In the recent decades, evidence has been accumulating concerning *in vivo* and *in vitro* anti-cancer activity of bisphosphonates. These effects are achieved through microevironmental changes, inhibition of tumor cell adhesion, invasion, neoangiogenesis and apoptosis induction. Zoledronic acid is known for its high potency with regard to antitumoral activity and has been to date studied in numerous clinical trials. In the adjuvant setting, postmenopausal patients benefit from zoledronate treatment; in the metastatic situation, zoledronate improves progression-free interval in patients with bone metastasis. Several authors hypothesized that bisphosphonates exhibit their oncologic effects through changes of bone marrow microenvironment making it less suitable for disseminated tumor cells; the presence of such cells in secondary sites is associated with higher risk of relapse and impaired prognosis. In the present review, the authors discuss experimental activity of bisphosphonates and review current data on the use of zoledronate acid in breast cancer patients.

Chapter 7 - Chronic inflammatory rheumatic diseases (CIRD) constitute a heterogeneous group of disorders that include rheumatoid arthritis (RA), systemic lupus erythematosus (SLE), ankylosing spondylitis (AS), psoriatic arthritis (PsA) and other diseases that affect a multiplicity of organs. Currently, it has been well recognized that a close link exists between the immune system and bone tissue, particularly in these disorders. CIRD have a high prevalence of osteoporosis (OP), observed between 25-59% in RA, 20-48% in SLE, 15-60% in AS and around 16% in PsA. Factors associated with OP in CIRD include the over-activation of osteoclasts by inflammatory cytokines, mainly tumor necrosis factor-alpha, and other interleukins (IL) including IL-1beta and IL-6, as well as other mechanisms such as impairment in joint function, and utilization of therapies that increase bone loss, mainly corticosteroids. OP is frequently underdiagnosed in CIRD; therefore, the onset of anti-osteoporotic therapy is delayed. Additionally, these patients have a high frequency of vertebral and non-vertebral fractures, with vertebral fractures being frequently asymptomatic or with non-severe symptoms leading to delays in treatment. Frequencies for vertebral fractures may vary; in RA around 21.7%, in SLE between 20-50%, in AS 19-65% and for PsA around 13%. According to the National Osteoporosis Foundation guidelines, adults with RA or any patient taking prednisone $\geq$5 mg/day or equivalent for $\geq$3 months should be evaluated for bone mineral density (BMD), and strategies to prevent fractures are required. Zoledronic acid (ZA) has been approved for the prevention and treatment of osteoporosis in patients expected to be on corticosteroid therapy for at least 12 months, as well as for the prevention of new clinical fractures. This review describes the current evidence of ZA to improve the BMD and as adjuvant therapy for controlling clinical inflammation in CIRD. In collagen-induced arthritis models, a combination of ZA plus methotrexate (MTX) prevents bone erosion, radiological damage and systemic bone loss, whereas clinical studies in patients with early RA suggest that this combination prevents bone erosions. On the other hand, the benefits of ZA in patients with established RA to prevent generalized bone loss are now recognized. Most of the evidence of ZA for OP is in postmenopausal women. Case reports in young patients and children with SLE describe how ZA decreases the incidence of bone fractures, although it is important to take into account the potential effects on growth. In animal models for AS, ZA prevents joint ankylosis; however, these preliminary data need to be evaluated in clinical studies. Patients with PsA treated with ZA have shown a decrease in the progression of bone edema, suggesting a suppression of osteitis that correlates with the improvement of disease activity in clinical measures. In tophaceous gout ZA increases BMD of the spine, neck of femur, total hip and total body, but does not influence bone erosions. In conclusion, ZA decreases generalized bone loss and focal bone damage, as well as improving some inflammatory parameters in some of the CIRD. The potential properties as immunomodulating need to be considered to define its possible role as adjuvant therapy directed against the mechanisms of inflammation in CIRD.

Chapter 8 - Bisphosphonates such as alendronate, risedronate and zoledronate have revolutionised the treatment of benign bone disease. Zoledronate (ZLD)/zoledronic acid is a nitrogen containing intravenous (IV) bisphosphonate which is a potent inhibitor of osteoclast mediated bone resorption via several possible mechanisms, but especially by inhibition of the enzyme farnesyl pyrophosphate synthase. Annual administration has been shown to increase bone mineral density at all sites measured, with a concomitant reduction in the risk of vertebral and hip fracture in patients with osteoporosis. Interestingly, IV ZLD has also been shown to lower mortality following hip fracture. The mechanism for this remains unclear, but may be related to a reduction in cardiovascular events. One of the main advantages of ZLD is the convenient annual IV dosing which improves patient compliance. This is of particular importance in the field of osteoporosis where poor compliance with bone protective therapy is well described. However, the long *in vivo* half-life and high potency of ZLD may be responsible for the reported association with delayed dental healing (DDH) and the rare, but potentially devastating complication of osteonecrosis of the jaw (ONJ). The possible association with atypical femoral fractures will also be discussed. This chapter will discuss the clinical use and therapeutic effects of ZLD in benign bone disease, focusing on the treatment of osteoporosis and Paget's disease. The advantages and disadvantages of ZLD relative to the other treatments for osteoporosis will be reviewed. A practical approach to the contentious issue of DDH and ONJ will also be discussed.

Chapter 9 - Zoledronic acid is the most potent bisphosphonate (BP) currently available for use in various clinical conditions. This increasing use of the high potency drug has led to an elevated incidence of a unique but well-documented oral adverse effect termed "bisphosphonate-related osteonecrosis of the jaws (BRONJ)".

BRONJ, as a clinical entity, is classically described as a non-healing ulcer on the jaw bone (maxillae or mandible) in a patient with a history of BP use in the absence of radiotherapy. Initially, the aetiology of BRONJ was considered to be related to direct suppression of osteoclastic activity in the jaw bone. However, recent literature suggests that a host of factors are involved in the pathogenesis of this complex condition and a wide variation exists in its occurrence, mainly based on the potency of the BP used. BRONJ is specifically reported in jaw bones and zoledronic acid, due to its high potency is the most commonly implicated drug. A thorough knowledge of BRONJ is important for a dental surgeon as it is essential for initial identification, prompt diagnosis and successful management of this unique condition.

This chapter comprises an overview of BRONJ as a clinical entity, classification and staging, various etio-pathological theories, and general guidelines in management of zoledronic acid induced BRONJ.

Chapter 10 - Zoledronic acid (ZA) is a potent nitrogen-containing bisphosphonate that was the first in its class to demonstrate efficacy in patients with bone metastases from solid tumors other than breast cancer. It is also used in multiple myeloma as well as non-malignant diseases associated with high bone turnover. This chapter focuses on the biology, pharmacokinetics, and toxicities of ZA and reviews efficacy data that lead to registration for its current clinical use.

In: Zoledronic Acid
Editor: Ronald Carman

ISBN: 978-1-63321-525-2

Chapter 1

USE OF ZOLEDRONIC ACID IN MEN AND WOMEN WITH LOW BONE MASS

Robin K. Dore *

David Geffen School of Medicine, University of California, Los Angeles, Los Angeles, CA US

ABSTRACT

Zoledronic acid is a bisphosphonate that was approved for the treatment of hypercalcemia of malignancy in 2001. Bisphosphonates are hydrolysis-resistant pyrophosphate derivatives that have a high affinity for bone and inhibit osteoclastic bone resorption. A once yearly infusion of zoledronic acid was approved for the treatment of post-menopausal osteoporosis in 2007; this therapy provides an alternative to oral bisphosphonate treatment of post-menopausal osteoporosis which is associated with an inconvenient mode of administration resulting in poor adherence and compliance. Since that time it has also been approved for the prevention of osteoporosis in post-menopausal women, to increase bone mass in men with osteoporosis, to decrease the incidence of new clinical fractures in patients at high risk of fracture (those with a recent low trauma hip fracture) and to treat and prevent glucocorticoid-induced osteoporosis in women and men who are expected to be on glucocorticoids for twelve months or longer. The data concerning combination use of zoledronic acid with other non-bisphosphonate therapy will be reviewed as will data concerning the long-term safety and head-to-head comparisons with other bone active drugs. The use of zoledronic acid in treating special populations will be discussed and suggestions for future research will be presented.

ZOLEDRONIC ACID, LOW BONE MASS AND OSTEOPOROSIS

Zoledronic acid is a third generation bisphosphonate which is administered intravenously once yearly at a dose of 5mg for multiple indications including the treatment of post-menopausal women with osteoporosis to reduce the incidence of vertebral, hip and non-

* Corresponding author: 12791 Newport Ave #201, Tustin CA 92780, Email: drdore@ robinkdoremd.com.

vertebral fractures and to increase bone mineral density (BMD), the prevention of clinical fractures after hip fracture in women and men, treatment of osteoporosis in men, prevention and treatment of glucocorticoid-induced osteoporosis (GIO), the prevention of post-menopausal osteoporosis (in the US) and the treatment of Paget's disease of bone [1]. This chapter will address all of the above indications except for Paget's disease of bone and its use in oncology.

Mechanism of Action

The effects of bisphosphonates on bone including zoledronic acid are characterized primarily by a reduction in resorption and by a secondary reduction in bone formation due to the normal coupling of bone resorption to formation. This reduction in bone resorption is accomplished by blockade of the mevalonate pathway as nitrogen-containing bisphosphonates target farnesyl pyrophosphate synthase (FPPS), a key regulatory enzyme in the mevalonate pathway [2]. Bergstrom et al. demonstrated that the more potent nitrogen-containing bisphosphonates such as zoledronic acid inhibit bone resorption by inhibiting FPPS, thus preventing the phrenylation of small GTPases (a group of enzymes that bind guanine triphosphate) such as Rho, Rac and Rabs that are considered essential for osteoclastic function [3]. The exact mechanism by which nitrogen-containing bisphosphonates inhibit FPPS is still being elucidated. Catalano et al. demonstrated that zoledronic acid increases sclerostin serum levels; sclerostin acts by competitive binding to Wnt coreceptor low-density lipoprotein receptor-related protein 5 (LRP5) and protein 6 (LRP6) and prevents interaction of Wnt ligands with the 7 transmembrane domain spanning frizzled receptors with a resulting decrease in bone formation [4]. The exact mechanism by which nitrogen-containing bisphosphonates modulate sclerostin levels is still being explored [5]. Pederson et al. have reported that osteoclast precursors express sclerostin, although mature osteoclasts do not, and it is possible that osteoclast precursor-derived sclerostin may have biologic significance. Gatti et al. have speculated that treatment with bisphosphonates is associated with an accumulation of osteoclast precursors that are able to secrete sclerostin [6].

Pharmokinetics

Maximum plasma concentrations of zoledronic acid are reached by the end of the 15 minute infusion. Blood levels rapidly decline to less than 10% at 4 hours after the infusion and to less than 1% by 24 hours after the infusion [1]. Approximately 61% of the intravenously administered dose is taken up rapidly by bone, localizing in areas of rapid bone turnover and then slowly released back into the circulation. The residual 39% is excreted unchanged in the urine via glomerular filtration without a significant component of tubular secretion. The elimination of zoledronic acid occurs in three phases composed of two rapid phases followed by a long terminal serum half-life of 146 hours. The clearance of zoledronic acid by the kidneys is dependent on a patient's creatinine clearance. When compared to subjects with a creatinine clearance above 80cc/min, the area under the concentration curve is about 15% higher for subjects with mild renal impairment (creatinine clearance 50-80 cc/min) and about 43% higher for subjects with moderate renal impairment (creatinine clearance of 30-50 cc/min). It is not recommended to treat patients with zoledronic acid who have a creatinine clearance below 35cc/min. It is recommended to exercise caution in patients on medications that have the potential to reduce the serum calcium levels, such as loop diuretics and aminoglycosides and potentially nephrotoxic medications such as non-steroidal anti-inflammatory medications.

CLINICAL STUDIES

Treatment of Post-Menopausal Osteoporosis

The use of zoledronic acid in the treatment of post-menopausal osteoporosis was initially assessed by Reid et al. in a one year, placebo-controlled, dose range finding study of 351 postmenopausal women aged 45-80 [7]; one of the doses was 4mg given once and another dose was 2 doses of 2 mg each six months apart. Increases in bone mineral density (BMD) were seen in all of the zoledronic acid group ranging from 4.3-5.1% higher compared to the placebo group in the lumbar spine and 3.1-3.5% higher in the femoral neck compared to the placebo group. Biochemical markers of bone resorption were significantly suppressed throughout the entire study in all of the zoledronic acid treated groups. This prolonged suppression of bone turnover is not a result of persistence of drug in the circulation as by 24 hours after administration, drug levels are less than one percent of the post-administration peak dose and 40 percent of the dose has been excreted in the urine. The remaining dose is bound to bone and slowly released back into the circulation resulting in a 167 hour terminal half-life in plasma. Evidence suggests that bisphosphonates are deposited on osteoclastic and osteoblastic surfaces in addition to the resting bone surfaces and remain on the latter for long periods of time [8,9] thus partly explaining the long-term effects of bisphosphonates on bone turnover.

This trial had two consecutive, open label, 2-year extension phases [10]. The objective of these long-term extension studies was to assess the long-term safety and efficacy of zoledronic acid for another four years. 119 women who completed the original study entered the first open label extension; these subjects received either 1 mg of zoledronic acid every 3 months for a total dose of 4mg yearly or 0.5mg of zoledronic acid every 3 months for a total dose of 2 mg yearly. Subjects who entered the second extension study had all received 4mg of zoledronic acid total yearly during the core study and in the first extension; during the second extension study, all of the subjects received either 4mg of zoledronic acid or calcium alone. The BMD increased in all three subgroups by the end of the five-year study period in the lumbar spine (6.4%-9%) and proximal femur (4.9%-5.5%). Markers of bone turnover decreased initially but levels of alkaline phosphatase (a bone formation marker) and C-telopeptide (CTx), a marker of bone resorption, both increased from month 24 on in patients treated for up to 5 years. This data suggested that the 4mg dose of zoledronic acid was not sufficient to adequately suppress bone turnover so that a higher intravenous dose of zoledronic acid might be required.

Black et al. presented data using 5mg of zoledronic acid yearly for 3 years in the treatment of postmenopausal osteoporosis with primary endpoints of new vertebral fracture (in subjects not on concomitant osteoporosis therapy) and hip fracture (in all subjects); secondary endpoints were bone mineral density, safety outcomes and markers of bone turnover [11]. The Health Outcomes and Reduced Incidence with Zoledronic Acid Once Yearly-Pivotal Fracture Trial (HORIZON-PFT) was an international, multicenter, double-blind, randomized, placebo-controlled trial of 3 years duration in which 7,765 postmenopausal women ages 65-89 years were randomized to either 5mg of intravenous zoledronic acid given over 15 minutes or a placebo. Concomitant use of non-bisphosphonate therapy was allowed at baseline and during follow-up; subjects were placed into two strata depending on whether they were taking osteoporosis therapy at baseline. Subjects in stratum 1 were not taking any osteoporosis medication at the time of randomization and subjects in stratum 2 were all taking an allowed medication; subjects who had previously taken bisphosphonate therapy and had undergone an appropriate washout, were randomly assigned to either stratum. Zoledronic acid reduced the risk of morphometric vertebral, clinical vertebral, hip and non-vertebral fractures by 70%, 77%, 41% and 25%, respectively. The BMD in the zoledronic acid group increased significantly at the lumbar spine, total hip and femoral neck by 6.1%, 6.02% and 5.06%, respectively. All three biochemical markers of bone turnover decreased significantly in those subjects in the zoledronic acid group as compared to those subjects in the placebo group. At 12 months, levels of CTx, bone specific alkaline phosphatase (bsAP) and N-telopeptide (NTx) were 59%, 30% and 58% lower, respectively, than those in the placebo group. Compared to the results with the 4mg yearly dose used in the Reid trial, the mean values were similar at 6 and 12 months without any progressive decline in the values of the bone turnover markers. There was not a statistically significant difference between the two treatment groups with regards to death, serious adverse events or study discontinuation due to adverse events but there were statistically more non-serious adverse events in the zoledronic acid treatment group most related to post-dose symptoms including nausea, bone pain, chills and back pain. Most of these non-serious adverse events were mild to moderate and resolved within a three-day period of time. No long- term adverse effects were observed regarding renal function. Arrhythmia was seen more commonly in the zoledronic acid treated subjects (6.9% compared to 5.4%, $p=0.003$). Serious atrial fibrillation was also more common in subjects treated with zoledronic acid (1.3% compared to 0.5%, $p<0.001$). This increased frequency of atrial fibrillation was not seen in a small electrocardiographic sub-study and it did not result in an excess death rate from cardiovascular causes. Primarily on the basis of this study, 5 mg of zoledronic acid infused once yearly was approved for the treatment of postmenopausal women with osteoporosis in the United States and Europe in 2007.

A bone biopsy sub-study was performed as part of the HORIZON trial [12]. One hundred fifty-two postmenopausal women underwent an iliac crest bone biopsy after double tetracycline labeling having received either zoledronic acid or placebo treatment for 3 years. One hundred forty-seven biopsies were suitable for microCT and histomorphometry (68 on placebo and 79 on active treatment). Results of the bone biopsies from the active treatment group revealed no evidence of marrow fibrosis, osteomalacia or woven bone. Subjects treated with zoledronic acid demonstrated decreased trabecular separation ($p=0.011$), a trend toward improved connectivity density ($p=0.062$) and higher trabecular numbers ($p=0.008$). MicroCT analysis of the bone structure revealed a higher trabecular bone volume (BV/TV) in the zoledronic acid treatment group (median, 16.6% versus 12.8%; $p=0.020$). All of these parameters suggest better preservation of trabecular bone structure after treatment with zoledronic acid. Tetracycline label was present in 81/82 biopsies from subjects treated with zoledronic acid and all 70 biopsies from the placebo patients showing evidence of continued bone remodeling. Treatment with zoledronic acid induced a 63% median reduction of the activation frequency, reduced volume referent bone formation rate and reduced mineralizing surface compared to placebo indicating reduced bone turnover. Also seen in this biopsy sub-study was a higher mineral apposition rate (MAR) with zoledronic acid that typically suggests that the activity of the individual osteoblasts at the basic multicellular unit (BMU) is stimulated.; this finding has not been seen with other bisphosphonates. Ebeling and Burr have suggested that this finding may have been influenced by technical issues with the biopsies as well as the statistical method used [13]. If this observation is confirmed in other studies, it would suggest that zoledronic acid may act via a different pathway of bone formation than other bisphosphonates.

Black et al. evaluated the effect of once yearly zoledronic acid on a sub-set of six types of non-vertebral fracture including hip, pelvis, leg, clavicle, wrist and humerus [14]. This data was derived from a post-hoc sub-analysis of the data from the HORIZON-PFT trial. At one year the reduction in the subset of these 6 non-vertebral fracture sites was 30% for zoledronic acid compared to placebo (2.3% versus 3.2%, p=<0.01) and at 3 years the incidence of these 6 types of non-vertebral fractures was 33% for zoledronic acid compared to placebo (5.9% versus 8.8%).

Eastell et al. studied the factors that influenced a response to zoledronic acid in the HORIZON-PFT [15]. A pre-planned post-hoc subgroup analysis was conducted which found that a greater effect of zoledronic acid on vertebral fracture risk was seen in subjects of younger age (p=0.05), normal creatinine clearance (p=0.04) and body mass index of greater than or equal to 25 kg/m2 (p=0.02). Femoral neck BMD and fracture risk factors were not found to influence the response to a yearly infusion of zoledronic acid.

Jacques et al. evaluated the relationship of changes in total hip BMD using the year-on-year approach to vertebral and non-vertebral fracture risk in women enrolled in the HORIZON-PFT [16]. Also studied were a subset of 1132 women in who procollagen type 1 amino-terminal propeptide (P1NP) was measured at baseline and 12 months to estimate the percentage of treatment effect explained by change in this bone turnover marker. The change in total hip BMD explained a large percentage of the effect of zoledronic acid on vertebral fracture risk reduction (40%, 95% CI, 30%-54%, for the three year analysis) regardless of the method used, that is year-on-year or the change over 3 years. The treatment effects for non-vertebral fracture were not statistically significant for the year-on-year analysis but the 3-year BMD change explained 61% of the treatment effect (95% CI, 24% to 154%). The change in P1NP explained 56% of the effect of zoledronic acid in reducing the risk of new vertebral fractures (95% CI, 15% to 22%).

Men and Women with a Recent Low Trauma Hip Fracture

The Health Outcomes and Reduced Incidence with Zoledronic Acid Once Yearly Recurrent Fracture Trial (HORIZON-RFT) was a multicenter, randomized, international, double-blind, placebo-controlled trial of subjects who had recently suffered a hip fracture [17]. Subjects were randomized to either zoledronic acid or a placebo infusion given over 15 minutes within 90 days of a surgical repair of a hip fracture with subsequent infusions given every 12 months for the duration of the study. Ambulatory women and men 50 years of age or older who had sustained a hip fracture with minimal trauma who were not candidates for oral bisphosphonate therapy were entered into the study. The primary end point of the study was a new clinical fracture. Secondary end points included new hip, vertebral and non-vertebral fractures; change in the BMD of the non-fractured hip; and pre-specified safety endpoints including death. A total of 2127 subjects were enrolled in the study; 1065 subjects were randomly assigned to receive zoledronic acid and 1062 subjects were assigned to receive the placebo infusion. Four hundred twenty-four fractures occurred in 231 subjects during the study; zoledronic acid was associated with a rate of new clinical fractures of 8.6% compared to 13.9% in the placebo group with a relative risk reduction of 35% and an absolute risk reduction of 5.3%. The rates of a new clinical non-vertebral fracture were 7.6% in the zoledronic acid group compared to 10.7% in the placebo group (P=0.03). The rates of a new clinical vertebral fracture were 1.7% in the zoledronic acid group and 3.8% in the placebo group (p=0.02). The rates of a new hip fracture in the zoledronic acid group were 2.7% compared to 3.5% in the placebo group, which was a non-significant risk reduction. Adverse and serious adverse events occurred with similar frequency in the two groups (38.3% in the zoledronic acid group versus 41.2% in the placebo group) however more patients in the zoledronic acid group compared to the placebo treated group reported myalgia (4.9% versus 2.7%), bone pain (3.2% versus 1.0%), musculoskeletal pain (3.1% versus 1.2%) and pyrexia (8.7% versus 3.1%). The incidence of cardiovascular events was similar between the two treatment groups including atrial fibrillation with 1.1% in the zoledronic acid group versus 1.3% in the placebo group. The incidence of renal adverse events was similar between the two groups. There were no adjudicated cases of osteonecrosis of the jaw and the rate of delayed or mal-union of the hip fracture was 3.2% in the zoledronic acid treated group versus 2.7% in the placebo group. A total of 242/2111 subjects died during the course of the study; 101/1054 in the zoledronic acid group (9.6%) and 141/1057 deaths occurred in the placebo group (13.3%) for a relative risk reduction in death of 28% for zoledronic acid. Further evaluation is being performed to determine the reason for this relative risk reduction that is most likely multifactorial.

Many post-hoc analyses of the HORIZON-RFT have been published. Eriksen et al. evaluated the relation of the timing of the first dose of zoledronic acid to reduction in hip fracture [18]. Median time to the first dose of zoledronic acid after the hip fracture surgery was approximately 6 weeks. Post-hoc analysis was performed and divided the study population into two-week intervals to examine the effects of zoledronic acid on BMD, mortality and fracture. This analysis demonstrated a significant increase in total hip BMD, reduction in overall clinical fractures and all-cause mortality in patients who received the first dose of zoledronic acid two weeks or later after surgical repair of their hip fracture.

Boonen et al. performed a post hoc subgroup analysis of data from both the HORIZON-PFT and the HORIZON-RFT to determine the efficacy and safety of once yearly zoledronic acid on the prevention of fractures in elderly post-menopausal women with osteoporosis aged 75 years of age or older [19]. This post-hoc analysis is felt to be very important as older women suffer the majority of hip and vertebral fractures and many of the prior studies with other osteoporosis therapies did not include women after the age of 80. There were 9354 postmenopausal women included in both of the HORIZON trials; 3887 aged 75 years of age and older and 5467 younger than 75. The results revealed a reduction in all three types of fractures (vertebral, non-vertebral and hip) in the younger group but in the older group there was not a significant reduction in hip fracture; this was interpreted to be due to factors other than BMD such as poor balance and eye sight leading to an increased risk of falls. Also, as this was a post-hoc analysis, the sample size used for the analysis was not powered statistically to detect a risk reduction in hip fracture for the older subgroup. The relative risk reduction in clinical vertebral fractures, clinical fractures and non-vertebral fractures was similar in both groups at both one and three years after treatment initiation. Post-dose infusion reactions, renal adverse events, deaths, atrial fibrillation and serious adverse events were similar in the treatment arms for both age groups.

The same authors analyzed the same two databases to determine the time to onset of anti-fracture efficacy and year-by-year persistence of the effect of zoledronic acid in women with osteoporosis [20]. The endpoints for the time-to-onset of anti-fracture effect analysis were the cumulative reductions in the rate of any clinical vertebral, non-vertebral or clinical fracture at 6, 12, 18, 24 and 36 months in the zoledronic acid group compared to the placebo group. The endpoints of the persistence of effect analysis were the year-by-year incidence of these 3 fracture types over the 3-year period of time. The risk of any clinical fracture was significantly reduced with zoledronic acid at 12 months and maintained at all subsequent time points (hazard ratio [HR], 0.75,p=0.0050). The risk for clinical vertebral fractures was also significantly reduced at 12 months (HR, 0.43, p=0.0035) with a trend towards risk reduction at 6 months (HR, 0.47, p=0.0553). The risk reduction for non-vertebral fractures did not become significant until 18 months (HR, 0.77, p=0.0049) although there was a trend towards risk reduction at 6 months. The incidence of clinical fractures and clinical vertebral fractures was significantly lower in the zoledronic acid treatment group than in the placebo group in each of the three years. Zoledronic acid also reduced the risk of non-vertebral fractures compared with placebo over the 3 years but this protective effect was not found in year one. This difference in time to onset of effect between clinical vertebral and non-vertebral fractures is also seen with other anti-resorptive agents [21]. A possible explanation is that the rapid reduction in bone resorption that is seen with potent anti-resorptive agents such as zoledronic acid is sufficient to decrease the risk of vertebral fractures but an increase in BMD is needed to reduce the risk of non-vertebral fractures [22].

IMAGING STUDIES

Eastell et al. published data that evaluated quantitative computed analysis (QCT) and dual energy x-ray absorptiometry (DXA) changes from baseline to 36 months in a subset comprised of 233 post-menopausal women who were enrolled in the HORIZON-PFT [23]. Mean percentage changes in lumbar spine BMD from baseline and between treatment differences (zoledronic acid versus placebo, t-test) were evaluated. Mean between treatment differences for lumbar spine BMD as measured by QCT (5.7%, p=0.0001) and DXA (7.0%, p<0.01) were significant. Between treatment differences were significant for trabecular trochanter (10.7%, p<0.0001), trochanter (14.1%, p<0.0001), total hip (10.8%, p<0.001) and compressive strength indices at the femoral neck (8.6%, p=0.001). These changes in trabecular bone resulted in increased indices of compressive strength.

Gamsjaeger et al. further investigated these changes in bone material properties using Raman microspectroscopy that is a vibrational spectroscopy technique that allows the analysis of bone tissue blocks with a spatial resolution of 0.6 to 1 micrometer [24]. The data this technique provides includes mineral/matrix ratio, lamellar organization, proteoglycan and mineral carbonate content in addition to information about the bone mineral maturity/crystallinity. These authors used this technique on the bone biopsies performed during the HORIZON-PFT trial; the biopsy technique was discussed earlier [12]. This study demonstrated that zoledronic acid influences matrix formation and mineralization quality compared to placebo which supports the data of increased mineral apposition rate that was seen in the study of Recker et al. [12] and cannot be explained by the effect of zoledronic acid on suppression of bone turnover. These authors conclude, as did Recker et al., that these results suggest a potential additional mechanism of action by which zoledronic acid may exert its anti-fracture effect during osteoporosis treatment.

Misof et al. evaluated the cancellous and cortical bone mineralization density distribution (BMDD) in the bone biopsy specimens discussed above; this was measured by quantitative back scattered electron imaging (qBEI) [25]. Comparison of zoledronic acid and placebo treated biopsy specimens revealed significantly higher average and mode calcium concentrations, lower heterogeneity of mineralization, increased percentages of highly mineralized bone areas and decreased percentages of low mineralized bone areas in the zoledronic acid treated group compared to placebo. These findings again suggest that other factors in addition to reduced bone turnover might contribute to the higher bone matrix mineralization that is seen after treatment with zoledronic acid.

Yang et al. used quantitative computed tomography to detect changes in bone mineral density in different regions of the hip after 3 years of zoledronic acid treatment in the HORIZON-PFT [26]. Volumetric BMD increased significantly from baseline with zoledronic acid compared to placebo ($p<0.05$). Cortical volumetric BMD increased at the proximal femoral neck (5.0%), the anterior femoral neck (2.3%), the middle trochanter (2.7%), the total trochanter (4.6%) and the total hip (3.8). The trabecular volumetric BMD increased at the femoral neck (5.4%), at the trochanter (6.5%) and the total hip (5.7%). Thus, after 3 years of treatment with zoledronic acid, volumetric BMD as measured by QCT increased at all sites measured but more at the trabecular sites.

Recently, the trabecular bone score (TBS) has been introduced as a means to measure bone microarchitecture which is calculated from the antero-posterior DXA scans of the lumbar spine; this score has been shown to predict fracture risk independent of BMD. Popp et al. evaluated the effects of zoledronic acid versus placebo on spine BMD and microarchitecture as measured by trabecular bone score in post-menopausal women [27]. These authors measured the changes in TBS in a subset of 107 women who were included in the HORIZON-PFT and treated with placebo or zoledronic acid. BMD was measured by DXA and TBS was assessed by TBS iNsight (v1.9) in both groups at 6, 12, 24 and 36 months after initiation of treatment. As expected, changes in the lumbar spine BMD were significantly greater in the zoledronic acid treatment group compared with the placebo at all time points ($p<0.0001$); at month 36 the lumbar spine BMD increased 9.58% compared to 1.38% for the placebo. Changes in TBS were also significantly greater with zoledronic acid compared to placebo as of 24 months; reaching +1.41% versus -0.49% at 36 months ($p=0.031$). There was no correlation between changes in BMD and TBS from baseline at any visit.

EXTENSION STUDIES

Black et al. presented the data from the HORIZON-PFT extension that compared the effect of three versus six years of zoledronic acid treatment of osteoporosis [28]. The goal of the study was to assess the safety and efficacy of six years of zoledronic acid versus three years of zoledronic acid followed by three years off therapy. Long- term safety and efficacy data for bisphosphonate therapy is scant except for the FLEX trial evaluating ten versus five years of alendronate therapy; this trial suggested that there was no significant difference in non-vertebral fracture reduction when taking alendronate for five versus ten years [29]. Although, atypical femoral fractures and ONJ were not reported in the FLEX trial, many case reports in the literature suggest a relationship between long term use of bisphosphonates and these adverse events. In the HORIZON-PFT, one case of ONJ occurred in the placebo and one in the zoledronic acid treatment groups [11]. In 2011, a Food and Drug Administration (FDA) advisory committee recommended that the FDA make changes to the bisphosphonate package inserts regarding long term use of these medications due to the lack of data regarding continued benefit of these drugs with long term use and the concern over adverse events such as ONJ and atypical femoral fractures with long term use [30].

In the extension of the HORIZON-PFT, subjects who were assigned to zoledronic acid in the core study were randomly assigned to receive yearly infusions of zoledronic acid or a yearly placebo infusion for three years in a 1:1 ratio [28]. The primary endpoint was percentage change in femoral neck BMD at year six compared to year three. Secondary endpoints included total hip and spine BMD, fractures (morphometric vertebral, clinical vertebral, non-vertebral and all clinical) and biochemical markers of bone turnover. The mean change from year 3 to year 6 for femoral neck BMD was +0.24% in the 6 year group compared to -0.80% in the 3 year group (difference =1.04%, p=0.0009). The difference in the total hip BMD was similar and significant. The difference in the lumbar spine BMD was slightly higher at 2.03% (p=0.002). The P1NP levels increased 33% in the year 3 group compared to a 19% increase in the year six group (difference=14%, p=0.0001). Morphometric vertebral fracture risk was significantly lower in the 6 year (n=14) compared to the 3-year group (n=30; 3.0% versus 6.2%, p=0.035). There was no significant difference, however, in the incidence of non-vertebral fracture (8.2% versus 7.6%), clinical vertebral, hip (1.3% versus 1.4%) or all clinical fractures between the 6-year and the 3 year groups. With regards to adverse events, significantly more of the 6- year subjects had a transient increase in the serum creatinine of more than 0.5 mg/dl (2.94% versus 0.65%). Atrial fibrillation was slightly more common in the year 6 group compared to the year 3-group but the difference was not significant. Several cardiovascular events including stroke occurred more commonly in the year 6 group but the difference was not significant. There was a statistically significant decrease in hypertension adverse events in the six-year group compared to the 3- year group (48 versus 93, p=0.0001). There were no cases of hip or knee avascular necrosis or atypical femoral fractures. There was one case of ONJ in the 6-year group that resolved with appropriate treatment. Overall these results suggest that after three years of zoledronic treatment, many patients may discontinue this therapy for up to 3 years but those patients who are at high risk of fracture, especially vertebral fracture, may benefit from continued yearly infusions.

Eastell et al. evaluated the relationship between the change in total hip BMD response to zoledronic acid and post-treatment change in total hip BMD in subjects enrolled in the HORIZON-PFT extension study [31]. The purpose of the study was to determine whether greater rates of bone loss after stopping therapy are associated with greater increases in bone density in response to initiation of anti-resorptive therapy, to baseline bone turnover or to change in bone turnover. Total hip BMD was measured by DXA at baseline, 1,2 and 3 years after the yearly infusion of zoledronic acid and at years 4, 5 and 6 after the annual placebo infusion. Total P1NP was measured at years 0, 3, 4, 5 and 6 (results were excluded if the subject had a fracture in the past year as P1NP can increase up to one year post-fracture). The results revealed that the change in the total hip BMD at years 0-3 was related to the change in total hip BMD on placebo at 3-6 years (r=-0.15,p=0.0015); subjects who had the greatest increases in BMD during years 0-3 had the greatest decreases in BMD in years 3-6. The P1NP value at baseline correlated with the change in total hip BMD at years 0-3 on zoledronic acid annually (r=0.32,p=0.002) and to the change in total hip BMD in years 3-6 after stopping therapy (r=-0.26,p=0.007). The change in P1NP at years 0-3 correlated with the change in total hip BMD at years 0-3 (r=-0.35,p=0.0003) on zoledronic acid and the change in P1NP at years 3-6 correlated with the change in total hip BMD in years 3-6 on zoledronic acid (r=-0.18,p=0.0005). The authors concluded that the decrease in BMD after stopping zoledronic acid is greater in those with the greatest increases in BMD on zoledronic acid therapy. The authors postulated that one possible mechanism of action for this association would be that a higher bone turnover before starting zoledronic acid therapy is associated with both greater increases in BMD response to zoledronic acid and a greater rate of bone loss when therapy is discontinued.

Black et al. randomized 190 subjects who had received zoledronic acid for six years in both the core and the extension studies to either 3 additional years of zoledronic acid (year 9) or placebo (year 6)[32]. The primary endpoint was comparison of the percentage change in total hip BMD at year 9 versus year 6. Secondary endpoints included total hip and femoral neck BMD and markers of bone turnover; exploratory endpoints included the incidence of vertebral and clinical fractures after year 6 and safety. At the present time the data is still blinded. This study will provide much needed data about longer-term bisphosphonate use with regards to efficacy and safety.

Data from a cohort study of 192 post-menopausal women with osteoporosis who were treated with one infusion of 5mg of zoledronic acid was analyzed in an effort to identify factors involved in predicting the response to intravenous zoledronic acid in elderly women with osteoporosis [33]. This was a retrospective study; women were followed up for 12-18 months after their first dose of zoledronic acid. Forty-three patients of this cohort who had DXAs performed at 12-18 months after the zoledronic acid infusion were entered into the analysis. The women were divided into 2 groups; women who did not achieve a 3% or more increase in BMD at the lumbar spine at 12-18 months were considered non-responders. There was no difference in the characteristics of both groups at baseline. A significant difference in bone density was observed between the responders (0.76 SD ±0.13) versus non-responders (0.87 SD ±0.19) (p=0.03). A significant trend was also observed towards an increase in response with lower baseline bone density at baseline (p=0.04). A higher baseline BMD was seen in patients with a higher baseline body mass index (BMI). Unfortunately, this analysis was not able to identify predictors of response but it did demonstrate that women with the lowest BMD at baseline in this study had the greatest response to treatment with zoledronic acid.

Borba et al. [34] evaluated bone turnover response 18 months after one dose of 4 mg of IV zoledronic acid. This study was performed before zoledronic acid 5mg became the approved dose for the treatment of osteoporosis. Male and female subjects with low BMD were treated with a single dose of 4mg of IV zoledronic acid. BMD was measured by DXA and bone turnover markers were measured at 12 and 18 months after the single infusion. The results revealed that the median serum carboxyterminal telopeptide of type I collagen (CTX-1) and bone specific alkaline phosphatase (bsAP) were suppressed at month 12 in comparison with baseline values for CTX-1(0.183-0.039 ng/ml, p=0.0002) and for bsAP (16.95-13.96 U/l,p=0.005). At 18 months, both CTX-1 and bsAP continued to be suppressed below baseline at 0.108 ng/ml (p=0.009) and 12.23 U/l (p=0.02). BMD also significantly improved at 18 months compared to 12 months with median increase of 6.1% for the lumbar spine and 2.0% for the total hip. The authors concluded that zoledronic acid inhibits bone turnover at 12 months with continued increase in BMD and continued suppression in bone turnover at 18 months.

Use in Women with Low Bone Mass

Grey et al. evaluated the anti-resorptive activity and BMD response to a single dose of zoledronic acid 5mg administered to 50 postmenopausal women with low bone mass rather than osteoporosis [35]. After 5 years, mean levels of beta-C-terminal telopeptide of type I collagen (beta-CTX) and P1NP were 277 ng/L (150,404) and 28mcg [16,40] lower in the zoledronic acid group, corresponding to reductions of 48% and 45%, respectively. After 5 years, the bone density in the zoledronic acid group was 4.2% higher at the lumbar spine (1.1,7.2), 5.3% higher at the total hip (2.7, 7.9) and 2.7% higher at the total body (1.1,4.2). These data suggest that the anti-resorptive effects and the BMD effects of a single dose of zoledronic acid persist for at least five years in postmenopausal women with low bone density. These authors suggest that clinical trial with longer dosing intervals (longer than one year)of zoledronic acid are justified.

These same authors [36] investigated the impact of dietary calcium intake and vitamin D status on the BMD and anti-resorptive effects of zoledronic acid and the frequency of acute phase reactions after one infusion in the population described above [35] as well as in 172 post-menopausal women also with low BMD who received a single dose of either 1, 2.5 or 5mg of zoledronic acid or placebo [37]. There were no significant differences in these variables between the two studies except that the 25 hydroxy Vitamin D level was slightly higher in the first study. The results revealed that there was no interaction between baseline dietary calcium intake and treatment or baseline Vitamin D level and treatment for either P1NP or CTX. There was also no interaction between baseline dietary calcium intake and treatment, or baseline Vitamin D level and treatment for lumbar spine or total hip BMD. There was also no interaction between baseline dietary calcium intake and treatment or baseline Vitamin D level and treatment for an acute phase reaction to zoledronic acid. It is important to note that these studies did not include subjects with Vitamin D deficiency so these results cannot be generalized to all post-menopausal women. As Vitamin D deficiency is common in elderly women and administration of IV zoledronic acid may cause significant hypocalcemia in women with Vitamin D deficiency, it is important to provide Vitamin D supplementation before treatment with IV zoledronic acid.

The women in the studies referenced above did not have osteoporosis but low bone mass defined as a T-score between -1.0 and -2.5 [35,37]. McClung et al. evaluated the efficacy of zoledronic acid in the prevention of bone loss in postmenopausal women with low bone mass [38]. In this two year randomized, double-blind, placebo-controlled, multicenter study, 581 postmenopausal women 45 years of age or older with low bone mass were treated with either 5mg of zoledronic acid at baseline and at 12 months (n=198), 5mg IV only at randomization and a placebo infusion at 12 months (n=181) or placebo at randomization and 12 months (n=202). The primary endpoint was the percentage change in lumbar spine BMD at 24 months compared to baseline; secondary endpoints included the percentage change in markers of bone turnover. Both groups treated with zoledronic acid regimens had significant increases in lumbar spine BMD compared to placebo at 24 months (5.18% and 4.42% respectively compared to -1.32%, both $p<0.001$). Both zoledronic acid groups also demonstrated a significant reduction in bone turnover markers compared to placebo (all $p<0.001$) but the changes seen with the 2 doses of zoledronic acid were sustained greater during the second year relative to the single dose group. The incidence of serious and overall adverse events was similar across all three treatment groups. Based on this study, the FDA in 2009 approved a bi-annual dose of 5mg of zoledronic acid for the prevention of bone loss in postmenopausal women with low bone mass.

Eskiyurt et al. studied the safety and efficacy of zoledronic acid in younger postmenopausal women between the ages of 50-65 [39]. One hundred twelve postmenopausal women ages 55-65 were enrolled in an open label, prospective, one year, multicenter study; one hundred one women (90.2%) completed the trial. The primary endpoints were the change in BMD in the lumbar spine and femoral neck as measured by DXA at 12 months. Secondary endpoints included the measurement of bone turnover markers (P1NP and CTX) at months 6 and 12. Safety evaluation was performed based on adverse event reporting. The results revealed that zoledronic acid increased the BMD at the lumbar spine and femoral neck at one year versus baseline by 13.1% and 5.2%, respectively ($p<0.001$). Serum P1NP and CTX levels decreased significantly at 6 and 12 months compared to pretreatment values. Forty-two patients (37.5%) developed 88 adverse events that were primarily mild and moderate in severity (77.3%). Arthralgia (n=10) and myalgia (n=29) were the most common adverse events. Seven serious adverse events occurred in 2 patients (1.8%). No cases of atrial fibrillation, ONJ or deterioration in renal function were observed. No subject withdrew due to adverse events. The safety and efficacy of a single infusion of zoledronic acid observed in this study was similar to the results of previous studies of older women age 65 years of age or older.

Osteoporosis in Men

Once yearly infusions of 5mg of zoledronic acid have also been studied in men with osteoporosis. Boonen et al. performed a multicenter, placebo-controlled, double-blind randomized study of 1199 men aged 50 to 85 with primary or hypogonadism-associated osteoporosis who received 5mg of zoledronic acid (n=588) or placebo (n=611) at baseline and 12 months [40] The primary endpoint was the proportion of subjects with one or more new morphometric vertebral fractures over a period of 24 months. Secondary endpoints included proportion of subjects with height loss and improvement in bone density. Approximately one-third of the subjects had a history of one or more vertebral fractures. At the end of the study, the relative risk reduction of new vertebral fracture was significantly higher in the zoledronic acid group compared to the placebo group (1.6% versus 4.9%, p=0.002) correlating to a relative risk reduction of 67% and an absolute risk reduction of 3.3%. Six men who received zoledronic acid (1.0%) and 11 men who received placebo (1.8%) had one or more non-vertebral or clinical vertebral fractures during the 24 months of the study. Given the small number of clinical fractures, the between-group difference was not significant. Height loss was also less in the zoledronic acid treated group (-2.34mm versus -4.49mm, p=0.0020). Compared to placebo, zoledronic acid was associated with sustained and significant increases in BMD at the lumbar spine, femoral neck and hip over the 24-month period (p<0.05 for all comparisons). Serum CTX, P1NP and bsAP levels were lower in men who received zoledronic acid compared to men who received placebo at all times measured (p<0.001 for all comparisons). The improvement in BMD and fracture reduction occurred to the same extent in hypogonadal and eugonadal men. With regards to adverse events, no significant differences were observed between the two treatment groups with respect to deaths or serious adverse events except for myocardial infarction in nine men in the zoledronic acid group (1.5%) and two in the placebo group (0.3%) (p=0.03). As expected, men who received zoledronic acid reported more adverse events of myalgia, arthralgia, headaches, pyrexia, chills, influenza-like symptoms and pain in the extremities. No cases of ONJ or atypical femoral fractures were reported. There were no significant differences between the groups in the incidence of cardiac arrhythmias, renal impairment or atrial fibrillation. On the basis of this data, the FDA and the European Medicines Agency (EMEA) granted approval for the use of zoledronic acid to treat osteoporosis in men.

GLUCOCORTICOID-INDUCED OSTEOPOROSIS

Zoledronic acid is also indicated for the prevention and treatment of glucocorticoid-induced osteoporosis. Reid et al. performed a double-blind, double-dummy, non-inferiority trial in which men and women were randomly assigned 1:1 to either 5mg of zoledronic acid given IV once yearly (n=416) or 5mg of risedronate daily by mouth (n=417)[41]. Sixty-two subjects did not complete the study due to multiple reasons. The groups were stratified by sex and allocated to a prevention or treatment subgroup; treatment was defined as receiving glucocorticoids for more than 3 months and prevention was defined as receiving glucocorticoids for less than 3 months. The primary endpoint was the percentage change from baseline in lumbar spine BMD. At study completion, zoledronic acid was both non-inferior and superior to risedronate with increases in lumbar spine BMD for the treatment group of 4.06% versus 2.71% (p=0.0001) and 2.6% versus 0.64% (p<0.0001) for the prevention group. Adverse events occurred more commonly in the zoledronic acid group most related to post-dose acute phase reactions. Two serious adverse events occurred; rheumatoid arthritis flared in the treatment group and pyrexia occurred in the prevention group.

SPECIAL POPULATIONS

Secondary Osteoporosis in Children

Although not an approved indication, zoledronic acid has been used to treat children with secondary osteoporosis. Simm et al. treated 20 children with secondary osteoporosis due to multiple primary conditions with every three-month infusions of zoledronic acid at doses of 0.1 mg/kg/yr for 2 years [42]. Seven of the children had vertebral wedging at baseline. At 12 months there was a significant improvement in the lumbar spine BMD by 1.88 SD ($p<0.001$) as measured by DXA. Bone turnover as measured by osteocalcin and alkaline phosphatase was suppressed. Skeletal architecture improved with increased second metacarpal cortical thickness from 2.44mm to 2.72mm ($p<0.001$). Some children had post-dose reactions but no serious adverse reactions were reported. No further fractures were reported during the study period. The authors suggest that long term follow up of this population is needed to confirm long-term efficacy and safety of zoledronic acid therapy in children.

Spinal Cord Injury

Zoledronic acid has also been used to prevent bone loss at the hip following acute spinal cord injury; it is know that BMD is lost rapidly following a spinal cord injury especially in the lower extremities. Bubbear et al. performed an open label study of 14 subjects with spinal cord injury who were randomized to either 4 mg of zoledronic acid or to standard treatment [43]. BMD was measured by DXA at 3, 6 and 12 months; markers of bone turnover were also measured. At 12 months, there was a significant difference in the BMD at the total hip between groups (12.4%, $p=0.005$) at the trochanter (13.4%, $p=0.028$) and at the lumbar spine (2.7%, $p=0.033$). The difference between treatment groups, however, was not significant (4.8%, $p=0.741$). Bone resorption was reduced in the zoledronic acid group and remained reduced for up to 12 months. No serious adverse events were reported; post-dose acute phase reactions were reported but did not result in subjects discontinuing the study. Schnitzer et al. studied the use of 5 mg of zoledronic acid or placebo in 10 patients all male who had suffered an acute spinal cord injury within 6 months of study entry [44]. Baseline demographics were similar between the two groups. Six months after the infusion, the change in BMD of the treatment group versus the placebo group at the lumbar spine was 2.0% ±1.6% versus -2.6%± 1.7% ($p=0.004$), at the left total hip -1.7% ± 2.8% versus -16.3%±0.3% ($p=0.002$), at the right total hip 2.0% ± 5.8% versus -11.2% ± 8.6% ($p=0.10$), at the left femoral neck 0.0% ± 6.7% versus -14.9% ± 12.9%($p=0.08$), and at the right femoral neck -1.0%±7.4% versus -21.7% ±4.2% ($p=0.005$). No serious adverse events felt related to the study drug were reported.

HIV

The use of zoledronic acid in HIV-associated osteopenia and osteoporosis has also been investigated. Huang et al. treated 30 HIV-infected men and women with osteopenia and osteoporosis with either 5 mg of zoledronic acid or placebo and were followed for 12 months

[45]. Median T-scores at baseline were -1.7 in the lumbar spine and -1.4 in the total hip. Ninety-seven percent of the subjects were taking anti-viral therapy. BMD improved significantly in the zoledronic acid treated subjects compared to the placebo and markers of bone turnover decreased significantly compared to the placebo subjects. No acute infusion reactions were reported but one subject did develop uveitis, which is a known adverse reaction to bisphosphonates. The authors suggested that a larger study be performed for a longer period of time as the results suggest that 5mg of zoledronic acid is an effective therapy for HIV-associated bone loss as measured by BMD and markers of bone turnover.

Frail Long Term Care Residents

Greenspan et al. studied the safety and efficacy of a single dose of zoledronic acid to treat osteoporosis in frail long-term care residents [46]. The ZEST study was a double blind, randomized, placebo controlled trial which enrolled female residents in long-term care facilities in the Pittsburgh, Pennsylvania area. This study enrolled women of any age including those with cognitive impairment, immobility, multiple medical problems and medications that can have adverse effects on bone. A total of 181 women were randomized to treatment and placebo in a 1:1 distribution. All participants were allowed to continue with raloxifene, calcitonin or hip protectors if these had been prescribed by the referring physicians. All study procedures were performed at the subjects own long-term care facility to encourage study participation and retention. The primary outcome was change in the BMD of the hip and spine at 12 months. Secondary outcomes included death, other adverse events, abnormal laboratory studies, participation, BMD changes at other skeletal sites, functional and cognitive assessments, survival for 24 months after enrollment and co-morbidities. An exploratory assessment included fragility fractures at months 12 and 24. The mean age of subjects at baseline was 85.3±5.1 years with a range from 70.4 to 98.9 years. Approximately 63% of the subjects reported a fracture as an adult; 29% of the subjects had been diagnosed with osteoporosis by a medical professional. Results of this study demonstrated that BMD changes were significantly greater in the active treatment group compared to the placebo group at months 12 and 24 ($p<0.01$ for all) with a 12-month absolute difference of 3.2% at the total hip and 1.8% at the spine. At 24 months, there was a 3.9% difference between treatment groups of the total hip BMD, 2.7% difference in the femoral neck BMD and a 3.6% difference in the lumbar spine BMD. At month 24, there was a 35% difference in the CTX and a 34% difference in the P1NP. There was no difference in vertebral or total fractures. Approximately 97% of subjects had an adverse event with 63% suffering a serious adverse event. Seventy-five percent of the subjects in the zoledronic acid group suffered a fall compared to 58% in the placebo group, this difference was statistically significant but when this data was adjusted for baseline frailty, previous falls and diabetes, the difference was no longer significant. This trial is the first study to demonstrate that an infusion of zoledronic acid 5mg is safe and effective in improving/preserving the skeletal integrity of long term care residents. Further study is needed to determine if these BMD improvements translate into fracture reduction [47].

Comparison of Different Agents

Jansen et al. performed a meta-analysis that compared the efficacy of bisphosphonates in the prevention of vertebral, hip and non-vertebral fractures in osteoporosis [48]. With a systematic literature review, eight randomized placebo controlled trials that investigated the effects of alendronate [3], risedronate [2], etidronate [1], ibandronate [1] and zoledronic acid [1] were identified. The results demonstrated that there is a 79% probability that zoledronic acid shows the greatest reduction in vertebral fractures of all of the bisphosphonates compared. Zoledronic acid demonstrated a relative risk reduction (RRR) of 0.30 relative to placebo (0.23-0.37), a RRR of 0.50 (0.36-0.70) compared to risedronate, a RRR of 0.55 (0.41-0.76) compared to alendronate and a RRR of 0.58 (0.37-0.92) compared to ibandronate. Risedronate demonstrated the greatest reduction in non-vertebral, non-hip fractures followed by zoledronic acid. With regards to hip fracture, there is a 47% probability that zoledronic acid demonstrates the greatest RRR followed by alendronate (36%) and risedronate (11%). Overall there was a 94% probability that zoledronic acid demonstrated the greatest reduction in any fracture.

McClung et al. studied a single infusion of 5mg of zoledronic acid versus weekly oral alendronate 70mg in postmenopausal women with low bone mineral density who had previously received alendronate [49]. This was a randomized double-blind, double-dummy, multicenter trial that compared the safety and efficacy of these two treatment regimens. In the zoledronic acid treatment group, the markers of bone turnover were reduced from baseline after 3 months, returned to baseline after 6 months and continued to increase but remained in the pre-menopausal range. The rate of adverse events in both treatment groups was similar. Bone biopsies from both treatment groups demonstrated a decrease in the excessive bone remodeling that is seen in osteoporosis. A preference question was also part of this study; seventy-eight percent of the subjects preferred a once yearly infusion compared to a weekly oral therapy.

Gauthier et al. evaluated the clinical effectiveness and harms of denosumab, raloxifene and zoledronic acid for the treatment of postmenopausal osteoporosis [50]. The authors identified six randomized controlled trials that assessed the efficacy and safety of raloxifene [4], denosumab [1] and zoledronic acid [1] in the treatment of postmenopausal women with osteoporosis. No direct treatment comparisons were available to assess the relative efficacy of these therapies. This review revealed that raloxifene, zoledronic acid and denosumab are all effective in reducing the risk of vertebral fractures, both morphometric and clinical. Zoledronic acid and denosumab both reduced the risk of multiple vertebral fractures, non-vertebral fractures and hip fractures. Raloxifene, zoledronic acid and denosumab all increased spine and hip BMD compared to placebo at 36 months of therapy and up to seven years of treatment with raloxifene in one trial; the significance of these findings is unknown, as fracture risk reduction does not directly correlate with changes in BMD. With regards to harm, denosumab was associated with an increased risk of cellulitis, raloxifene with venous thromboembolism and hot flashes and zoledronic acid with atrial fibrillation. The authors note that the FDA has stated that there is not a clear association between overall bisphosphonate exposure and the rate of serious and non-serious atrial fibrillation. The incidence of atypical fracture and ONJ was not significantly different between the active drug and the placebo in these trials. The authors note that zoledronic acid has been associated with renal impairment but that no evidence of toxicity was seen in the study that was included in this review. The authors also note that raloxifene is associated with a reduced incidence of invasive cancer and that this information might influence choice of therapy in some postmenopausal women.

Hadji et al. compared the effect of zoledronic acid 5 mg once yearly with alendronate 70mg weekly on bone metabolism in postmenopausal women with low bone mass as measured by markers of bone turnover [51]. A greater reduction in levels of P1NP was demonstrated in the zoledronic acid group compared to the alendronate group (28.21 versus 25.53 ng/ml, p=0.0024) at month 12. A significantly greater reduction in urine NTx levels from baseline to 12 months was observed in subjects treated with zoledronic acid (n=408) compared to those receiving alendronate (n=196) (0.282ng/ml versus 0.270ng/ml, p=0.012). The incidence of adverse events was similar between the two groups from days 4-360, as more subjects developed influenza-like symptoms after the infusion of zoledronic acid up to day 3. Alendronate therapy was associated with more frequent gastro-intestinal adverse events than zoledronic acid therapy. In summary, once yearly zoledronic acid therapy was associated with a greater and more rapid reduction in the markers of bone turnover compared to once weekly alendronate.

Dempster et al. compared the differential effects of teriparatide and zoledronic acid on the outer and inner surfaces of cortical bone in postmenopausal women with osteoporosis [52]. These authors performed a randomized, double-blind, active comparator controlled study in which after double tetracycline labeling, trans-iliac bone biopsies were obtained from 58 subjects receiving teriparatide 20mcg daily or zoledronic acid 5mg yearly. At 6 months, the proportion of samples with tetracycline labels was significantly higher in all three envelopes measured in the teriparatide group compared to the zoledronic acid group (p<0.001). One hundred percent of samples from the teriparatide group displayed labels on the endocortical surface all of which were double labels compared to 52% of the zoledronic acid group of which only 21% had double labels. Mineralizing surface/bone surface, bone formation rate, osteoid surface, osteoid thickness, wall thickness and mineral apposition were all significantly higher in the teriparatide group compared to the zoledronic acid group in both endocortical and cancellous envelopes. In both envelopes, eroded surface was lower in the zoledronic acid group than in the teriparatide group. On the periosteal surface, 70% of samples displayed labels in the teriparatide group of which 26% had double labels compared to 17% of the samples from the zoledronic acid group of which 7% had double labels. These changes seen in the bone biopsy specimens confirm the different mechanisms of action of teriparatide compared to zoledronic acid.

Invernizzi et al. described the effects of denosumab on bone turnover markers compared to zoledronic acid in severe osteoporotic women one month after administration [53]. Seventy-seven post-menopausal women were randomized 1:1 to either denosumab (n=37) or zoledronic acid (n=40). Inclusion criteria were age greater than 70, a T-score of less than -3.0 at the lumbar spine or hip and the presence of one or more vertebral or hip osteoporotic fractures. The percentage of subjects who were treatment naive in the denosumab group was 40.5% and in the zoledronic acid was 48%. Bone turnover markers were assessed at baseline and one month after treatment. Tolerability was captured in adverse event reporting. At one month, denosumab treatment was found to decrease osteocalcin by 19.8%, serum CTX by 77.8% and bsAP by 11% compared to baseline values. At one month, treatment with zoledronic acid was associated with a decrease in osteocalcin of 10%, serum CTX 42% and bsAP by 7.2% compared to baseline values. There was no significant difference in the change in bone turnover markers between treatment naïve and previously treated subjects. Two subjects (5.4%) complained of myalgia and arthralgia after denosumab treatment and 18 subjects (45%) complained of an acute phase reaction after the infusion of zoledronic acid. The authors concluded that, based on the above data that demonstrates a more rapid onset of reduction in bone turnover and a greater suppression of bone turnover, perhaps denosumab should be considered before zoledronic acid in patients with severe osteoporosis although other factors may play a role in this decision making process. Nevertheless, as has been stated for increases in BMD, more rapid reduction in bone turnover markers does not necessarily correlate with greater fracture reduction.

Sheedy et al. compared the efficacy, adverse effects and cost of zoledronic acid and denosumab in a retrospective chart review of patients at Loyola University Medical Center in Chicago, USA [54]. The study cohort consisted of 107 patients, 56 in the zoledronic acid group and 51 in the denosumab group. A subset of 29 patients responded to a questionnaire. The change in the femoral neck T-score BMD and the change in the spine T-score at one year were not statistically different between the two groups at one year. The denosumab treated patients had a greater mean increase in the lumbar spine BMD at one year of 0.060g/cm2 compared to the increase in the zoledronic acid group of 0.021g/cm2 (p=0.04). There were no significant differences in the bsAP, back pain, muscle pain or patient satisfaction. As expected, the zoledronic acid treated patients had a significantly greater incidence of mild flu-like symptoms compared to the denosumab group (29% versus 0%, p=0.04). All of the zoledronic acid treatments were covered by the patients' insurance compared to 93% of the denosumab treated patients. In summary, although more zoledronic acid treated patients complained of flu-like symptoms post-dose and greater BMD increases occurred in the denosumab treated patients, patient satisfaction and cost were similar. It is not known if the greater increase in BMD in the denosumab treated group corresponds to greater fracture protection.

Combination Therapy

Cosman et al. evaluated the effects of intravenous zoledronic acid plus subcutaneous terparatide in women with post-menopausal osteoporosis [55]. Previous studies of combination therapy with alendronate and (1-84) PTH showed a blunting of the bone formation effect of the PTH analog [56]. These authors conducted a one-year multi-center, randomized, multi-national, partial double-blinded, controlled trial. Four hundred twelve post-menopausal women were randomized to receive either 5mg zoledronic acid alone (n=137), teriparatide 20 mcg daily alone (n=138) or a combination of a single infusion of zoledronic acid 5mg plus daily teriparatide 20mcg subcutaneously daily (n=137). The primary endpoint was the percentage increase in the lumbar spine BMD as measured by DXA at 52 weeks compared to the baseline DXA. Secondary endpoints were change in the lumbar spine BMD at earlier time points and change in the femoral neck, total hip and trochanteric BMD at all time points measured. Eligible women were 45 to 89 years of age with BMD T-scores at the lumbar spine, total hip or femoral neck of -2.5 or lower or a BMD T-score of -2.0 or lower at any of these 3 sites in addition to one or more documented vertebral or non-vertebral fractures. The results demonstrated at 52 weeks increases in lumbar spine BMD of 7.5% with combination therapy, 7.0% with teriparatide alone and 4.4% for zoledronic acid monotherapy. This was not a significant difference between the teriparatide and combination therapy groups at week 52 but lumbar spine BMD increments were greater with combination therapy versus teriparatide montherapy at weeks 13 and 26, for combination therapy versus zoledronic acid monotherapy at all time points measured and for teriparatide monotherapy compared to zoledronic acid monotherapy at week 52 (all $p<0.001$). Increments in femoral neck and trochanteric BMD with combination therapy were greater than with teriparatide monotherapy throughout the study. Increases in total hip BMD at 52 weeks were 2.3% with combination therapy, 1.1% with teriparatide monotherapy and 2.2% with zoledronic acid monotherapy. This study was not powered to compare anti-fracture efficacy so clinical fractures were captured as adverse events. Clinical fractures occurred in 13 subjects on zoledronic acid monotherapy, in 8 subjects on teriparatide monotherapy and in 4 subjects on combination therapy. Serum CTX, a marker of bone resorption, was reduced to its nadir at week 4 in the zoledronic acid monotherapy group whereas in the teriparatide monotherapy group serum CTX levels were unchanged at week 4 then increased to maximal levels by week 26 and decreased slightly thereafter. In the combination therapy group, there was an initial reduction in CTX similar to that seen in the zoledronic acid monotherapy group followed by a gradual increase after week 8, with levels remaining above baseline throughout the second half of the study. P1NP, a bone formation marker, declined until week 8 with little change thereafter in the zoledronic acid monotherapy group. In the teriparatide monotherapy group, P1NP was elevated by week 4. In the combination group, P1NP increased through week 4, decreased slightly between the 4th and 8th week, then progressively increased from months 6 to 12 with levels above baseline. The decrease in P1NP in the combination therapy group was much less than the decrease in P1NP in the zoledronic acid monotherapy group. As expected, short- term post-infusion symptoms occurred in the zoledronic acid monotherapy group (58.4%) and the combination therapy group 68.6% but adverse events three days after the infusion were comparable across all three treatment groups. In summary, combination therapy with zoledronic acid and teriparatide resulted in rapid reduction of bone resorption that was maintained over the first 8 weeks followed by a gradual resolution of this decrease and a subsequent increase of resorption over the last 6 months of treatment. The authors suggested that the duration of reduction of bone resorption, as measured by CTX, induced by zoledronic acid that is shorter in the presence of teriparatide compared to when zoledronic acid is given as monotherapy could be due to rapid removal of zoledronic acid from the bone surface in the presence of teriparatide. They also concluded that based on the P1NP results that zoledronic acid did not interfere with the osteoblastic response to teriparatide. As hip BMD in the combination group was greater than that in the teriparatide group, the authors hypothesized that co-treatment with teriparatide and zoledronic acid may prevent the increase in cortical porosity that is seen with teriparatide monotherapy. The authors hypothesized further that the lack of continued increase in the BMD at the hip during the second sixth months of the study in the combination therapy group perhaps is due to increased cortical remodeling and resulting increases in cortical porosity as the effects of the zoledronic acid waned. The authors suggested that the differing results of their study compared to that of Black [56] could be due to several causes including the fact that a different form of PTH was used (1-84 compared to 1-34), a different bisphosphonate was used (alendronate compared to zoledronic acid) and daily administration of alendronate may impair the osteoblastic response to PTH, an effect that may be avoided by a once yearly infusion. In conclusion, this study only demonstrated that combination therapy with zoledronic acid and teriparatide was non-inferior to teriparatide alone in increasing BMD. Again, as there is not a direct correlation between increase in BMD and fracture reduction, further studies need to be performed with fractures as an end point before combination therapy can be recommended as superior to monotherapy with teriparatide. Nevertheless, as teriparatide monotherapy has not been shown to reduce the risk of hip fracture, combination therapy may be appropriate therapy for patients at increased risk of hip fracture.

Adverse Events

The post-dose acute phase reactions have been discussed in the above studies. Although worsening renal function was not seen in the randomized controlled clinical trials other than age-related changes, the FDA notified patient and healthcare professionals on September 1, 2011 about an update to the prescribing information with regards to the risk of renal failure [57]. This update was prompted by cases of acute renal failure that required dialysis or resulted in death following administration of zoledronic acid. This revised package information states that in patients with a creatinine clearance less than 35cc/min or in patients with evidence of acute renal impairment, zoledronic acid is contra-indicated. This updated label also suggests that healthcare professionals, prior to administering zoledronic acid, screen patients to identify those who are at risk of developing acute renal damage and monitor renal function in patients who are undergoing treatment with zoledronic acid. Listed risk factors for developing acute renal failure associated with administration of zoledronic acid include use of nephrotoxic drugs or diuretics while receiving zoledronic acid, pre-existing moderate to severe renal impairment and severe dehydration occurring before or after zoledronic acid is infused. Advancing age in patients with pre-existing renal impairment also increases the risk of developing acute renal failure. This update suggests that patients be appropriately hydrated prior to infusion of zoledronic acid to prevent renal impairment from occurring. It is also suggested that serum creatinine be measured before each administration of zoledronic acid and consideration should be given to interim monitoring of serum creatinine in patients who are at increased risk of renal impairment.

Hicks et al. performed a retrospective chart review of 237 charts of receiving osteoporosis therapy [58] to evaluate the effect of zoledronic acid infusions on renal function and serum calcium levels. One hundred forty-one patients received two zoledronic acid infusions and 58 patients had received 3 infusions. No significant difference was found between pre- and post-infusion estimated glomerular filtration rates for all infusions ($p=0.07$) or pre- and post-creatinine clearance values ($p=0.4269$). Two hundred forty-four pre-and post-serum calcium levels (corrected for albumin) and eighty-six pre- and post-ionized calcium levels showed a significant difference with the first infusion but not with the second or third infusion ($p=<0.0001$ for corrected calcium and $p=0.0272$ for ionized calcium). This chart review indicates that in this population zoledronic acid did not alter renal function but that significant changes in serum calcium occurred during the first infusion but serious hypocalcemia did not occur in the Vitamin D replete population.

Adherence, Compliance and Persistence

Lee et al. evaluated the proportion of patients who had second infusions of zoledronic acid after the first administration and the factors that contributed to discontinuation; the data was collected via questionnaire at an outpatient clinic [59]. Two hundred fifty-nine patients received one zoledronic acid infusion; 192 patients returned to the clinic one year later but only 94 underwent a second infusion. Of the 192 patients, 136 patients completed the questionnaire, 47 patients refused a second infusion and 18 patients asked to change to an oral osteoporosis medication. Of the 47 patients who refused a second infusion, 41 experienced adverse events; the remaining 6 refused the second infusion despite not having an adverse event. Thirty-nine of the 47 patients (83%) reported the reason that they refused a second infusion was due to a post-infusion reaction. Univariate analysis showed that adverse events ($p<0.001$), gender ($p=0.001$), cost ($p<0.001$), explanation of IV zoledronate ($p<0.001$), explanation of osteoporosis ($p<0.001$) and history of oral bisphosphonate therapy ($p=0.007$) were associated with discontinuation. This data suggests that persistence with a second infusion of zoledronic acid is 36.3% which is comparable to persistence with oral bisphosphonates after one year [60]. The limitation of this study was the low follow up rate (74.1%, 192/259) and the large difference in non-response rates between the persistent group and the discontinuation group (5/94 versus 51/98) which could and perhaps did affect the results.

Lee et al. evaluated the factors that determine patient adherence with anti-osteoporosis treatments by reviewing published articles from 1970-2009 [61]. As expected patient adherence and preference at 12 months were higher with weekly than daily bisphosphonates. Preference was 84% or greater for weekly therapy with medication possession ratio of 60-76% versus 46-64% and persistence 43.6-69.7% versus 31.7-55.7%. The medication possession ratio at 12 months for oral bisphosphonates were 68-71% but at 2 years only 43% of patients had a medication possession rate of $\geq$ 80% for daily and weekly bisphosphonates. Observational studies that included data from 6-12 months reported discontinuation rates of 7% for weekly bisphosphonates and 18-22% for daily bisphosphonates. Data on monthly bisphosphonates was confounded by manufacturer-sponsored patient support programs and cost differences. Studies suggested patient preference for yearly infusions of zoledronic acid over weekly bisphosphonates (66.4-78.8% versus 9.0-19.7%) but no compliance or persistence data was available during this time period. This literature review demonstrated that medication effectiveness, side effects and route of administration were more important than frequency of administration in determining patient preference.

Conclusion

The goal of osteoporosis therapy is to reduce fractures; zoledronic acid has demonstrated fracture risk reduction of vertebral, non-vertebral and hip fractures. This once yearly infusion offers women with low bone mass and osteoporosis and men with osteoporosis an alternative to oral daily, weekly and monthly bisphosphonate therapy and an alternative to every 3-month infusions of ibandronate. It is hoped that a once yearly infusion will increase adherence and persistence. Patient preference data suggests that this once yearly infusion is preferred to daily, weekly and monthly bisphosphonate therapy. The most common adverse event is a post-dose infusion reaction that occurs less frequently with subsequent infusions. Older patients with renal impairment or taking potentially nephrotoxic drugs are at increased risk of acute renal failure. Combination therapy with teriparatide is intriguing for patients at high risk of all types of fracture but especially hip fracture. Hopefully future studies will clarify the optimum frequency of zoledronic acid infusions and long-term safety data will continue to be published.

References

[1] Reclast Prescribing Information, Novartis Pharmaceutical Corp. East Hanover NJ, April 2013

[2] Rogers, MJ. New insights into the Molecular Mechanism of Action of Bisphosphonates, *Curr Pharm*, 2003, 2643-2658.

[3] Bergstrom, JD; Bostedor, RG; Masarachia, PJ; et al. Alendronate is a Specific, Nanomolar Inhibitor of Farnesyl Diphosphate Synthase, *Biochem Biophys*, 2000, 373, 231-234

[4] Catalano, A; Morabito, N; Basile, G; et al. Zoledronic Acid Acutely Increases Sclerostin Serum Levels in Women with Postmenopausal Osteoporosis, *J Clin Endocrinol Metab*, May 2013, 98(5), 1911-1915

[5] Pederson, L; Ruan, M; Westerdorf, JJ; et al. Regulation of Bone Formation by Osteoclasts Involves Wnt/BMP Signaling and the Use of Chemokine Sphingosine-1-phosphate. *Proc Natl Acad Sci USA*, 2008, 105, 20764-20769.

[6] Gatti, P; Viapiana, O; Adami, S; et al. Treatment of Postmenopausal Osteoporosis is Associated with a Dose-Dependent Increase in Serum Sclerostin. *Bone*, 2012, 50, 739-742

[7] Reid, IR; Brown, JP; Burckhardt, P; et al. Intravenous Zoledronic Acid in Post Menopausal Women with Low Bone Mineral Density, *N Engl J Med*, 2002, 346, 653-661

[8] Sato, M; Grasser, W; Endo, N; et al. Bisphosphonate Action: Alendronate Localization in Rat Bone and Effects on Osteoclast Ultrastructure. *J Clin Invest*, 1991, 88, 2095-2105

[9] Masarachia, P; Weinreb, M; Balena, R; Rodan, GA. Comparison of the Distribution of 3-Alendronate and 3-Etidronate in Rat and Mouse Bones. *Bone*, 1996, 19-281-290

[10] Devogelaer, JP; Brown, JP; Burkhardt, P; et al. Zoledronic Acid Efficacy and Safety Over Five Years in Postmenopausal Osteoporosis. *Osteoporos Int*, 2007, 18 (9), 1211-1218

[11] Black, DM; Delmas, PD; Eastell, R; et al. Once-Yearly Zoledronic Acid for Treatment of Postmenopausal Osteoporosis, *N Engl J Med*, 2007, 356, 1809-1822

[12] Recker, RR; Delmas, PD; Halse, J; et al. Effects of Intravenous Zoledronic Acid Once Yearly on Bone Structure. *J Bone Min Res*, 2008, 23 (1), 6-16

[13] Ebeling, RR; Burr, DB. Positive Effects of Intravenous Zoledronic Acid on Bone Remodeling and Structure: Are Different Effects on Osteoblastic Activity to Other Oral Bisphosphonates Responsible? *J Bone Min Res*, 2008, 23 (1), 2-5

[14] Black, CB; Eastell, R; Cosman, F; et al. Effect of Once-Yearly Zoledronic Acid 5mg on a Subset of Six Non-vertebral Fractures. Annual Meeting ASBMR 2009, Denver, Colorado, Sunday September 13, presentation number sU0360

[15] Eastell, R; Black, CM; Boonen, S; et al. Effect of Once-Yearly Zoledronic Acid 5mg on Fracture Risk and Change in Femoral Neck Bone Mineral Density. *J ClinEndocrinol Metab*, 2009 Sept, 94(9), 3215-3225

[16] Jacques, RM; Boonen, S; Cosman, F; et al. Relationship of Changes in the Total Hip Bone Mineral Density to Vertebral and Non-vertebral Fracture Risk in Women with Postmenopausal Osteoporosis Treated with Once-yearly Zoledronic Acid: The HORIZON-PFT. *J Bone Miner Res*, 2012 August, 27 (8), 1627-1634

[17] Lyles, KW; Colon-Emeric, CS; Magaziner, JS; et al. Zoledronic Acid in Reducing Clinical Fracture and Mortality after Hip Fracture, *N Engl J Med*, 2007, 357, 1799-1809

[18] Ericksen, EF; Lyles, KW; Colon-Emeric, CS; et al. Anti-Fracture Efficacy and Reduction of Mortality in Relation to Timing of the First Dose of Zoledronic Acid After Hip Fracture. *J Bone Miner Res*, 2009 Jul, 24(2), 1308-1313

[19] Boonen, S; Black, DM; Colon-Emeric, CS; et al. Efficacy and Safety of a Once-Yearly Intravenous Zoledronic Acid 5mg for Fracture Prevention in Elderly Postmenopausal Women with Osteoporosis Aged 75 or Older, *J Am Geriatr Soc*, 2010, 58, 292-299

[20] Boonen, S; Eastell, R; Su, G; et al. Time-to-Onset of Anti-fracture Efficacy and Year-by-Year Persistence of Effect of Zoledronic Acid in Women with Osteoporosis, *J Bone Miner Res*, 2012 July, 27 (7), 1487-1493

[21] Black, DM; Thompson, DE; Bauer, DC; et al. Fracture Intervention Trial, Fracture Risk Reduction with Alendonate in Women with Osteoporosis: the Fracture Intervention Trial. Fit Research Group. *J Clin Endocrinol Metab*, 2000, 85, 4118-4124

[22] Saag, K; Lindsay, R; Kriegman, A; et al. A Single Zoledronic Acid Infusion Reduces Bone Resorption Markers More Rapidly than Weekly Oral Alendronate in Postmenopausal Women with Low Bone Mineral Density. *Bone*, 2007, 40, 1238-1243

[23] Eastell, R; Lang, T; Boonen, S; et al. Effect of Once-Yearly Zoldronic Acid on the Spine and Hip as Measured by Quantitative Computed Analysis: Results of the Horizon-PFT. *Osteoporos Int*, 2010 Jul, 21 (7), 1277-1285

[24] Gamsjaeger, S; Buchinger, B; Zwettler, E; et al. Bone Mineral Properties in Actively Bone-Forming Trabeculae in Postmenopausal Women with Osteoporosis After Three Years of Treatment with Once-Yearly Zoledronic Acid. *J Bone Min Res*, 2011, 26 (1), 12-18

[25] Misof, BM; Roschger, P; Gabriel, D; et al. Annual Intravenous Zoledronic Acid for Three Years Increased Cancellous Bone Matrix Mineralization Beyond Normal Values in the HORIZON Biopsy Cohort. *J Bone Miner Res*, 2013, 28(3), 442-448

[26] Yang, L; Sychera, AV; Black, DM; Eastell, R. Site-Specific Differential Effects of Once-Yearly Zoledronic Acid on the Hip Assessed with QCT: Results from the HORIZON-PFT. *Osteoporos Int*, 2013 Jan, 24 (1), 329-338

[27] Popp, AW; Guler, S; Larny, O; et al. Effects of Zoledronate Versus Placebo on Spine Bone Mineral Density and Microarchitecture Assessed by the Trabecular Bone Score in Postmenopausal Women with Osteoporosis: A Three-Year Study. *J Bone Miner Res*, 2013 March, 28 (3), 449-454

[28] Black, DM; Reid, IR; Boonen, S; et al. The Effect of Three versus Six Years of Zoledronic Acid Treatment of Osteoporosis: A Randomized Extension of the HORIZON-PFT. *J Bone Min Res*, 2012 Feb, 27(2), 243-254

[29] Black, DM; Bauer, DC; Cummings, SR; et al. Efficacy of Continued Alendronate for Fractures in Women With and Without Prevalent Vertebral Fractures: The FLEX Trial. *J Bone Miner Res*, 2010, 25 (5), 976-982

[30] FDA, September 9, 2011. Joint Meeting of the Reproductive Health Drug Advisory Committee and the Drug Safety and Risk Assessment Advisory Committee Meeting Announcement. Available from http://www.fda.gov/AdvisoryCommittees/Calendar /ucm262477.htm

[31] Eastell, R; Palermo, L; McNabb, B; et al. The Relationship Between the Change in Total Hip Bone Mineral Density: The HORIZON-PFT Extension study, ASBMR Annual Meeting, Minn, Minn, Friday Oct 12, 2012, presentation RR0376

[32] Black, DB; Reid, I; Cauley, J; et al. The Effect of Six Versus Nine Years of Zoledronic Acid Treatment in Osteoporosis: A Randomized Extension to the HORIZON-PFT, ASBMR Annual Meeting, Baltimore MD, Sat Oct 5, 2013,presentation SA0389

[33] Siddique, N; Cheuny, NK; Carroll, KM; et al. Identifying Factors Involved in Predicting Response to Intravenous Zoledronic Acid in Elderly Patients with Osteoporosis. ASBMR Annual Meeting Minn, Minn, Sat Oct 13, 2012, presentation SA 0370

[34] Borba, VZ; Paz-Filho, G; Kulak; CA; et al. Bone Turnover Eighteen Months After a Single Intravelous Dose of Zoledronic Acid. *Int J Clin Prac*, 2007, 61, 1058-1062

[35] Grey, A; Bolland; MJ; Horne, A; et al. Five Years of anti-Resorptive Activity After a Single Dose of Zoledronate-Results from a Randomized Double-blind, Placebo-controlled Trial. *Bone*, 2012 June, 50(6), 1389-1393

[36] Bourke, S; Bolland, MJ; Grey, A. The Impact of Dietary Calcium Intake and Vitamin D Status on the Effects of Zoledronate. *Osteoporos Int*, 2013, 24, 349-354

[37] Grey, A; Bolland; Hong, S; et al. Low Dose Zoledronate in Osteopenic Postmenopausal Women: A Randomized Controlled Trial *J Clin Endocrinol Metab*, 2012, 97, 286-292

[38] McClung, M; Miller, P; Recknor, C; et al. Zoledronic Acid for the Prevention of Bone Loss in Postmenopausal Women with Low Bone Mass, *Obstet Gynecol*, 2009 Nov, 114 (5), 999-1007

[39] Eskiyurt, N; Gunaydin, R; Erhan, B; et al. Efficacy and Safety of Zoledronic Acid in Postmenopausal Osteoporosis Patients Between 50-65 Years Old. ASBMR Annual Meeting. Baltimore MD, Sat Oct 5, 2013 presentation SA 0385

[40] Boonan, S; Reginster; J-Y; Kaufman, J-M; et al. Fracture Risk and Zoledronic Acid Therapy in Men with Osteoporosis, *N Engl J Med*, 2012, 367, 1714-1723

[41] Reid, DM; Devogelaer, J-P; Saag, K; et al. Zoledronic Acid and Risedronate in the Prevention and Treatment of Glucocorticoid-Induced Osteoporosis (HORIZON: A Multicentre, Double-blind, Double-dummy, Randomized Controlled Trial. *Lancet*, 2009 Apr, 373(9671), 1253-1263

[42] Simon, PJ; Johannesen, J; Brody, J; et al. Zoledronic Acid Improves Bone Mineral Density, Reduces Bone Turnover and Improves Skeletal Architecture over Two Years of Treatment in Children with Secondary Osteoporosis. *Bone*, 2011 Nov, 49 (5), 939-943

[43] Bubbear, JS; Gall, A; Middleton, FRI; et al. Early Treatment with Zoledronic Acid Prevents Bone Loss at the Hip Following Acute Spinal Cord Injury. *Osteoporos Int.*, 2011, 22, 271-279
[44] Schnitzer, T, ; Barkema, D; Herrman, K; Kim, K. Effect of Zoledronic Acid on Acute Bone Loss after a Spinal Cord Injury. ASBMR Annual Meeting, Minn, Minn, Fri Oct 12, 2012. Presentation FR 0370
[45] Huang, J; Meixner, L; Fernandez, S; McCutchon, JA. A Double-blind, Randomized Controlled Trial of Zoledronate Treatment for HIV Associated Osteopenia and Osteoporosis. *AIDS*, 2 Jan 2009, 23 (1), 51-57
[46] Greenspan, SL; Nace, D., Perera, S; et al. Lessons Learned from the Osteoporosis Trial in Frail Long Term Care Residents, *Clin Trials,* 2012 April, 9 (2), 247-256
[47] Greenspan, SL; Ferchak, MA; Perera, S; et al. Against All Odds: Results from the ZEST Trial in Long Term Care Residents, ASBMR Annual Meeting, Baltimore, MD, Sat Oct 5, 2013, presentation SA1025
[48] Jansen, JD; Bergman, GJD; Huels, J; Olson, M. The efficacy of Bisphosphonates in the Prevention of Vertebral, Hip and Nonvertebral-Non-hip Fractures in Osteoporosis. *Sem Arth Rheum*, 2011 Feb, 40 (4), 275-284
[49] McClung, M; Recker, R; Miller, P; et al. Intravenous Zoledronic Acid 5mg in the Treatment of Postmenopausal Women with Low Bone Mineral Density Previously Treated with Alendronate. *Bone*, 2007 July, 41 (1), 122-128
[50] Gauthier, K; Bai, A; Perras, C; et al. Denosumab, Raloxifene and Zoledronic Acid for the Treatment of Postmenopausal Osteoporosis: Clinical Effectiveness and Harms (Internet). Ottawa: Canadian Agency for Drugs and Technologies in Health, 2012 (Rapid Response: Systematic Review)
[51] Hadji, P; Gamerdeinger, D; Spieler, W; et al. Rapid Onset and Sustained Efficacy (ROSE) Study: Results of a Randomized, Multicentre Trial Comparing the Effect of Zoledronic Acid or Alendronate on Bone Metabolism in Postmenopausal Women with Low Bone Mass. *Osteoporous Int*, 2012 Feb, 23 (2), 625-633
[52] Dempster, D; Shou, H; Recker, R; et al. Differential Effects of Teriparatide and Zoledronic Acid on the Outer and Inner Surfaces of Cortical Bone in Postmenopausal Women with Osteoporosis: Results from the SHOTZ Trial, ASBMR Annual Meeting Minn, Minn, Mon Oct 15, 2012, presentation MO 1170
[53] Invernizz, M; Barich, A; Bevilacqua, M; et al. Effects of Denosumab on Bone Turnover Markers Compared to Zoledronic Acid in Severe Osteoporotic Women: A Randomized Head-to-Head Study. ASBMR Annual Meeting, Minn, Min, Mon Oct 15, 2012, presentation MO 0369
[54] Sheedy, K; Camara, I; Camacho, P. Comparison of the Efficacy, Adverse Effects and Cost of Zoledronic Acid and Denosumab in the Treatment of Osteoporosis. ASBMR Annual Meeting, Baltimore MD, Mon Oct 7, 2013, presentation MO 0378
[55] Cosman, F; Eriksen, EF; Recknor, C; et al. Effects of Intravenous Zoledronic Acid plus Subcutaneous Teriparatide [rhPTH(1-34)] in Postmenopausal Osteoporosis. *J Bone Min Res*, 2011 Mar, 26 (3), 503-511
[56] Black, DM; Greenspan, SL; Ensrud, KE; et al. The Effects of PTH and Alendronate Alone or in Combination in Postmenopausal Osteoporosis, *N Engl J Med*, 2003, 249(13), 1207-1215

[57] Reclast (Zoledronic acid): Drug Safety Communication-New Contra-indication and Updated Warning on Kidney Impairment. Med Watch, Safety Information, posted 09/01/2011

[58] Hicks, H; Camacho, P. The Occurrence of Renal Insufficiency and Hypocalcemia After Zoledronic Acid Infusion, ASBMR Annual Meeting, Baltimore MD, Mon Oct 7, 2013, presentation MO 0391

[59] Lee, YK; Nho, JH; Ha, KC; Koo, KH. Persistence with Intravenous Zoledronic Acid in Elderly Patients with Osteoporosis, *Osteoporos Int*, 2012, 23, 2329-2333

[60] Lee, S; Glendenning, P; Inderjeeth, CA. Efficacy, Side Effects and Route of Administration Are More Important than Frequency of Dosing of Anti-Osteoporosis Treatments in Determining Patient Adherence: A Critical Review of Published Articles from 1970-2009. *Osteoporos Int*, 2011, 22, 741-753

[61] Cramer, JA; Gold, DT; Silverman, SL; Lewiecki, EM. A Systematic Review of Persistence and Compliance with Bisphosphonates for Osteoporosis. *Osteoporos Int*, 2007, 18, 1023-1031

In: Zoledronic Acid
Editor: Ronald Carman
ISBN: 978-1-63321-525-2

Chapter 2

Clinical and Experimental Evidences of Anti-Myeloma Activities of Zoledronic Acid

R. Ria, A. Reale, A. Melaccio and A. Vacca
Department of Biomedical Sciences and Human Oncology,
Section of Internal Medicine and Clinical Oncology,
University of Bari Medical School, Bari, Italy

Abstract

The biphosphonate zoledronic acid is indicated for the treatment of patients with osteolytic lesions from multiple myeloma for the prevention of skeletal related events. In patients with multiple myeloma the clonal expansion of plasma cells in the bone marrow results in the disruption of the homeostasis within the bone marrow microenvironment. Interactions between myeloma cells and bone marrow stromal cells directly increase growth and survival of myeloma cells through the dysregulation of growth factors and cytokines and accelerate the destruction of the bone.

Thus, most of multiple myeloma patients develop osteolytic bone lesions, which are often associated with bone pain and skeletal-related events which include spinal cord compression, pathologic fractures, or the need for surgery or radiation to the bone. Bisphosphonates are effective inhibitors of osteoclastic bone resorption. *In-vitro* evidences suggest that bisphosphonates may also have an antimyeloma activity.

Furthermore, they may synergize with anticancer agents used in the treatment of myeloma. Recent clinical data show a survival advantage for high-risk patients receiving zoledronic acid concurrently with antimyeloma therapies. This review summerizes the antimyeloma benefits of zoledronic acid combined with new drugs for the treatment of multiple myeloma patients.

Keywords: Multiple myeloma, novel agents, progression-free survival, skeletal-related events, zoledronic acid

INTRODUCTION

Multiple myeloma (MM) is characterised by a clonal expansion of malignant plasma cells in the bone marrow, where they proliferate and acquire resistance to apoptosis and eventually lead to osteolysis, renal dysfunction and anaemia [1]. Since the disease mainly progresses in the bone marrow, signals from its microenvironment play a pivotal role in maintaining plasma cell growth, migration and survival [2]. Interactions between myeloma cells and bone cells and the extracellular matrix proteins within the bone microenvironment underlie this progression and are mediated through cell surface receptors—for example, integrins, cadherins, selectins, syndecans and the immunoglobulin superfamily of cell adhesion molecules [3].

These interactions trigger a self-amplifying cascade of events that result in the secretion of cytokines and growth factors (such as vascular endothelial growth factor [VEGF], insulin-like growth factor-1, interleukin [IL]-6 and IL-1β) and members of the tumor necrosis factor superfamily (transforming growth factor [TGF]β1, CCL3, hepatocyte growth factor [HGF] and IL-10) that promote the growth and proliferation of myeloma cells, increase bone resorption and enhance drug resistance by inducing antiapoptotic pathways [3, 4]. The role of bisphosphonates for patients with myeloma may go beyond simply inhibiting bone resorption and the resulting skeletal complications. Radl et al. [5] suggest that pamidronate might reduce myeloma tumor burden in treated mice. In vitro studies also suggest that pamidronate may possess antimyeloma properties as shown by its ability to induce the apoptosis of myeloma cells [6] and the suppression of IL-6 production [7] and antiangiogenesis [8, 9].

Interestingly, the antitumor effects of bisphosphonates are not only observed alone but seem to be synergistic with other drugs [10-14].

MYELOMA BONE DISEASE

Patients with MM commonly experience skeletal-related complications that result from a shift in the normal balance between bone formation and bone resorption toward enhanced bone loss [15]. As a result, diffuse osteopenia, focal lytic lesions, pathologic fractures, hypercalcemia, and bony pain are common clinical manifestations in patients with MM. These complications are major causes of morbidity and mortality [16]. The lytic process observed in MM is different from other cancers that metastasize to the bone in which bone destruction is followed by new bone formation.

Even when patients with MM respond to anti-MM therapies, they may still have progression of skeletal events [17, 18] without repair of osteolytic lesions. These patients frequently require radiation therapy, surgery, and use of analgesics to overcome pain and improve their quality of life.

Bone destruction in MM results from asynchronous bone turnover wherein increased osteoclastic bone resorption is not accompanied by a comparable increase in bone formation. A dramatic increase in osteoclast function, in addition to an inhibition of osteoblast ability to produce new bone, leads to the development of lytic lesions [19-22].

Increased osteoclast activity can be detected by the production of type I collagen breakdown products as well as by the release osteoclast-specific enzymes. Further changes in the cytokine milieu also contribute to bone loss [19, 20, 22-26]. A variety of markers of bone resorption and formation have been used to assess bone disease in patients with myeloma.

Patients with MM have increases in bone resorption markers such as COOH-terminal telopeptide of type I collagen, NH terminal telopeptide of collagen I, pyridinoline, and deoxypyridinoline, and decreases in bone formation markers such as osteocalcin [27-30]. In recent clinical trials [29, 31, 32], changes in these markers were shown to predict the development of new skeletal complications and were associated with survival.

Apoptosis of osteoblasts is mediated by increased expression of the Fas ligand and tumor necrosis factor (TNF)-related apoptosis inducing ligand on myeloma cells, which activate the Fas receptor and the death receptor-4/5 on cells of the osteoblast lineage [33]. Osteoblast function is also impeded by the rapid growth of myeloma cells [22], which attach to bone marrow stromal cells (BMSCs) stimulating the production of osteoclast-activating factors such as receptor activator of nuclear factor-kappa B ligand (RANKL), macrophage colony stimulating factor as well as an assortment of cytokines (IL-6, IL-1b, IL-11) [34, 35].

The secretion of TNFa and other cytokines into the myeloma bone microenvironment induces osteoblasts and BMSCs to produce additional RANKL and decrease the production of osteoprotegerin, the decoy receptor for RANKL [36-38]. Furthermore, macrophage inflammatory protein 1-alpha, hepatocyte growth factor, and vascular endothelial growth factor are increased in the bone microenvironment, further stimulating osteoclastogenesis and bone digestion [36-40]. Finally, transforming growth factor-β inhibits osteoblast maturation and mineralization. It is release by activated osteoclasts [23, 41].

Near osteoclast activation and osteoblast inhibition, suppression of osteoblast precursor differentiation and induction of apoptosis in mature osteoblasts further result in decreased bone formation [34, 42-50].

Increased production of dickkopf-1 and secretion of frizzled-related protein 2, [51, 52] are also responsible for the osteoblast dysfunction in MM, acting as Wingless-type signaling antagonists. Moreover, interleukin (IL)-7 and IL-3 have been shown to inhibit osteoblastic differentiation in vitro [53, 54].

BISPHOSPHONATES

BPs are synthetic, stable and resistant to hydrolysis by blood phosphatases analogues of inorganic pyrophosphate (PPi) [55, 56]. There are two main types of BPs, nitrogen and non-nitrogen containing, each of which has a different mechanism of action for preventing bone resorption. The nitrogen-containing BPs (N-BPs) such as ibandronate (IBA), risedronate (RIS), pamidronate (PAM), and zoledronic acid (ZOL) bind and inhibit the enzyme farnesyl pyrophosphate synthase, in the mevalonate pathway, disrupting the formation of farnesyl diphosphate and geranylgeranyl diphosphate [57-59] and inhibit prenylation [60]. This post-translational modification of proteins, is important for the activity of a range of proteins including the small GTPases, Ras, Rac, and Rho,because tethering them to the cell membrane with a hydrophobic anchor. This is critical for allowing proteins to be localized to the appropriate parts of the cell in order to mediate their biological activity, which play key roles in regulating osteoclast function and events in bone resorption [61]. Nitrogen-containing BPs have a much greater potency in vitro than first generation non-nitrogen-containing BPs etidronate (ETI) and clodronate (CLO) that are compounds [62] which are metabolized to cytotoxic ATP analogues, which induce osteoclast cell death [63-65].

BPs have high affinity to Ca2 allowing them to bind quickly and specifically to hydroxyapatite, the major calcium-containing mineral in bone, especially in regions where resorption is occurring.

When osteoclasts break down bone, BPs accumulate in the resorption space under these cells, exposing them to high BP concentrations [66, 67].

The in vivo efficacy of BPs seems to correlate with the in vitro potency. Generally, with regards to potency, etidronate < clodronate < pamidronate < alendronate < risendronate < ibandronate < zoledronate [68, 69].

Only clodronate, pamidronate and zoledronate have been approved for use in MM patients in Europe, and clodronate is not approved in many EU countries.

The majority of MM patients suffer debilitating pain due to osteolytic bone disease [70, 71]. Reduction and control of pain is a crucial aspect in maintaining a high QoL. BPs have been shown to reduce bone pain and maintain it at a lower level, improve QoL in myeloma patients, and reduce analgesic consumption though it is uncertain if this effect is a direct one or if it is due to amelioration of bone disease [72-75].

Pain is one of the most distressing symptoms of MM, and pain control is deemed as important as prolonging OS.

Treatment of MM patients with BPs has been evaluated in several studies. Assessment of skeletal-related events (SREs), such as pathological fracture, radiation therapy, and surgery to bone, hypercalcemia, and spinal cord compression, are common end points in clinical trials of BPs in cancer treatment [73]. Impact on bone pain and bone resorption markers are also often examined as secondary end points.

In a randomized double-blind study of patients with newly diagnosed MM of the Cross Cancer Institute in Canada the administration of daily etidronate versus placebo, showed a lack of effectiveness in preventing SREs, bone pain, and fracture [17]. The GERM group confirmed these data, showing that etidronate therapy did not have a clinically significant effect in MM [76].

Ibandronate also failed to show any effect on bone morbidity and in prolonging patient survival in a phase III double-blind trial comparing monthly injections of 2 mg of ibandronate versus placebo in addition to antineoplastic therapy [77]. This monthly dose of i.v. ibandronate did not show significant benefits in reducing skeletal complications in patients with myeloma with lytic bone disease.

Oral clodronate has been evaluated in three large randomized trials in comparison to placebo in patients with MM showing variable clinical results [72, 78, 79].

In the study conducted by the Medical Research Council a significant reduction in nonvertebral fractures (6.8% versus 13.2%; $P = 0.04$) and vertebral fractures rates (38% versus 55%; $P = 0.01$) has benn obtained in the clodronate arm compared with the placebo arm. After a 1-year follow-up, and at 2 years, the clodronate-treated patients also had less myeloma-related pain than patients treated with placebo [72].

On the contrary, the Finnish trial reported no differences in the reduction of overall pathologic fractures, as well as vertebral and nonvertebral fractures [78]. In this last trial clodronate has been shown to reduce the development of new osteolytic lesions by 50% after 2 years of administration, as well as to reduce the degree of hypercalcemia and hypercalciuria, and to decrease bone pain (24% versus 12%; $P = 0.026$) [78].

Moreover, McCloskey et al. showed that among the subgroup of patients without skeletal fractures at presentation, there was a significant survival advantage (P = 0.006) in favor of patients receiving clodronate, with median survival time reported as 59 months [95% confidence interval (CI) 43–71 months] and 37 months (95% CI 31–52 months) and 5-year survivals of 46% and 35%, respectively [80]. The Finnish study established that there was no difference in OS of MM patients treated with clodronate [81]. However, [78] clodronate has never been directly compared with other BPs.

Daily oral pamidronate (300 mg/d) was evaluated in a double-blind randomized trial versus placebo by a Danish-Swedish cooperative group, in 300 patients with newly diagnosed myeloma. [82].

After a median duration of 18 months, no significant reduction was detected in the primary end points defined as skeletal-related morbidity, hypercalcemic episodes, or survival between the treatment arms.

In another trial conducted to determine the effect of monthly 90-mg infusions of pamidronate in MM patients, with lytic lesions. Pamidronate showed a reduced number of SREs (41% versus 24%; P < 0.001) and a decrease in the time to the first skeletal event [73].

Confirming the results of a small open-label trial that lasted up to 24 months suggested that i.v. pamidronate disodium might be effective in reducing skeletal complications for patients with MM [83].

At the preplanned primary end point after nine cycles of therapy [73], the proportion of patients with myeloma having any skeletal event was 41% in patients receiving placebo, but only 24% in pamidronate-treated patients.

The patients who received pamidronate also had a significant decrease in bone pain without increasing its analgesic use, and did not have deterioration in performance status and quality of life at the end of 9 months.

The proportion of patients developing any skeletal event and the skeletal morbidity rate continued to remain significantly lower in the pamidronate group than the placebo group during the additional 12 cycles of treatment [84]. While there were no differences in survival time in the treatment groups, a subgroup of patients who had received more than one previous antimyeloma treatment displayed increased survival time (14 versus 21 months, P = 0.041). In addition, pain scores and QoL were improved in the PAM group [84].

Zoledronic acid is an imidazole-containing bisphosphonate that shows more potency than any other bisphosphonate currently available in preclinical studies [85].

A phase II trial [86] evaluated two doses of zoledronic acid (4 and 8 mg) compared with 90 mg pamidronate infused every 3 to 4 weeks for the treatment of patients with myeloma or breast cancer with metastatic bone disease. Both BPs significantly reduced SREs. The doses and infusion times (5 minutes) of zoledronate were selected based on the safety and superiority of these doses in reversing hypercalcemia of malignancy compared with 90 mg pamidronate [87].

During the clinical trial, increases in creatinine level were more frequently observed in the zoledronic acid treatment arms. Because of the renal toxicity, the infusion time of zoledronic acid was increased to 15 minutes, and patients in the 8 mg zoledronic acid group subsequently had their dosage reduced to 4 mg. Long-term follow-up data are now available and do not show differences in the renal profile between patients receiving 4 mg of zoledronic acid infused during 15 minutes and 90 mg of pamidronate infused during 120 minutes. The potential risk of increased creatinine levels from long-term administration of zoledronic acid

[88] has prompted a risk-adapted approach to dose this bisphosphonate considering calculated creatinine clearance. Whether this is either necessary or will reduce the low risk of renal toxicity from this bisphosphonate is still unknown.

The skeletal morbidity rate and normalization of the bone resorption marker, N-telopeptide of collagen type I (NTX), were improved in the zoledronate group. The results of the study showed that the proportion of patients with any skeletal event did not differ among the three treatment arms. In addition, the time to first skeletal event and analgesic use was similar in the three groups (12-13 months). Moreover, after 25 months of follow-up, the overall proportions of patients developing skeletal events remained similar between the zoledronic acid (4 mg) and pamidronate-treated patients.

A large phase III trial [89] showed an increase in time to first SRE in both groups (zoledronate and pamidronate).

However, in an additional preplanned analysis, the multiple-events analysis, zoledronic acid – treated patients showed a 16% reduction in the risk of developing skeletal complications compared with those patients who received pamidronate. A follow-up study [90] showed that zoledronate was more effective than pamidronate in reducing the risk of skeletal complications in patients with bone metastases from breast carcinoma by an additional 20% ($P = 0.025$), while confirming the similar efficacies of zoledronate and pamidronate in MM patients.

These long-term results show the efficacy and convenience of this more potent bisphosphonate for treating patients with myeloma with skeletal involvement [84].

Based on these studies, BPs appear to be effective in preventing the development of osteolytic bone disease in patients with myeloma and have become key agents in treating MM patients.

Another complication that may result from bisphosphonate therapy is osteonecrosis of the jaw (ONJ). Over the past 2 to 3 years, a number of case reports in the medical and dental literature suggest that this potential complication develops among cancer patients receiving either long-term zoledronic acid or pamidronate treatments [91]. ONJ has also been observed in patients treated with oral alendronate and risedronate for postmenopausal osteoporosis [91-94]. The mean time to onset of ONJ among patients receiving zoledronic acid was 18 months and 3 to 6 years for patients receiving pamidronate [95]. Most cases are associated with exposed mandibular bone with minimal symptoms, but patients slightly require extensive intervention, including surgical procedures to treat this problem. Necrotic bone is sometimes associated with Actinomyces colonization. Risk factors for ONJ may be multifactorial. To date, no reliable, predictive pattern has been clearly identified to allow a risk evaluation for ONJ. It is now recommended that patients receiving bisphosphonates, including most patients with myeloma, should be evaluated early in their treatment for dental problems and encouraged to maintain excellent dental hygiene.

It has not been demonstrated that the discontinuation of the bisphosphonate or the replacement with other bisphosphonates would change the course of this complication. Therefore, it is critical for clinicians to evaluate both the risks and the benefits of the continued use of bisphosphonates among patients with this complication. In conclusion, the choice of a BP for the treatment of myeloma bone disease is defined by several factors including efficacy, patient's compliance, choice of route of administration, safety profile as well as costs and availability.

EXPERIMENTAL EVIDENCE OF ANTI-CANCER ACTIVITY BY ZOLEDRONIC ACID

In solid tumors and multiple myeloma, increased osteoclastogenesis or the process of bone resorption is a consequence and a necessity ate the same time for tumor growth and clonal expansion [96, 97].

The bone marrow microenvironment is a rich source of bone-derived growth factors including Transforming Growth Factor-Beta (TGF-ß) and Insulin-Like Growth Factor (IGF) that are released during osteolysis [98].

BPs are the current standard of care for the prevention and treatment of malignant bone disease in solid Tumors [69, 99].

In soft tissue mouse tumors and metastases, N-BPs may exert anticancer activity by interacting with monocytes, macrophages, and tumor cells. For example, zoledronic acid inhibits breast cancer cell invasion in visceral organs (lung, liver) in vivo [100, 101].

N-BPs also synergize with cytotoxic drugs such as doxorubicin to prevent tumor cell growth and survival in vivo [102].

They also reduce tumor-associated angiogenesis in different mouse models of cancer (myeloma, melanoma, and breast, ovarian, and cervical carcinomas) [100, 103].

CD11b (also known as integrin, alpha M [complement component 3 receptor 3 subunit]) and Vascular Endothelial Growth Factor (VEGF; also known as VEGFA) are known to have key roles in cell adhesion [104] and angiogenesis, respectively [105].

In some models, N-BP treatment of tumor xenograft-bearing mice induced a profound reduction in CD11b-positive (CD11b+) macrophages infiltrating mammary or cervical carcinoma lesions, which was accompanied by decreased VEGF and Matrix Metalloproteinase (MMP)-9 levels in the tumor microenvironment [106].

This may be explained by the fact that MMP-9 produced by CD11b+ macrophages regulates the mobilization of VEGF from the extracellular matrix. Interestingly, the bone marrow is a reservoir for proangiogenic CD11b+ myelomonocytic cells that contribute to the vascularization of primary tumors [107].

N-BPs could therefore inhibit tumor-associated angiogenesis by blocking the recruitment of bone marrow-derived myeloid cells to the site of tumors.

ANTI-MYELOMA ACTIVITY OF ZOLEDRONIC ACID

There is strong preclinical evidence from various mouse models of MM using injection of primary myeloma cells or the 5T2 MM cell line, that N-BPs such as zoledronic acid have anticancer activity including inhibition of angiogenesis, enhancement of antitumor immune responses, and direct or indirect modulation of the proliferation and survival of myeloma cells [108-110].

By inhibiting bone resorption, zoledronic acid deprives tumor cells of bone-derived growth factors (e.g., TGF-β) that are required for the seeding and growth of tumor cells in the bone marrow [108]. N-BPs might also alter the retention of calcium-sensing receptor-expressing tumor cells in the bone marrow by inhibiting the release of ionic calcium from bone mineral [111].

Preclinical mouse models of myeloma indicate that the antimyeloma effects of BPs may be mediated via the inhibition of protein prenylation and consequent inhibition of the RAS-RAF-MAPK pathway [112], a mechanism of action not shared by non-BPs.

These findings further support the notion that the interaction between myeloma cells and the surrounding bone marrow microenvironment (Figure 1) constitutes an important factor that needs to be taken into account in the development of novel therapeutic strategies.

In vivo, N-BPs may also affect progression of myeloma by blocking the release of cytokines and growth factors from the bone matrix, thereby breaking the "vicious cycle" of bone destruction and cancer growth [113]. In addition, the anticancer effects of BPs have been demonstrated to have synergy with agents that are used in the treatment of myeloma, including dexamethasone, thalidomide, and bortezomib [114-116].

Myeloma Plasma Cells/Microenvironment Interactions

MM is the ideal disease model for studying tumor–microenvironment interactions [97, 117].

Myeloma cells induce changes in several cell types that are intimately involved in the induction of bone lesions, including bone marrow stem cells, bone marrow endothelial cells, immune cells, and osteoblasts and osteoclasts which control the bone formation and resorption equilibrium [97].

The induced changes, in turn, provide myeloma cells a supportive stromal environment, accessing to vascular networks, and locally produced growth factors and cytokines [97], all favoring cancer cell growth.

Cell adhesion-mediated drug resistance, a feature of the myeloma cell interaction with osteoclasts, could also be responsible for maintaining myeloma stem cells within a stromal cell niche in the bone marrow, mediating chemoresistance and subsequent disease relapses [96].

Additionally, genetic lesions associated with subgroups of myeloma have been identified. They increase the risk of bone disease through increasing myeloma cell proliferation and adhesion to stromal cells [118].

Zoledronate-Mediated Antiangiogenesis

In MM, bone marrow stromal cells increase the concentration of angiogenic factors and matrix degrading enzymes in the bone marrow microenvironment by direct secretion or by the stimulation of myeloma cells or endocrine cells through paracrine interactions [2, 119].

Corso et al. [120] have explored the treatment of bone marrow stromal cells derived from the bone marrow of myeloma patients with zoledronic acid. They observed a reduction in cell proliferation; an increased apoptosis; decreased production of IL-6, tumor necrosis factor-α and IL-1β; and a modified pattern of expression of adhesion molecules, especially those involved in plasma cell binding. These effects on bone marrow stromal cells suggest that the anticancer activity of zoledronic acid may in part result from its ability to disrupt the vicious cycle of signaling that promotes myeloma growth and progression.

Pathologic angiogenesis is a constant hallmark of bone marrow microenvironment in MM [121], but mechanisms of its induction are not well established. Plasma cells are the primary inducers since they secrete major angiogenic factors such as VEGF, Basic Fibroblast Growth Factor (bFGF), and Hepatocyte Growth Factor (HGF) [48, 121, 122].

MM Patient-Derived Endothelial Cells (MMECs) behave as secondary inducers following recruitment and activation by plasma cells [2, 123], being a huge source of these growth factors too [124]. The VEGF/VEGF Receptor-2 (VEGFR2) pathway greatly contributes to MM angiogenesis and progression [125], and mediates proliferation and capillarogenesis in MMECs through an autocrine loop [126], supporting the view that effective antiangiogenesis could be achieved via VEGF-VEGFR2 inhibition [127].

Zoledronic acid as other Nitrogen-containing bisphosphonates shows a direct cytotoxic activity on tumor cells and suppresses angiogenesis [8, 128, 129]. It inhibits bFGF-induced proliferation [8], adhesion, migration, and survival of human umbilical vascular endothelial cells [130]; it decreases bone tumor–associated angiogenesis in the murine 5T2 MM model [131]; it inhibits revascularization of the ventral prostate gland in castrated rats treated with testosterone [9]; modulates αvβ3 and αvβ5 integrins [132]; inhibits MMP-2 and MMP-9 [133]; and modulates in cancer patients serum levels of proangiogenic growth factors including VEGF and bFGF [134].

In vivo, zoledronic acid antiangiogenic activity may be also mediated via inhibition of osteoclasts, which actually produce angiogenic factors [40].

The antiangiogenic activity of Zoledronic acid in MM is mediated by abrogation of VEGF/VEGFR2 autocrine loop in MMECs and thus induces an indirect antitumor activity [135].

Proliferative response of bone marrow endothelial cells is significantly reduced by zoledronic acid in a dose-dependent fashion.

Moreover, zoledronic acid exerts an inhibitory effect on the bone marrow endothelial cells migration in chemotaxis assays, markedly inhibit the capillarogenesis on Matrigel and the angiogenic response to VEGF165 and bone marrow endothelial cells conditioned media in the chic embryo corioallantoic membrane assay.

These data provide direct evidence that zoledronic acid exerts antiangiogenic activity on MMECs by specifically blocking the over-angiogenic response to VEGF165 [127] in opposition to the selective activity on bFGF-dependent normal human umbilical vascular endothelial cells [8].

Zoledronic acid down-regulates VEGF165 and VEGFR2 expression at mRNA and protein level in bone marrow endothelial cells from active multiple myeloma. Thus, in turn, strongly inhibit the VEGF/VEGFR2 autocrine loop responsible to automaintain the angiogenesis process in these patients [126].

Another evidence of the antiangiogenic activity of zoledronic acid is related to its ability to modulate circulating endothelial cells and circulating endothelial precursor cells in early prostate cancer patients [136].

In MM patients the bone marrow neovascularisation is also partially sustained by bone marrow macrophages through their angiogenic and vasculogenic activities.

Macrophages, in fact, are key cells for these activities [119], they form capillary-like lumina and branching patterns in vitro, thus participating to the de novo formation of neovessels in a process named vasculogenic mimicry [137].

Moreover, they express and release major cytokines (i.e. VEGF, bFGF, HGF, platelet derived growth factor (PDGF) and MMPs) which promote angiogenesis, hence plasma cell growth and invasion [137].

These data agree with those obtained on the vasculogenic mimicry of osteosarcoma cells in vitro [138].

Zoledronic acid and bortezomib are synergic for their antiangiogenic activity [116]. Particularly, zoledronic acid down-regulates the VEGF/VEGF receptor 2 (VEGFR2) autocrine system through the inhibition of the farnesyl diphosphate synthase, [135] while bortezomib inhibits angiogenic genes, including VEGF, IL-6, Angiopoietin-2 (Ang-2) and Insulin-Like Growth Factor (IGF-1) [139].

Both drugs act synergistically and impact several angiogenic and vasculogenic activities at clinically achievable concentrations [128, 140].

Immunomodulation by Zoledronate

Recent in vivo data using a panel of human breast cancer cell lines injected into Non-Obese Diabetic Severe Combined Immunodeficient (NOD/ SCID) mice indicate that N-BPs stimulate the expansion of Vγ9Vδ2 T cells, a subset of human T cells with antitumor activity [109, 141]. For example, upon adoptive transfer into immunodeficient mice, purified human Vγ9Vδ2 T cells given together with alendronate (a drug given to postmenopausal women for the treatment of osteoporosis) plus the cytokine interleukin-2 showed a statistically significantly prolonged survival of mice bearing human melanoma or pancreatic carcinoma cells [109].

Similarly, treatment with zoledronic acid enhanced Vγ9Vδ2 T-cell cytotoxicity in experimental models of chronic myelogenous leukemia and breast, lung, and bladder carcinomas [109, 141]. The inhibition of FPP sythase in the mevalonate pathway, results in zoledronic acid-induced intracellular accumulation and secretion of the ATP analogues isopentenyl pyrophosphate (IPP) and 1-adenosin-5′-yl ester 3-(3-methylbut-3-enyl) ester triphosphoric acid (ApppI) in tumor cells in vitro and in vivo, thus promoting chemotaxis of Vγ9Vδ2 T cells to tumors and triggering their destruction [141].

Moreover, zoledronic acid enhances direct natural killer cytotoxicity against tumor cells [110]. Thus, there is a growing interest and a substantive dataset to support the use of N-BPs for cancer immunotherapy.

BPs also repress cancer progression by stimulating the host anticancer response and/or by inhibiting proangiogenic signaling by immune cells.

BP treatment has been shown to induce the accumulation of IPP and dimethylallyl bisphosphonate, phosphoantigens that activate Vγ9Vδ2 T cells.

Indeed, they appear to induce or activate Vγ9Vδ2 subset T cells by mimicking phosphoantigens and/or by increasing circulating phosphoantigen levels [142]. Several studies have demonstrated that zoledronic acid treatment causes the expansion of Vγ9Vδ2 T-cell populations and increases sensitivity of cancer cells to the cytotoxic effects of Vγ9Vδ2 T cells [143, 144].

The Vγ9Vδ2 T cells have antitumor activity and appropriate cell surface antigens to target secondary lymphoid organs and exert costimulatory activity [145]. In a small clinical study, patients infused with zoledronic acid-activated Vγ9Vδ2 T cells generated from the culture of peripheral blood mononuclear cells, maintained their M-protein levels in the serum at baseline, demonstrating that activation of the innate host antitumor response by BPs can successfully control the expansion of myeloma cells [146].

In MM, cells belonging to the monocyte-macrophage lineage form part of an inflammatory circuit which promotes tumor progression, invasion and metastasis, mainly through their proangiogenic activity [119, 137].

These cells express a broad array of MMPs, proangiogenic cytokines and growth factors.

The combination of factors facilitates matrix breakdown and tunneling that promote neovascularization and invasion. A recent study evaluating the effect of clinically relevant doses of zoledronic acid on bone metastasis in a constitutionally active ErbB-2 transgenic mouse model reported that zoledronic acid treatment resulted in M2 (anti-inflammatory and proangiogenic) to M1 (antitumor) reversion of tumor-associated macrophages [107]. This study also reported that zoledronic acid treatment resulted in a profound reduction in CD11+ macrophages infiltrating mammary lesions and was accompanied by reduced vascularization of the tumor and decreased VEGF levels in the tumor microenvironment.

Moreover, this study also showed that Ras prenylation and Ras-GTP levels were suppressed by the zoledronic acid treatment. Overall, the study demonstrated that zoledronic acid improved disease-free and OS.

These data are consistent with decreases in VEGF levels observed in cancer patients treated with low-dose therapy with zoledronic acid [147]. These results show that N-BPs affect the immune system by both increasing host antitumor activity and reducing tumor-associated neovascularization.

Finally, bortezomib and zoledronic acid showed distinct and synergistic inhibitory effects on cell proliferation, adhesion, migration and expression of angiogenic cytokines as well as on capillarogenic organization and expression of vascular markers in cells that became vasculogenic. Activation of VEGFR2, ERK1/2 and NF-κB activities were also inhibited [116].

DIRECT ANTIMYELOMA ACTIVITY BY ZOLEDRONATE

Pamidronate and incadronate induce apoptosis and significantly decrease the cell number in the human myeloma cell line JJN-3 and the EBV transformed Burkitt lymphoma cell line HS-Sultan ($P<0.001$) [148, 149]. Moreover, these two BPs increase the proportion of cells with altered nuclear morphology ($P<0.05$) and fragmented DNA, in both JJN-3 and HS-Sultan cells. In contrast, clodronate, a BP that does not contain any nitrogen and does not inhibit the mevalonate pathway, have little effects on cell number and do not cause apoptosis at the concentrations examined.

Roelofs AJ et al. [150] have demomstrated the critical role of mevalonate pathway inhibition by BPs and the consequent impairment of the function of small GTPases in mediating the observed anticancer effects. In this study they showed that risedronate is able to inhibit prenylation of Rap1A and Rab6 two ras in brain (RAB)-GTPases, in a dose dependent manner.

Thus eliciting a dose-dependent apoptotic response in human myeloma cells and arresting these cells in the S phase. Moreover, geranylgeraniol prevented inhibition of prenylation, induction of apoptosis and cell-cycle arrest in response to risedronate. Indeed, treatment with incadronate and mevastatin (a known inhibitor of the mevalonate pathway) caused apoptosis in JJN-3 myeloma cells and inhibited cell proliferation [10]. The mevalonate pathway intermediates such as geranylgeraniol and farnesol prevented incadronate-induced apoptosis of JJN-3 myeloma cells and had a partial effect on cell-cycle arrest, suggesting that the anticancer effects of incadronate are a direct consequence of its known mechanism of action, the mevalonate pathway inhibition.

The role of isoprenylation of proteins in mediating these events is also supported by data from a more recent study in the 5T2MM model of MM which showed that 3-PEHPC (2-[3-Pyridinyl]-1-Hydroxyethylidene-1,1-Phosphonocarboxylic Acid), a novel geranylgeranyl-transferase II inhibitor, prevented bone loss, inhibited the development of osteolytic bone lesions and reduced myeloma burden in bone [151].

In contrast to other agents that inhibit the mevalonate pathway or post-translational prenylation, BPs have a natural affinity toward bone mineral that limits the effects of mevalonate pathway inhibition to select cellular components (mainly osteoclasts, and non-osteoclast cells including tumor cells and lymphocytes) within the bone microenvironment. This is particularly desirable in a disease such as MM which progression is primarily driven within the bone.

In a study conducted by Baulch-Brown et al. [152], the authors showed that myeloma cells treated with zoledronic acid, or other mevalonate pathway antagonists such as fluvastatin (an HMG-CoA reductase inhibitor) or SCH663-36 (a farnesyl transferase inhibitor) suppressed the proliferation of myeloma cells (RPMI 8226, U266, OMP2, LP1 and NCI-H929), and that combinations of zoledronic acid and fluvastatin, but not zoledronic acid and SCH66336 acted synergistically. The study also showed that the antiproliferative effect of mevalonate pathway inhibitors is principally mediated by prevention of geranylgeranylation and is the result of both cell-cycle arrest and apoptosis induction. Indeed, microarray and quantitative real-time PCR analyses further demonstrated that genes related to apoptosis, cell-cycle control and the mevalonate pathway were particularly affected by zoledronic acid and fluvastatin, and that some of these transcriptional effects were synergistic.

In-vivo experiments in animal models of MM, provide additional evidence of the antimyeloma activity of BPs. For example, zoledronic acid significantly prolonged survival in severe combined immunodeficiency mice inoculated with human INA-6 plasma cells [112]. Importantly, this study used clinically relevant doses of zoledronic acid, and histological analysis of INA-6 tumors from the peritoneal cavity revealed extensive areas of apoptosis associated with poly (ADP ribose) polymerase cleavage.

Furthermore, western blot analysis of tumor homogenates demonstrated the accumulation of unprenylated Rap1A, which is indicative of the uptake of zoledronic acid by non-skeletal tumors and inhibition of the mevalonate pathway.

Myeloma cells may be dependent on osteoclast activity and vice versa [153, 154]. Zoledronic acid has been shown to prevent the development of osteolytic bone disease and decrease bone tumor burden in bone in an established MM animal model [131]. It prevented the formation of skeletal lesions, loss of bone mineral density, and reduced osteoclast perimeter in mice injected with 5T2MM murine myeloma cells [131].

Zoledronic acid also decreased paraprotein concentration, decreased tumor burden and reduced angiogenesis. In separate experiments, Kaplan–Meier analysis demonstrated a significant increase in disease-free survival after treatment with zoledronic acid when compared with control (P<0.005).

Thus, these data are consistent with the antimyeloma effects observed with other mevalonate pathway inhibitors. The antimyeloma activity by zoledronic acid is increased by the association with other drugs acting on the mevalonate pathway or on other pathways active in myeloma cells. Schmidmaier et al. demonstrated that sequential treatment with zoledronic acid and simvastatin resulted in the synergistic induction of apoptosis and reversal of cell adhesion-mediated drug resistance in cancer cells [115]. Moreover, treatment with the combination of zoledronic acid and dexamethasone demonstrated synergistic induction of apoptosis in vitro in myeloma cell lines [12, 114].

Clinical Evidence of Zoledronic Acid Antimyeloma Activity

Traditionally, bone-targeted agents have been used as a supplementary therapy to prevent or reduce the incidence of SREs in patients with malignant bone diseases. However, there might be a greater role for the use of these agents. Recent data suggest that they may act as antitumor agents [155], that they are able to delay disease progression and prolong survival in MM [156] and in solid tumors [157, 158]. Bone disease contributes substantially to morbidity and mortality in patients with cancer. Approximately 70% of patients with Myeloma have overt lytic metastases at diagnosis, and approximately 60% of patients report a pathological bone fracture over the course of their disease [159]. Data from clinical trials on the use of BPs in MM patients provided the clinical evidence of their antimyeloma activity [80, 84, 160]. In a long-term follow-up (8.6 years) of a placebo-controlled trial (N=619), the subset of clodronate-treated patients who did not have vertebral fractures at baseline had significantly longer OS vs patients who received placebo (median OS, 59 months vs 37 months, respectively; P=0.006). Similarly, in patients with newly diagnosed or relapsed/refractory MM (N=392), long-term treatment with pamidronate significantly increased survival in the subset of MM patients receiving second-line antimyeloma therapy (14 months vs 21 months; P=0.041 compared with placebo). In a retrospective analysis of MM patients with bone marker assessment (N=353), in a phase III trial comparing zoledronic acid (4 mg) with pamidronate (90 mg), patients with high baseline bone-specific alkaline phosphatase levels had significantly better 25-month survival with zoledronic acid than with pamidronate (82 vs 53%, respectively; P=0.041) [160].

The antimyeloma potential of zoledronic acid has also been provided by similar clinical studies. 94 patients with MM treated with cyclophosphamide, vincristine, melphalan and prednisone were randomized to receive 4 mg intravenous infusion of zoledronic acid every 28 days. 5-year event-free survival was 80% in the zoledronic acid group vs 52% in the control group (P<0.01); 5-year OS was 80% in the zoledronic acid group vs 46% in the control group (P<0.01) showing significantly greater benefit for the zoledronic acid-treated group after 49.6 months median follow-up [161].

A large, randomized, controlled trial demonstrating an antimyeloma benefit from zoledronic acid treatment in patients with newly diagnosed MM has been conducted by the Medical Research Council Myeloma IX trial [156].

This phase III trial compared the efficacy and safety of 4 mg/15 min monthly intravenous infusion of zoledronic acid vs 1600 mg daily oral clodronate. Patients were assigned to myeloma treatment according to standard indications: younger, transplant-eligible patients were assigned to the intensive therapy (induction therapy randomized between standard cytotoxic and thalidomide-based regimens followed by autologous stem-cell transplantation); non-transplant eligible patients were assigned to a less intensive therapy (randomized between melphalan/prednisone and a thalidomide-based regimen). Within each treatment schedule, patients were randomized to oral clodronate or zoledronic acid until disease progression or death.

981 received zoledronic acid and 979 received clodronate. The median time of treatment was ~1 year across all treatment groups and at the median follow-up of 3.7 years, 24% and 19% of patients, respectively, discontinued study before disease progression. Zoledronic acid significantly prolonged both progression-free (P=0.0179) and overall survival (P=0.0118). However, it should be pointed out that the effects of zoledronic acid relative to clodronate occurred in the first 4 months, whereas the curves were parallel during followup probably due to the better bioavailability of zoledronic acid since the intravenous application possibly results in a stronger inhibition of FPPS and subsequent protein prenylation [162], and the markedly higher relative activity of zoledronic acid [163].

Moreover, the proportion of patients with a skeletalrelated event was reduced by Zoledronic acid (27.0 vs 35.3%, respectively; P=0.0004) vs clodronate and zoledronic acid halved the incidence of new osteolytic lesions, regardless of treatment pathway.

Finally, the improvement in OS was maintained after adjustment for time to first skeletal-related event in a Cox model (P=0.0178), suggesting that antimyeloma effects likely underlie the overall survival benefit [156].

In a retrospective analysis of clinical practice, the hearly initiation of zoledronic acid treatment and its prolonged use has been demonstrated to delay disease progression in patients with MM.

Moreover, zoledronic acid treatment was well tolerated in association with a broad array of antimyeloma agents and regimens [164].

As reported below, bisphosphonates may synergize with anticancer agents used in the treatment of myeloma, including dexamethasone, thalidomide, and bortezomib [114-116]. The analysis conducted by Ria R. et al. [164] demonstrated the safety and efficacy of combining zoledronic acid with first- and/or second-line antimyeloma therapy, which included both bortezomib and immunomodulatory agents (IMIDs) such as lenalidomide.

Our group shows that patients who received zoledronic acid therapy at diagnosis or throughout treatment had longer disease-free intervals compared with patients who received zoledronic acid therapy later or not at all, consistent with the early benefits reported in the MRC Myeloma IX trial, and the reported antimyeloma effects of zoledronic acid with bortezomib [156].

Overall, adding zoledronic acid to either first- or second-line treatment numerically improved the 1-year PFS rate regardless the type of antimyeloma therapy received at relapse. Moreover, patients who received zoledronic acid throughout the study period had a better 1-

year PFS rate (71%) compared with patients who received zoledronic acid only at diagnosis or at relapse (58% and 54%, respectively).

In addition, patients receiving zoledronic acid plus bortezomib had fewer SREs than any other treatment group, which is not surprising given previous clinical evidence of increased bone mineral density in a subset of patients with relapsed MM who received the combination of bortezomib, dexamethasone, and zoledronic acid [165].

These effects are consistent with preclinical data showing that bortezomib promotes bone formation in myelomatous and nonmyelomatous bone tissue by simultaneously inhibiting osteoclastogenesis and stimulating osteoblastogenesis, thus having an overall anabolic effect on bone [166].

Bortezomib exerts a direct cytotoxic activity on plasma cells by blocking the activation of nuclear factor kB, an inducer of gene transcription [167], and by preventing the activa-tion of caveolin1, a promoter of plasma cell growth and migration. Zoledronic acid inhibits farnesyl diphosphate (FFP) synthase, a key enzyme in the meva-lonate pathway, thus preventing prenylation of several proteins, including the GTP-binding Ras, Rho, Rac and Rab leading to cellular apoptosis, antiangio-genesis and activation of gamma/delta T-cells.

In contrast, there are also reports that suggest that BPs do not have any clinically meaningful effect on the progression of MM. For example, in an updated indirect meta-analysis of 17 trials with ~3000 patients [168], the authors concluded that BP treatment was not significantly associated with any survival benefit. However, it should be noted that this study included several different BPs, which in individual studies have shown differences in their antimyeloma activity.

Overall, zoledronic acid and pamidronate have proven to be more effective than other BPs in terms of the clinical benefit they provide. Moreover, it should be noted that these analyses did not include the Medical Research Council Myeloma IX study [156] and that did include the study by Aviles et al. [41] that showed survival benefits.

It comprised only a small fraction of the pooled population and the effect might therefore be masked. Similarly, McCloskey et al. [72, 80] did not observe survival benefit in the overall study population, but subgroup analysis showed significant survival benefit in the subset of patients without skeletal involvement at diagnosis.

Finally, Musto et al. [169], showed that zoledronic acid treatment did not effect the progression from asymptomatic to symptomatic MM disease.

All these data suggest that to gain clinically meaningful benefits, it may be needed to both evaluate the specific type of BP and the disease stage.

Conclusion

BPs have an important role in the treatment of MM bone disease. In addition to the established benefit on bone health, there are both in-vitro and in-vivo evidences that BPs have potential antimyeloma effects, decrease osteolysis, tumor burden, and angiogenesis and increase survival.

In addition to the direct effects of BPs on myeloma cells, BPs may indirectly affect tumor growth by preventing bone resorption and inhibiting further release of tumor stimulating factors. BPs inhibit the survival of stromal cells and block the interaction between plasma cells and stromal cells, thus interfering with bone microenvironment.

In addition, inhibition of angiogenesis and immunomodulatory effects of BPs including activation of Vγ9Vδ2 T cell-mediated innate immunity may contribute to their negative effects on tumor progression.

The in-vitro evidence of the antimyeloma effects of BPs is further confirmed by several clinical studies that demonstrate the efficacy of BPs in the reduction of skeletal events in MM patients with a concomitant antimyeloma effect. Although other studies suggest that BPs do not improve mortality in the overall study population, the majority of data provide evidence for the antimyeloma effects of BPs.

Furthermore, several studies have proven the reduction of skeletal-related events in MM patients treated with either pamidronate or zoledronic acid.

Although the optimal duration of BP treatment is still unknown, the potential antimyeloma benefits justify further evaluation of the risk/benefit ratio of BPs in conjunction with primary treatment for MM.

References

[1] Kyle, R. A. and Rajkumar, S. V. (2004). Multiple myeloma. *New Engl. J. Med.*, 351, 1860–73.

[2] Ribatti, D., et al. (2006). Importance of the bone marrow microenvironment in inducing the angiogenic response in multiple myeloma. *Oncogene*, 25, 4257–66.

[3] Corso, A., et al. (2005). Zoledronic acid exerts its antitumor effect in multiple myeloma interfering with the bone marrow microenvironment. *Hematology*, 10, 215–24.

[4] Raab, M. S., et al. (2009). Multiple myeloma. *Lancet*, 374, 324–39.

[5] Radl, J., et al. (1985). Influence of treatment with APD-bisphosphonate on the bone lesions in the mouse 5T2 multiple myeloma. *Cancer*, 55, 1030-40.

[6] Aparicio, A., et al. (1998). In vitro cytoreductive effects on multiple myeloma cells induced by bisphosphonates. *Leukemia*, 12, 220-9.

[7] Savage, A. D., et al. (1996). Pamidronate reduces IL-6 production by bone marrow stroma from multiple myeloma patients. *Blood*, 88, 105a.

[8] Wood, J., et al. (2002). Novel antiangiogenic effects of the bisphosphonate compound zoledronic acid. *J. Pharmacol. Exp. Ther.*, 302, 1055–61.

[9] Fournier, P., et al. (2002). Bisphosphonates inhibit angiogenesis in vitro and testosterone-stimulated vascular regrowth in the ventral prostate in castrated rats. *Cancer Res.*, 62, 6538–44.

[10] Shipman, C. M., et al. (1998). The bisphosphonate incadronate (YM175) causes apoptosis of human myeloma cells in vitro by inhibiting the mevalonate pathway. *Cancer Res.*, 58, 5294–7.

[11] Takahashi, R., et al. (2001). A newly developed bisphosphonate,YM529, is a potent apoptosis inducer of human myeloma cells. *Leuk. Res.*, 25, 77-83.

[12] Tassone, P., et al. (2000). Growth inhibition and synergistic induction of apoptosis by zoledronate and dexamethasone in human myeloma cell lines. *Leukemia*, 14, 841–4.

[13] Ochiai, N., et al. (2005). Nitrogen containing bisphosphonate incadronate augments the inhibitory effect of farnesyl transferase inhibitor tipifarnib on the growth of fresh and cloned myeloma cells in vitro. *Leuk. Lymphoma*, 46, 1619-25.
[14] Ochiai, N., et al. (2005). Combination therapy with thalidomide, incadronate, and dexamethasone for relapsed or refractory multiple myeloma. *Int. J. Hematol.*, 82, 243-7.
[15] Mundy, G. R. and Bertoline, D. R. (1986). Bone destruction and hypercalcemia in plasma cell myeloma. *Semin. Oncol.*, 13, 291-9.
[16] Kyle, R. A. (1975). Multiple myeloma: review of 869 cases. *Mayo Clin. Proc.*, 50, 29-40.
[17] Belch, A. R., et al. (1991). Effect of daily etidronate on the osteolysis of multiple myeloma. *J. Clin. Oncol.*, 9, 1397–402.
[18] Kyle, R. A., et al. (1975). Multiple myeloma bone disease: the comparative effect of sodium fluoride and calcium carbonate or placebo. *N. Engl. J. Med.*, 293, 1334-8.
[19] Terpos, E. and Dimopoulos, M. A. (2005). Myeloma bone disease: pathophysiology and management. *Ann. Oncol.*, 16, 1223–31.
[20] Heider, U., et al. (2005). Novel aspects of osteoclast activation and osteoblast inhibition in myeloma bone disease. *Biochem. Biophys. Res. Commun.*, 338, 687–93.
[21] Terpos, E., et al. (2007). The effect of novel anti-myeloma agents on bone metabolism of patients with multiple myeloma. *Leukemia*, 21, 1875–84.
[22] Giuliani, N., et al. (2006). Multiple myeloma bone disease: pathophysiology of osteoblast inhibition. *Blood*, 108, 3992–6.
[23] Hayashi, T., et al. (2004). Transforming growth factor beta receptor I kinase inhibitor down-regulates cytokine secretion and multiple myeloma cell growth in the bone marrow microenvironment. *Clin. Cancer Res.*, 10, 7540–6.
[24] Terpos, E., et al. (2003). New insights into the pathophysiology and management of bone disease in multiple myeloma. *Br. J. Haematol.*, 123, 758–69.
[25] Sezer, O., et al. (2003). RANK ligand and osteoprotegerin in myeloma bone disease. *Blood*, 101, 2094–8.
[26] Vanderkerken, K., et al. (2003). Multiple myeloma biology: lessons from the 5TMM models. *Immunol. Rev.*, 194, 196–206.
[27] Nawawi, H., et al. (1996). Biochemical bone markers in patients with multiple myeloma. *Clin. Chim. Acta*, 253, 61-77.
[28] Abildgaard, N., et al. (1997). Serum markers of bone metabolism in multiple myeloma: prognostic significance of the carboxy-terminal telopeptide of type 1 collagen (ICTP). *Br. J. Haematol.*, 96, 103-10.
[29] Abildgaard, N., et al. (2003). Comparison of five biochemical markers of bone resorption in multiple myeloma: elevated pre-treatment levels of S-ICTP and U-Ntx are predictive for early progression of the bone disease during standard chemotherapy. *Br. J. Haematol.*, 120, 235-42.
[30] Alexandrakis, M. G., et al. (2003). Urinary N-telopeptide levels in multiple myeloma patients, correlation with TC-99M-sesta MIBI scintigraphy and other biochemical markers of disease activity. *Hematol. Oncol.*, 21, 17-24.
[31] Elomaa, I., et al. (1996) Monitoring the action of clodronate with type I collagen metabolites in multiple myeloma. *Eur. J. Cancer*, 32, 1166-70.

[32] Roux, C., et al. (1994). Biologic, histologic and densitometric effects of oral risedronate on bone in patients with multiple myeloma. *Bone*, 15, 41-9.

[33] Berenson, J. R., et al. (2006). Bone complications in multiple myeloma. *Cancer Biol. Ther.*, 5, 1082-5.

[34] Chauhan, D., et al. (1996). Multiple myeloma cell adhesioninduced interleukin-6 expression in bone marrow stromal cells involves activation of NF-kappa B. *Blood*, 87, 1104–12.

[35] Uchiyama, H., et al. (1993). Adhesion of human myelomaderived cell lines to bone marrow stromal cells stimulates interleukin-6 secretion. *Blood*, 82, 3712–20.

[36] Sati, H. I. A., et al. (1999). Expression of interleukin-1b and tumour necrosis factor-alpha in plasma cells from patients with multiple myeloma. *Br. J. Haematol.*, 104, 350–7.

[37] Roux, S. and Mariette, X. (2004). The high rate of bone resorption in multiple myeloma is due to RANK (receptor activator of nuclear factor-Kb) and RANK ligand expression. *Leuk. Lymphoma*, 45, 1111–8.

[38] Oyajobi, B. O. and Mundy, G. R. (2003). Receptor activator of NF-kappaB ligand, macrophage inflammatory protein-1alpha, and the proteasome: novel therapeutic targets in myeloma. *Cancer*, 97 (3 Suppl.), 813–7.

[39] Mitsiades, C. S., et al. (2006). Proteasome inhibition as a new therapeutic principle in hematological malignancies. *Curr. Drug Targets*, 7, 1341–7.

[40] Tanaka, Y., et al. (2007). Myeloma cell-osteoclast interaction enhances angiogenesis together with bone resorption: a role for vascular endothelial cell growth factor and osteopontin. *Clin. Cancer Res.*, 13, 816–23.

[41] Franchimont, N., et al. (2000). Transforming growth factor-beta increases interleukin-6 transcripts in osteoblasts. *Bone*, 26, 249–53.

[42] Cozzolino, F., et al. (1989). Production of interleukin-1 by bone marrow myeloma cells. *Blood*, 74, 380-7.

[43] Kawano, M., et al. (1989). Interleukin-1 accelerates autocrine growth of myeloma cells through interleukin-6 in human myeloma. *Blood*, 73, 2145-8.

[44] Lacy, M. Q., et al. (1999). Comparison of interleukin-1h expression by in situ hybridization in monoclonal gammopathy of undetermined significance and multiple myeloma. *Blood*, 93, 300-8.

[45] Garrett, I. R., et al. (1987). Production of lymphotoxin,a bone-resorbing cytokine, by cultured human myeloma cells. *N. Engl. J. Med.*, 317, 526-32.

[46] Hjertner, O., et al. (1999). Hepatocyte growth factor (HGF) induces interleukin-11 secretion from osteoblasts: a possible role for HGF in myeloma-associated osteolytic bone disease. *Blood*, 94, 3883-9.

[47] Choi, S. J., et al. (2000). Macrophage inflammatory protein1-a is a potential osteoclast stimulatory factor in multiple myeloma. *Blood*, 96, 671-8.

[48] Börset, M., et al. (1996). Hepatocyte growth factor and its receptor c-met in multiple myeloma. *Blood*, 88, 3998–4004.

[49] Suzuki, A., et al. (1994). Production of parathyroid hormone-related protein by cultured human myeloma cells. *Am. J. Hematol.*, 45, 88-96.

[50] Oyajobi, B. O., et al. (2003). Dual effects of macrophage inflammatory protein-1a on osteolysis and tumor burden in the murine 5 TGM1 model of myeloma bone disease. *Blood*, 102, 311-9.

[51] Tian, E., et al. (2003). The role of the Wnt-signaling antagonist DKK1 in the development of osteolytic lesions in multiple myeloma. *N. Engl. J. Med.*, 349, 2483–94.

[52] Oshima, T., et al. (2005). Myeloma cells suppress bone formation by secreting a soluble Wnt inhibitor, sFRP-2. *Blood*, 106, 3160–5.

[53] Giuliani, N., et al. (2005). Myeloma cells block RUNX2/CBFA1 activity in human bone marrow osteoblast progenitors and inhibit osteoblast formation and differentiation. *Blood*, 106, 2472–83.

[54] Ehrlich, L. A., et al. (2005). IL-3 is a potential inhibitor of osteoblast differentiation in multiple myeloma. *Blood*, 106, 1407–14.

[55] Rogers, M. J., et al. (2000). Cellular and molecular mechanisms of action of bisphosphonates. *Cancer*, 88 (12 Suppl.), 2961–78.

[56] Russell, R. G., et al. (1970). Inorganic pyrophosphate in plasma, urine, and synovial fluid of patients with pyrophosphate arthropathy (chondrocalcinosis or pseudogout). *Lancet,* 2, 899–902.

[57] Dunford, J. E., et al. (2001). Structure-activity relationships for inhibi-tion of farnesyl diphosphate synthase in vitro and inhibition of bone resorption in vivo by nitrogen-containing bisphosphonates. *J. Pharmacol. Exp. Ther.*, 296, 235–42.

[58] Russell, R. G., et al. (2007). Bisphosphonates: an update on mechanisms of action and how these relate to clinical efficacy. *Ann. N Y Acad. Sci.*, 1117, 209–57.

[59] Van Beek, E., et al. (1999). Nitrogen-containing bisphosphonates inhibit isopentenyl pyrophosphate isomerase/farnesyl pyrophosphate synthase activity with relative potencies corresponding to their antiresorptive potencies in vitro and in vivo. *Biochem. Biophys. Res. Commun.*, 255, 491–4.

[60] Luckman, S. P., et al. (1998). Nitrogen-containing bisphosphonates inhibit the mevalonate pathway and prevent post-translational prenylation of GTP-binding proteins, including Ras. *J. Bone Miner. Res.*, 13, 581–9.

[61] Dunford, J. E., et al. (2006). Inhibition of protein prenylation by bisphosphonates causes sustained activation of Rac, Cdc42, and Rho GTPases. *J. Bone Miner. Res.*, 21, 684–94.

[62] Coleman, R. E. (2004). Bisphosphonates: clinical experience. *Oncologist*, 9 (Suppl. 4), 14–27.

[63] Frith, J. C., et al. (1997). Clodronate and liposomeencapsulated clodronate are metabolized to a toxic ATP analog, adenosine 5#-(beta, gammadichloromethylene) triphosphate, by mammalian cells in vitro. *J. Bone Miner. Res.*, 12, 1358–67.

[64] Hughes, D. E., et al. (1995). Bisphosphonates promote apoptosis in murine osteoclasts in vitro and in vivo. *J. Bone Miner. Res.*, 10, 1478–87.

[65] Selander, K. S., et al. (1996). Characteristics of clodronateinduced apoptosis in osteoclasts and macrophages. *Mol. Pharmacol.*, 50, 1127–38.

[66] Boonekamp, P. M., et al. (1986). Two modes of action of bisphosphonates on osteoclastic resorption of mineralized matrix. *Bone Miner.*, 1, 27–39.

[67] Rowe, D. J., et al. (1999). Relationship between bisphosphonate concentration and osteoclast activity and viability. *In Vitro Cell. Dev. Biol. Anim.*, 35, 383–8.

[68] Green, J. R. (2004). Bisphosphonates: preclinical review. *Oncologist*, 9 (Suppl. 4), 3–13.

[69] Aapro, M., et al. (2008). Guidance on the use of bisphosphonates in solid tumours: recommendations of an international expert panel. *Ann. Oncol.*, 19, 420–32.

[70] Vogel, C. L., et al. (2004). Safety and pain palliation of zoledronic acid in patients with breast cancer, prostate cancer, or multiple myeloma who previously received bisphosphonate therapy. *Oncologist*, 9, 687–95.

[71] Gralow, J. and Tripathy, D. (2007). Managing metastatic bone pain: the role of bisphosphonates. *J. Pain Symptom Manage.*, 33, 462–72.

[72] McCloskey, E. V., et al. (1998). A randomized trial of the effect of clodronate on skeletal morbidity in multiple myeloma. MRC Working Party on Leukaemia in Adults. *Br. J. Haematol.*, 100, 317–25.

[73] Berenson, J. R., et al. (1996). Efficacy of pamidronate in reducing skeletal events in patients with advanced multiple myeloma. Myeloma Aredia Study Group. *N. Engl. J. Med.*, 334, 488–93.

[74] Wong, R. and Wiffen, P. J. (2002). Bisphosphonates for the relief of pain secondary to bone metastases. *Cochrane Database Syst. Rev.*, 2, CD002068.

[75] Terpos, E., et al. (2000). Effect of pamidronate administration on markers of bone turnover and disease activity in multiple myeloma. *Eur. J. Haematol.*, 65, 331–6.

[76] Daragon, A., et al. (1993). Treatment of multiple myeloma with etidronate: results of a multicentre double-blind study. Groupe d'Etudes et de Recherches sur le Myelome (GERM). *Eur. J. Med.*, 2, 449–52.

[77] Menssen, H. D., et al. (2002). Effects of long-term intravenous ibandronate therapy on skeletal-related events, survival, and bone resorption markers in patients with advanced multiple myeloma. *J. Clin. Oncol.*, 20, 2353-9.

[78] Lahtinen, R., et al. (1992). Randomised, placebo-controlled multicentre trial of clodronate in multiple myeloma. Finnish Leukaemia Group. *Lancet*, 340, 1049–52.

[79] Heim, M. E., et al. (1995). Prospective randomized trial of dicholoromethylene bisphosphonate (clodronate) in patients with multiple myeloma requiring treatment: a multicenter study. *Onkologie*, 18, 439-48.

[80] McCloskey, E. V., et al. (2001). Long-term follow-up of a prospective, double-blind, placebo-controlled randomized trial of clodronate in multiple myeloma. *Br. J. Haematol.*, 113, 1035–43.

[81] Laakso, M., et al. (1994). Subgroup and cost-benefit analysis of the Finnish multicentre trial of clodronate in multiple myeloma. Finnish Leukaemia Group. *Br. J. Haematol.*, 87, 725–9.

[82] Brincker, H., et al. (1998). Failure of oral pamidronate to reduce skeletal morbidity in multiple myeloma: a double-blind placebo-controlled trial. Danish-Swedish cooperative study group. *Br. J. Haematol.*, 101, 280–6.

[83] Man, Z., et al. (1990). Use of pamidronate for multiple myeloma osteolytic lesions. *Lancet*, 335, 663-8.

[84] Berenson, J. R., et al. (1998). Long-term pamidronate treatment of advanced multiple myeloma patients reduces skeletal events. Myeloma Aredia Study Group. *J. Clin. Oncol.*, 16, 593–602.

[85] Green, J. R., et al. (1994). Preclinical pharmacology of CGP 42 446, a new, potent, heterocyclic bisphosphonate compound. *J. Bone Miner. Res.*, 9, 745-51.

[86] Rosen, L. S., et al. (2001). Zoledronic acid versus pamidronate in the treatment of skeletal metastases in patients with breast cancer or osteolytic lesions of multiple myeloma: a phase III, double-blind, comparative trial. *Cancer J.*, 7, 377–87.

[87] Major, P., et al. (2001). Zoledronic acid is superior to pamidronate in the treatment of hypercalcemia of malignancy: a pooled analysis of two randomized, controlled clinical trials. *J. Clin. Oncol.*, 19, 558-67.
[88] Chang, J.T., et al. (2003). Renal failure with the use of zoledronic acid. *N. Engl. J. Med.*, 349, 1676-9.
[89] Berenson, J. R., et al. (2001). Zoledronic acid reduces skeletal-related events in patients with osteolytic metastases. *Cancer*, 91, 1191–200.
[90] Rosen, L. S., et al. (2003). Long-term efficacy and safety of zoledronic acid compared with pamidronate disodium in the treatment of skeletal complications in patients with advanced multiple myeloma or breast carcinoma: a randomized, double-blind, multicenter, comparative trial. *Cancer*, 98, 1735–44.
[91] Ruggiero, S. L., et al. (2004). Osteonecrosis of the jaws associated with the use of bisphosphonates: a review of 63 cases. *J. Oral Maxillofac. Surg.*, 62, 527-34.
[92] Van Poznak, C. H., et al. (2004). Osteonecrosis of the jaw in patients with metastatic breast cancer. *Breast Cancer Res. Treat.*, 88, S131, 3057.
[93] Hoff, A. O., et al. (2005). Osteonecrosis of the jaw in patients receiving intravenous bisphosphonate therapy. *J. Bone Miner. Res.*, 20, S55, 1218.
[94] Durie, B. G. M., et al. (2005). Osteonecrosis of the jaw and bisphosphonates. *N. Engl. J. Med.*, 353, 99.
[95] Maerevoet, M., et al. (2005). Osteonecrosis of the jaw and bisphosphonates. *N. Engl. J. Med.*, 353, 100-1.
[96] Zipori, D. (2010). The hemopoietic stem cell niche versus the microenvironment of the multiple myeloma-tumor initiating cell. *Cancer Microenviron.*, 3, 15–28.
[97] Mitsiades, C. S., et al. (2007). The role of the bone marrow microenvironment in the pathophysiology of myeloma and its significance in the development of more effective therapies. *Hematol. Oncol. Clin. North Am.*, 21, 1007–34.
[98] Schmidt-Kittler, O., et al. (2003). From latent disseminated cells to overt metastasis: genetic analysis of systemic breast cancer progression. *Proc. Natl. Acad. Sci. US*, 100, 7737–42.
[99] Kyle, R. A., et al. (2007). American Society of Clinical Oncology 2007 clinical practice guideline update on the role of bisphosphonates in multiple myeloma. *J. Clin. Oncol.*, 25, 2464–72.
[100] Ottewell, P. D., et al. (2008). Antitumor effects of doxorubicin followed by zoledronic acid in a mouse model of breast cancer. *J. Natl. Cancer Inst.*, 100, 1167–78.
[101] Korpal, M., et al. (2009). Imaging transforming growth factor-beta signaling dynamics and therapeutic response in breast cancer bone metastasis. *Nat. Med.*, 15, 960–6.
[102] Ottewell, P. D., et al. (2008). Differential effect of doxorubicin and zoledronic acid on intraosseous versus extraosseous breast tumor growth in vivo. *Clin. Cancer Res.*, 14, 4658–66.
[103] Woodward, E. J. and Coleman, R. E. (2010). Prevention and treatment of bone metastases. *Curr. Pharm. Des.*, 16, 2998–3006.
[104] Malinin, N. L., et al. (2012). Integrin signaling in vascular function. *Curr. Opin. Hematol.*, 19, 206–11.
[105] Carmeliet, P. and Jain, R. K. (2011). Molecular mechanisms and clinical applications of angiogenesis. *Nature*, 473, 298–307.

[106] Dudley, A. C., et al. (2010). Bone marrow is a reservoir for pro-angiogenic myelomonocytic cells but not endothelial cells in spontaneous tumors. *Blood*, 116, 3367–71.

[107] Coscia, M., et al. (2010). Zoledronic acid repolarizes tumor-associated macrophages and inhibits mammary carcinogenesis by targeting the mevalonate pathway. *J. Cell. Mol. Med.*, 14, 2803–15.

[108] Clézardin, P. (2011). Bisphosphonates' antitumor activity: an unravelled side of a multifaceted drug class. *Bone*, 48, 71–9.

[109] Clézardin, P. and Massaia, M. (2010). Nitrogen-containing bisphosphonates and cancer immunotherapy. *Curr. Pharm. Des.*, 16, 3007–14.

[110] Maniar, A., et al. (2010). Human gammadelta T lymphocytes induce robust NK cell-mediated antitumor cytotoxicity through CD137 engagement. *Blood*, 116, 1726–33.

[111] Li, X., et al. (2011). Drugs which inhibit osteoclast function suppress tumor growth through calcium reduction in bone. *Bone*, 48, 1354–61.

[112] Guenther, A., et al. (2010). The bisphosphonate zoledronic acid has antimyeloma activity in vivo by inhibition of protein prenylation. *Int. J. Cancer*, 126, 239–46.

[113] Terpos, E., et al. (2010). Prognostic variables for survival and skeletal complications in patients with multiple myeloma osteolytic bone disease. *Leukemia*, 24, 1043–49.

[114] Ural, A. U., et al. (2003). The bisphosphonate zoledronic acid induces cytotoxicity in human myeloma cell lines with enhancing effects of dexamethasone and thalidomide. *Int. J. Hematol.*, 78, 443-9.

[115] Schmidmaier, R., et al. (2006). Synergistic antimyeloma effects of zoledronate and simvastatin. *Anticancer Drugs*, 17, 621–9.

[116] Moschetta, M., et al. (2010). Bortezomib and zoledronic acid on angiogenic and vasculogenic activities of bone marrow macrophages in patients with multiple myeloma. *Eur. J. Cancer*, 46, 420-9.

[117] Morgan, G. J. (2011). Can bisphosphonates improve outcomes in patients with newly diagnosed multiple myeloma? *Crit. Rev. Oncol. Hematol.*, 77(suppl. 1), S24–S30.

[118] Jagannath, S. (2008). Pathophysiological underpinnings of multiple myeloma progression. *J. Manag. Care Pharm.*, 14(suppl. 7), 7–11.

[119] Ribatti, D. and Vacca, A. (2009). The role of monocytes-macrophages in vasculogenesis in multiple myeloma. *Leukemia*, 23, 1535–6.

[120] Corso, A., et al. (2005). Zoledronic acid down-regulates adhesion molecules of bone marrow stromal cells in multiple myeloma: a possible mechanism for its antitumor effect. *Cancer*, 104, 118–25.

[121] Vacca, A. and Ribatti, D. (2006). Bone marrow angiogenesis in multiple myeloma. *Leukemia*, 3, 193–9.

[122] Bellamy, W. T., et al. (1999). Expression of vascular endothelial growth factor and its receptors in hematopoietic malignancies. *Cancer Res.*, 59, 728–33.

[123] Dankbar, B., et al. (2000). Vascular endothelial growth factor and interleukin-6 in paracrine tumor-stromal cell interactions in multiple myeloma. *Blood*. 95, 2630–6.

[124] Vacca, A., et al. (2003). Endothelial cells in the bone marrow of patients with multiple myeloma. *Blood*, 102, 3340–8.

[125] Podar, K. and Anderson, K. C. (2005). The pathophysiologic role of VEGF in hematologic malignancies: therapeutic implications. *Blood*, 105, 1383–95.

[126] Ria, R., et al. (2004). A VEGF-dependent autocrine loop mediates proliferation and capillarogenesis in bone marrow endothelial cell of patients with multiple myeloma. *Thromb. Haemost.*, 92, 1438–45.

[127] Vacca, A., et al. (2006). Loss of inhibitory semaphorin 3A (SEMA3A) autocrine loops in bone marrow endothelial cells of patients with multiple myeloma. *Blood*, 108, 1661–7.

[128] Clezardin, P. (2002). The antitumor potential of bisphosphonates. *Semin. Oncol.*, 29, 33–42.

[129] Stresing, V., et al. (2011). Nitrogen-containing bisphosphonates can inhibit angiogenesis in vivo without the involvement of farnesyl pyrophosphate synthase. *Bone*, 48, 259-66.

[130] Hasmim, M., et al. (2007). Zoledronate inhibits endothelial cell adhesion, migration and survival through the suppression of multiple, prenylation-dependent signaling pathways. *J. Thromb. Haemost.*, 5, 166–73.

[131] Croucher, P. I., et al. (2003). Zoledronic acid treatment of 5T2MM-bearing mice inhibits the development of myeloma bone disease: evidence for decreased osteolysis, tumor burden and angiogenesis, and increased survival. *J. Bone Miner. Res.*, 18, 482–92.

[132] Bezzi, M., et al. (2003). Zoledronate sensitizes endothelial cells to tumor necrosis factor-induced programmed cell death. Evidence for the supperssion of sustained activation of focal adhesion kinase and protein kinase B/Akt. *J. Biol. Chem.*, 278, 43603–14.

[133] Corey, E., et al. (2003). Zoledronic acid exhibits inhibitory effects on osteoblastic and osteolytic metastases of prostate cancer. *Clin. Cancer Res.*, 9, 295–306.

[134] Santini, D., et al. (2003). Zoledronic acid induces significant and long-lasting modifications of circulating angiogenic factors in cancer patients. *Clin. Cancer Res.*, 9, 2893–7.

[135] Scavelli, C., et al. (2007). Zoledronic acid affects over-angiogenic phenotype of endothelial cells in patients with multiple myeloma. *Mol. Cancer Ther.*, 6, 3256-62.

[136] Santini, D., et al. (2013). Zoledronic acid induces a significant decrease of circulating endothelial cells and circulating endothelial precursor cells in the early prostate cancer neoadjuvant setting. *Oncology*, 85, 342-7.

[137] Scavelli, C., et al. (2008). Vasculogenic mimicry by bone marrow macrophages in patients with multiple myeloma. *Oncogene*, 27, 663–74.

[138] Fu, D., et al. (2011). Zoledronic acid inhibits vasculogenic mimicry in murine osteosarcoma cell line in vitro. *BMC Musculoskelet. Disord.*, 12, 146-51.

[139] Roccaro, A. M. et al. (2006). Bortezomib mediates antiangiogenesis in multiple myeloma via direct and indirect effects on endothelial cells. *Cancer Res.*, 66, 184–91.

[140] Podar, K., et al. (2004). Caveolin-1 is required for vascular endothelial growth factor-triggered multiple myeloma cell migration and is targeted by bortezomib. *Cancer Res.*, 64, 7500–6.

[141] Benzaïd, I., et al. (2011). High phosphoantigen levels in bisphosphonate-treated human breast tumors promote Vgamma9Vdelta2 T-cell chemotaxis and cytotoxicity in vivo. *Cancer Res.*, 71, 4562–72.

[142] Casetti, R. and Martino, A. (2008). The plasticity of gamma delta T cells: innate immunity, antigen presentation and new immunotherapy. *Cell. Mol. Immunol.*, 5, 161–70.

[143] Sato, K., et al. (2005). Cytotoxic effects of gammadelta T cells expanded ex vivo by a third generation bisphosphonate for cancer immunotherapy. *Int. J. Cancer*, 116, 94–9.

[144] Yuasa, T., et al. (2009). Intravesical administration of gammadelta T cells successfully prevents the growth of bladder cancer in the murine model. *Cancer Immunol. Immunother.*, 58, 493–502.

[145] Fiore, F., et al. (2007). Enhanced ability of dendritic cells to stimulate innate and adaptive immunity upon short-term incubation with zoledronic acid. *Blood*, 110, 921–7.

[146] Abe, Y., et al. (2009). Clinical and immunological evaluation of zoledronate-activated Vgamma9gammadelta T-cell-based immunotherapy for patients with multiple myeloma. *Exp. Hematol.*, 37, 956–68.

[147] Santini, D., et al. (2007). Repeated intermittent low-dose therapy with zoledronic acid induces an early, sustained, and long-lasting decrease of peripheral vascular endothelial growth factor levels in cancer patients. *Clin. Cancer Res.*, 13, 4482–6.

[148] Shipman, C. M. and Rogers, M. J. (1997). Apperley, J. F., Russell, R. G., Croucher, P. I. Bisphosphonates induce apoptosis in human myeloma cell lines: a novel anti-tumour activity. *Br. J. Haematol.*, 98, 665–72.

[149] Drexler, H. G., et al. (2001). Cross-contamination: HS-Sultan is not a myeloma but a Burkitt lymphoma cell line. *Blood*, 98, 3495–6.

[150] Roelofs, A. J., et al. (2006). Selective inhibition of Rab prenylation by a phosphonocarboxylate analogue of risedronate induces apoptosis, but not S-phase arrest, in human myeloma cells. *Int. J. Cancer*, 119, 1254–61.

[151] Lawson, M. A., et al. (2008). Geranylgeranyl transferase type II inhibition prevents myeloma bone disease. *Biochem. Biophys. Res. Commun.*, 377, 453–7.

[152] Baulch-Brown, C., et al. (2007). Inhibitors of the mevalonate pathway as potential therapeutic agents in multiple myeloma. *Leuk. Res.*, 31, 341–52.

[153] Yaccoby, S., et al. (2002). Myeloma interacts with the bone marrow microenvironment to induce osteoclastogenesis and is dependent on osteoclast activity. *Br. J. Haematol.*, 116, 278–90.

[154] Yaccoby, S., et al. (2006). Inhibitory effects of osteoblasts and increased bone formation on myeloma in novel culture systems and a myelomatous mouse model. *Haematologica*, 91, 192–9.

[155] Costa, L., et al. (2011). Anticancer evidence for zoledronic acid across the cancer continuum. *Crit. Rev. Oncol. Hematol.*, 77(suppl. 1), S31–S37.

[156] Morgan, G. J., et al., National Cancer Research Institute Haematological Oncology Clinical Study Group. (2010). First-line treatment with zoledronic acid as compared with clodronic acid in multiple myeloma (MRC Myeloma IX): a randomised controlled trial. *Lancet*, 376, 1989-99.

[157] Gnant, M., et al. (2009). Endocrine therapy plus zoledronic acid in premenopausal breast cancer. *N. Eng. J. Med.*, 360, 679–91.

[158] Smith, M. R., et al. (2012). Denosumab and bone-metastasis-free survival in men with castration-resistant prostate cancer: results of a phase 3, randomised, placebo-controlled trial. *Lancet*, 379, 39–46.

[159] Melton, L. J. III, et al. (2005) Fracture risk with multiple myeloma: a population-based study. *J. Bone Miner. Res.*, 20, 487–93.

[160] Berenson, J. R., et al. (2006). Zoledronic acid may improve survival compared to pamidronate in patients with MM and high BALP levels: univariate and multivariate models of hazard ratios, *Blood*, 108 Abstract, 3589.

[161] Aviles, A., et al. (2007) Antitumor effect of zoledronic acid in previously untreated patients with multiple myeloma. *Med. Oncol.*, 24, 227–30.

[162] Kavanagh, K. L., et al. (2006). The molecular mechanism of nitrogen-containing bisphosphonates as antiosteoporosis drugs. *Proc. Natl. Acad. Sci. US*, 103, 7829–34.

[163] Kellinsalmi, M., et al. (2005). In vitro comparison of clodronate, pamidronate and zoledronic acid effects on rat osteoclasts and human stem cell-derived osteoblasts. *Basic Clin. Pharmacol. Toxicol.*, 97, 382–91.

[164] Ria, R., et al. (2013). A retrospective study of skeletal and disease-free survival benefits of zoledronic acid therapy in patients with multiple myeloma treated with novel agents. *Int. J. Clin. Exp. Med.*, 6, 30-8.

[165] Terpos, E., et al. (2010). Increased bone mineral density in a subset of patients with relapsed multiple myeloma who received the combination of bortezomib, dexamethasone and zoledronic acid. *Ann. Oncol.*, 21, 1561-2.

[166] Pennisi, A., et al. (2009). The proteasome inhibitor, bortezomib suppersses primary myeloma and stimulates bone formation in myelomatous and nonmyelomatous bones in vivo. *Am. J. Hematol.*, 84, 6-14.

[167] Sun, X. F. and Zhang, H. (2007). NFKB and NFKBI polymorphisms in relation to susceptibility of tumour and other diseases. *Histol. Histopathol.*, 22, 1387–98.

[168] Mhaskar, R., et al. (2010). Bisphosphonates in multiple myeloma. *Cochrane Database Syst. Rev.* (Online). p. CD003188.

[169] Musto, P., et al. (2008). A multicenter, randomized clinical trial comparing zoledronic acid versus observation in patients with asymptomatic myeloma. *Cancer*, 113, 1588–95.

In: Zoledronic Acid
Editor: Ronald Carman

ISBN: 978-1-63321-525-2

Chapter 3

THE USE OF ZOLEDRONIC ACID IN OSTEOARTHRITIS: FROM ANIMAL MODELS TO CLINICAL STUDIES

Nidhi Sofat[1,•], Anasuya Kuttapitiya[1] and Toby Smith[2]
[1]Institute of Infection and Immunity, St. George's University of London, Cranmer Terrace, London, UK
[2]Faculty of Medicine and Health Sciences, University of East Anglia, Norwich Research Park, Norwich, UK

ABSTRACT

Zoledronic acid is a bisphosphonate drug administered as an intravenous infusion which is licensed internationally for the treatment of osteoporosis. Pharmacologically, it can slow down bone resorption, potentiates an anabolic effect on bone-forming cells and promotes bone remodelling. Bone and cartilage turnover are affected in other musculoskeletal conditions including osteoarthritis (OA) and rheumatoid arthritis (RA). OA is the most common arthritic disease worldwide, with an increasing prevalence due to a rising ageing population and the epidemic of obesity worldwide. The most common joints affected in OA include the larger weight-bearing hip and knee joints, the hands and spine. Radiographic examination of affected joints often reveals joint space narrowing, cartilage degradation and bone marrow lesions observed by magnetic resonance imaging (MRI) scans.

Recent interest has focused on evaluating the therapeutic effects of bisphosphonate drugs to target OA pain and structural damage. This chapter presents the results of a systematic review assessing the currently available evidence on zoledronic acid in human and animal studies. In this chapter, we report the rationale for using zoledronic acid for OA from animal model data in the studies so far reported, discussing the effects of this drug on bone remodelling and inhibition of cartilage degradation.

We discuss how zoledronic acid could target lesions observed in the pathophysiology of OA, which include damage to the components of cartilage extracellular matrix (ECM) and peri-articular bone. We then report the effect of zoledronic acid in the clinical studies

• E-mail: nsofat@sgul.ac.uk.

published so far for people with OA, including data on the use of this bisphosphonate as an adjunct to high tibial osteotomy surgery. We also discuss the impact of the use of zoledronic acid on improving knee pain in clinical trials and its effect on reducing the size of bone marrow lesions detected by magnetic resonance imaging (MRI) scans in the same studies.

In summary, this chapter outlines emerging data on the use of the bisphosphonate drug zoledronic acid in OA. Clinical trials published to date have shown an improvement in OA pain in the short term, coupled with an effect on the size of bone marrow lesions following infusion of zoledronic acid. It is possible that treatment with bisphosphonate drugs at earlier stages of the condition, as suggested by animal models of OA, may have a greater impact on modulating disease activity in this chronic, common arthritic disease.

Abbreviations

ACR	American College of Rheumatology
BMD	Bone mineral density
CGRP	Calcitonin gene related peptide
CT	Computerised tomography
CTX-1	Collagen C terminal telopeptide
DRG	Dorsal root ganglion
FG	Fluoro gold
GFAP	Glial fibrillalary acidic protein
HCO	Hemicallotosis
Iba-1	Ionized calcium binding adaptor molecule 1
KOOS	Knee injury and osteoarthritis outcome score
MIA	Monoiodoacetate
MMT	Medial Meniscectomy model
MRI	Magnetic Resonance Imaging
NS	Normal saline
NTX-1	Collagen N terminal telopeptide
OA	Osteoarthritis
SC	Subcutaneous
TRAP	Tartrate resistant alkaline phosphatase
VAS	Visual analogue scale
VRS	Visual Rating Scale
WOMAC	Western Ontario and McMaster Universities Arthritis
ZOL	Zoledronic acid

Introduction

Zoledronic acid is a third generation bisphosphonate drug [1]. It is currently licensed for the treatment of osteoporosis. Its mechanisms of action include inhibition of osteoclast function, thereby resulting in delayed bone resorption [2]. Zoledronic acid potentiates its anabolic effects on bone and enhanced bone remodelling [2]. Zoledronic acid is administered by intravenous infusion over a minimum of 15 minutes. It is already licensed for the prevention of skeletal fractures in people with malignancy such as multiple myeloma and prostate cancer, and in the treatment of osteoporosis [3, 4]. Zoledronic acid is also used to treat hypercalcaemia of malignancy and can be useful for treating pain emanating from bony metastases. Since zoledronic acid is excreted via the kidneys, it is therefore contraindicated in people with impaired renal function.

Osteoarthritis (OA) is the most common arthritic joint disorder worldwide and is associated with significant pain and reduced function [5]. There are currently no treatments that have been shown to demonstrate a sustained effect on halting the progression of the disease in the long-term [6]. Recent work from animal models has focussed on assessing the effect of zoledronic acid on bone and cartilage in OA. Potentially beneficial results on bone and cartilage in such animal models have provided momentum to conduct clinical trials in people with OA. The aim of these studies has been to potentially improve pain outcomes and structural changes at early time points in OA. This chapter outlines results from these animal model studies utilising zoledronic acid and some of the early clinical trials of this drug in the treatment of people with OA.

Methods

The identification of papers was undertaken in accordance with the PRISMA recommendations for systematic review reporting [7, 8].

Search Strategy

The principle search undertaken was an electronic search of the databases: AMED, CINAHL, EMBASE, MEDLINE, PUBMED, and the Cochrane Library. In addition, secondary searches were conducted of the unpublished and grey evidence. Databases searches were: the WHO International Clinical Trials Registry Platform, Current Controlled Trials, the United States National Institute of Health Trials Registry, OpenGrey (System for Information on Grey Literature in Europe). The search terms adopted and Boolean operators used for the MEDLINE search strategy are presented in Table 1. These were modified for each individual database. Finally, all reference lists of each potentially relevant papers identified from the search strategy were scrutinised to identify any outstanding papers.

Study Eligibility

The first part of this chapter aimed to assess the results surrounding zoledronic acid in animal models. Accordingly, papers published investigating the use of zoledronic acid in animal models of OA were included. Papers assessing other pathological disorders in any animal model were therefore excluded from this analysis.

To answer the question regarding understanding of zoledronic acid in people with osteoarthritis, a separate eligibility criteria were constructed. In this, studies were deemed eligible if they were:

1. Randomised controlled trials (RCT) comparing bisphosphonate therapy to: a non-treatment control, a placebo, another bisphosphonate therapy. Alternatively bisphosphonate therapy could be compared to an alternative pharmacological intervention.
2. Participants recruited with symptomatic OA of any anatomical region. For example: knee, hips, spine and hand, in isolation or multi-joint.

Table 1. Search strategy (MEDLINE) for the systematic review

1.	Osteoarthritis
2.	Degenerate changes
3.	Arthritis
4.	OR/1-3
5.	Joint
6.	Hip
7.	Knee
8.	Ankle
9.	Foot
10.	Shoulder
11.	Elbow
12.	Wrist
13.	Hand
14.	Fingers
15.	Thumb
16.	OR/5-15
17.	Zoledronate
18.	Zoledronic Acid
19.	Aclasta
20.	Zometa
21.	Reclast
22.	OR/17-22
23.	AND/4,16,22

3. However, trials where the principle anatomical region of osteoarthritis was spinal were excluded. This was based on the premise that the relationship between radiographic OA and back pain is unclear [8].
4. Trials were not excluded based on dosage or delivery method of medication or follow-up periods.
5. Trials were not excluded based on severity or duration of symptomatic OA.
6. Trials were not excluded based on age of publication or language of study.
7. Trials were excluded if based on *in vitro*, animal studies or where participant's predominant pathology was not OA.

STUDY IDENTIFICATION

All titles and/or abstract from the search strategy were reviewed independently by two authors (NS/AK) against the pre-defined eligibility criteria above. The full-texts of all potentially eligible papers were then reviewed by two authors (NS and AK), and all papers meeting these criteria were included in the review.

DATA EXTRACTION AND OUTCOME MEASURES

Data extracted from all eligible papers included: medication therapy under investigation (name, dose, timing), diagnosis of OA, participant eligibility criteria, cohort size, cohort age, cohort gender, duration of medications, primary and secondary outcomes, data collection intervals, and follow-up period. For the animal-study papers, data extracted included: animal model investigated, cohort size, cohort age, animal gender, anatomical joint investigated, status and nature of induced osteoarthritis, trauma, medication therapy under investigation (name, dose, timing and duration), follow-up period, all results of presenting paper.

For the human cohort studies, *a priori* primary and secondary outcomes were identified. Perceived pain as measured using a validated pain assessment scoring system such as the visual analogue scale (VAS), visual rating scale (VRS) or evaluation with the *Western Ontario And Mcmaster Universities Arthritis* (WOMAC) index were considered the primary outcome measures.

This review's secondary outcomes included:

- Evaluation of joint structural changes
- Indirect pain, such as assessment via skin impedance studies
- Administration of analgesics post-therapy
- Blood and urine analyses of cartilage and bone turnover biomarkers e.g. CTX-II/NTX-I

Data Analysis

After undertaking the search strategy, there appeared to be a small and varied evidence base on the use of zoledronic acid in OA. The evidence was divided into a single randomised controlled trial [9] and a series of papers exploring animal models. Accordingly, based on this heterogeneity, it was considered inappropriate to pool any data as part of a meta-analysis, but a narrative review of the clinical paper and the animal models was undertaken to report these findings.

Results

Data from Animal Models

Although there is not a large amount of clinical data available as yet on the use of zoledronic acid for OA treatment in humans, we identified a total of 6 studies using animal models from our searches. The studies reported data which revealed data is available for use of zoledronic acid from animal models of OA and is discussed further in the section below. A summary of the identified animal study papers is presented in Table 2.

Use of the Monoiodoacetate Model to Assess Efficacy of Zoledronic Acid

The monoiodoacetate model is a chemically-induced animal model of OA [10]. In this model, Sprague Dawley rats can be utilised in order to inject monoiodoacetic acid in the knee joint.

Table 2. Animal models testing effects of zoledronic acid

Study	Animal model	Method/Effect of zoledronic acid
Strassle et al., (2010)	Monoiodoacetate (Rat)	Treatment: Zoledronate administered every 3 days before and during model induction at a dose of 10, 30 or 100ug/kg Outcome measures: Histological analysis Radiographic analysis Hind limb pain testing Effect: Joint degradation and pain prevented by zoledronate treatment, delayed treatment reduced efficacy

Study	Animal model	Method/Effect of zoledronic acid
Yu et al., (2013)	Monoiodoacetate (Rat)	Treatment: Zoledronate administered post model induction twice weekly at 100ug/kg Outcome measures: Weight-bearing asymmetry Micro-CT imaging Histological analysis Immunofluorescence analysis Effect: Zoledronate treatment reduced weight bearing deficit and over-expression of CGRP in DRG neurons and GFAP and Iba-1 in spinal dorsal horns
Muehlman et al., (2002)	Chymopapain (Rabbit)	Treatment: Zoledronate administered 24hrs prior to model induction thrice weekly at a dose of 10ug/kg Outcome measures: Histological analysis Proteogylcan content analysis Effect: Bone resorption inhibited via treatment along with a level of chonroprotection
Yu et al., (2012)	Medial Meniscectomy (Rat)	Treatment: Zoledronate administered immediately, 4 weeks and 8 weeks post model induction at a dose of 100ug/kg Outcome measures: Weight-bearing asymmetry Micro-CT imaging Histological analysis Immunofluorescence analysis Effect: Early treatment improved subchondral microstructural parameters, cartilage degradation, reduced pain and CGRP expression in DRG neurons

Table 2. (Continued)

Study	Animal model	Method/Effect of zoledronic acid
Dearmin et al., (2014)	Cranial cruciate ligament transection (Dog)	Treatment: Zoledronate administered every 3 months post model induction at a dose of 10ug/kg or 25ug/kg Outcome measures: Radiographic analysis Biomarker analysis (bone-specific alkaline phosphatase, type I and II collagen, carboxy-propepide of type II collagen and chondroitin sulphate 846) Effect: High dose group had fewer articular defects, lower severity scores, less change in collagenase cleavage of type I and II collagen, greater changes in bone alkaline phosphatase. Zoledronate has a condroprotective effect
Agnello et al., (2005)	Cranial cruciate ligament transection (Dog)	Treatment: Zoledronate administered 3 monthly post model induction at a dose of 10ug/kg or 25ug/kg Outcome measures: Biomarker analysis (osteocalcin, bone-specific alkaline phosphatase, pyridinoline and deocypyridinoline) Bone mineral density Effect: Treatment inhibited osteocalcin, decreased bone alkaline phosphatase, increased bone mineral density after 3 months. Zoledronate may reduce subchondral bone loss

Control animals are injected with saline. Animals can then be assessed by behavioural testing for pain using hind limb testing of weight-bearing using a Linton Incapacitance meter.

The percent of weight borne on the ipsilateral hind limb can be determined using the following formula:

$$\frac{\text{Weight on ipsilateral hindlimb}}{\text{Weight on ipsilateral hindlimb + weight on contralateral hindlimb}}$$

In this study described [11], pharmacological testing was conducted using zoledronic acid (disodium tetrahydrate). Zoledronic acid was administered by subcutaneous (sc) administration. Five different dosing regimens were used as outlined below:

1. Pre-emptive chronic (10, 30 or 100 micrograms per kg) every third day from Day 1 to 21
2. Early sub-chronic (100 micrograms per kg), every third day from Day 14 to 21
3. Early chronic (100 micrograms per kg), every third day from Day 14 to 35
4. Delayed chronic (100 micrograms per kg), every third day from Day 21 to 35
5. Curative sub-chronic (100 micrograms per kg), every third day from Day 28 to 35.

Samples from rats subjected to this model were taken for histological analysis from the pre-emptive chronic group on Day 5 and from the pre-emptive chronic and early sub-chronic groups on Day 22: weight-bearing and bone densitometry analysis was performed weekly.

Bone mineral density analysis showed a significant reduction in bone mineral density for all three concentrations of MIA used i.e. 0.3, 1.0 or 3.0 mg MIA one week post-injection. The effect was concentration-dependent and was maintained for the 1.0 and 3.0 mg dose two to four weeks post-injection. In later experiments, treatments did not significantly affect body weight. Since the treatments were being administered in actively growing animals, it is important to note that it is normal for bone mineral density to increase in control animals over time. Radiographs were performed (three weeks post-1.0 mg MIA) which demonstrated that the joint degeneration characterized by osteolysis at the medial and lateral condyles of the knee was induced as expected in this animal model. The influence of zoledronic acid at varying intervention times was then evaluated.

Zoledronic Acid Inhibits MIA-Induced Loss of Bone Mineral Density and Pain

The group of rats that were treated pre-emptively with zoledronic acid at 10-100 micrograms per kg showed significant and dose-dependent increases in bone mineral density (BMD) above the level of control animals and prevented MIA-induced bone loss ($p<0.0001$). To determine if zoledronic acid could reverse established changes in the animal model, early treatment started two weeks after the model was induced showed, that at 100 micrograms per kilogram, zoledronic acid significantly elevated bone mineral density.

In studies where the dosing was delayed, when zoledronic acid was administered every third day at Week 2, 3 or 4 post-MIA at a dose of 100 micrograms per kilogram, zoledronic acid significantly increased bone mineral density loss in a time-dependent manner in all treatment groups. The largest effect was noted in animals treated for the longest period. Zoledronic acid also reduced the weight-bearing deficits in all treatment groups ($p<0.0001$).

Histological evaluation of tissue obtained from rats treated in this model was assessed by cartilage thinning, loss of chondrocytes, decreased proteoglycan and areas of total loss of cartilage. Three weeks after inducing the MIA model, rats showed cartilage thinning and loss of chondrocytes. Large, multi-nucleated osteoclasts were observed at the bone-cartilage interface and bone and cartilage had been resorbed in the weight-bearing regions of the joint. Early sub-chronic MIA treatment, initiated two weeks post-MIA, led to a partial reduction in resorption of both the non-calcified and calcified cartilage and subchondral bone. In comparison, pre-emptive chronic zoledronic acid resulted in a preservation of the joint. When such findings were quantified they showed that erosion of bone and cartilage was significantly reduced with early sub-chronic zoledronic acid and was prevented by pre-emptive chronic treatment. The authors also found that zoledronic acid protected toluidene blue staining and cartilage integrity without affecting synovitis. These findings reported in a quantified method demonstrate that erosion of bone, cartilage and tidemark was significantly increased with MIA treatment, which was significantly reduced by zoledronic acid.

Clinically in OA there is often evidence of bone remodelling, with evidence of osteophyte formation and bone sclerosis visible on plain radiography in people with OA. The use of bisphosphonates has therefore attracted attention as a potential therapeutic agent in OA. This animal model aimed to treat animals early even before their joint damage had developed in the MIA model, or during early stages of the damage. It is interesting to note that most clinical studies of bisphosphonates, and of zoledronic acid for that matter, have initiated the drug intervention during established phases of the disease [9]. However, results from this animal model have shown that cartilage and bone damage as well as pain can be inhibited by 'pre-emptive' administration of zoledronic acid.

The authors postulate three potential mechanisms whereby zoledronic acid may directly inhibit MIA-induced chondrocyte cell death, thereby preserving joint integrity and reducing pain. Secondly, at early time points after the MIA model induction, cell and proteoglycan loss was only observed close to areas of osteoclast-mediated cartilage resorption. These pre-clinical findings are consistent with a recent study demonstrating that cartilage loss was only observed close to areas of osteoclast-mediated cartilage resorption. Inhibiting osteoclasts could therefore be chondroprotective and prevent cartilage resorption. The authors suggest that this may explain why the effect of pre-emptive chronic dosing and when dosing was delayed for two weeks. However, at four weeks post-MIA, cartilage damage was severe, which could be a stage where cartilage-sparing therapies may be less relevant. The authors propose that a third mechanism may be whereby there is a direct analgesic action of zoledronic acid via the central and/or peripheral nervous system. It could explain the efficacy of the drug in the MIA model when it was dosed at late time points. Since bone is heavily innervated, cartilage and trabecular bone degeneration may result in exposure of sensory nerve terminals to chemical or mechanical stimulation not normally present in joints. Bisphosphonate-induced increases in bone mineral density may help to protect these exposed nerve fibres, shielding them from excitatory stimuli.

A more recent study has also demonstrated the effects of zoledronic acid on inhibiting subchondral bone lesions in the MIA model of OA pain [12].The authors also reported that zoledronic acid inhibited the overexpression of CGRP in DRG neurons, GFAP and Iba-1 in the spinal dorsal horn of treated animals [12]. This study utilised the MIA model to investigate the inhibition of subchondral bone lesions on OA joint pain. The investigators evaluated pain behaviour, knee joint histomorphometry and the expression of pain-related neurochemical indices in the DRGs and spinal cord dorsal horns that innervate OA joints in MIA-injected rats in the presence and absence of zoledronic acid.

The authors evaluated three groups of animals: sham treatment with normal saline, MIA treatment with normal saline and MIA with zoledronic acid. In assessing pain behaviour, weight-bearing asymmetry between the ipsilateral and contralateral hind limbs was measured as an index of pain behaviour. Intra-articular MIA markedly reduced hind limb weight bearing throughout the course of the experiment. Zoledronic acid treatment with 100 micrograms per kilogram body weight subcutaneously twice per week showed significant reversal of weight-bearing deficits compared to MIA/normal saline animals at three weeks ($p< 0.01$). The study group also conducted micro-Computer Tomography scans which showed intra-articular MIA-induced significant alterations in the subchondral bone. Changes observed included bone-cartilage interface collapse and subchondral bone loss, which were most prominent at three to six weeks post-MIA injection. Zoledronic acid reduced the subchondral bone loss and preserved the bone quantity. Of note, osteosclerosis was also observed at the tibial metaphysis in zoledronic acid treated animals. On histological evaluation of knee joints in this MIA study, MIA-ijected joints showed significant changes including articular cartilage loss, subchondral bone collapse and synovial reaction. Full thickness and extensive cartilage loss was found at three and six weeks post-induction of the model. Zoledronic acid treatment appeared to preserve joint shape, inhibited subchondral bone loss and delayed cartilage loss in treated animals. However, no significant difference in the synovial reaction of MIA/ZOL animals compared to MIA/NS animals was observed. The group also assessed osteoclast activity by tartrate resistant alkaline phosphatase staining (TRAP). They observed a large number of TRAP-positive multinucleated osteoclasts that were present at the surface of the subchondral bone in the MIA/NS animals at three and six weeks. Zoledronic acid treatment significantly inhibited osteoclast activity in MIA/Zoledronic acid treated animals. In the same study, the investigators evaluated alterations in the peripheral neurons of DRGs using the expression of a pain-related neuropeptide, CGRP. The total neuron numbers were similar between groups ($p>0.05$) at three and six weeks. The percentage of CGRP-positive Fluorogold labelled neurons in MIA/NS animals was significantly greater than sham/NS animals.

The study also looked at spinal astrocytes and microglia using immunofluorescence of Iba-1 and GFAP expression. Zoledronic acid treatment appeared to reduce the number of activated microglia at three weeks ($p< 0.01$) and six weeks ($p< 0.05$). Whereas intra-articular (IA) injections increased GFAP immunoreactivity, zoledronic acid treatment significantly attenuated the MIA-induced increase in GFAP immunoreactivity. No significant differences were observed in the expression of Iba-1 or GFAP in the contralateral spinal cords between groups ($p>0.05$).

Investigations using the MIA model data outlined above suggest that several potential mechanisms may contribute to pain relief. Zoledronic acid appears to target cartilage and bone changes in the MIA model, with effects of reverising changes being most marked the earlier the treatment is used. Both the studies outlined above showed that subchondral bone can be modulated by treatment with zoledronic acid. The subchondral bone is richly innervated [13, 14] and the neurovasculature invades the osteochondral junction in OA [15]. The mechanical properties of subchondral bone are significantly reduced in OA [16, 17]. Therefore, subchondral nociceptors can be activated due to pathological changes in OA tissue and mechanical forces on the unstable joint. The animal model data outlined above suggests that targeting subchondral bone by treatment with zoledronic acid could inhibit the development of subchondral bone lesions and the neurovascular invasion of damaged OA tissue. A critical consideration in the treatment of OA with potential bisphosphonate therapy will include the timing of treatment, since clinical studies have shown that a critical window of intervention occurs following which changes may be irreversible.

Medial Meniscectomy Model of Osteoarthritis

The medial meniscal tear model is a widely used model for the assessment of mechanical injury in animal models of OA [18]. In a study by [19], Sprague Dawly rats were subjected to the medial meniscal tear model (MMT). Adult male rats were treated with zoledronic acid (100 micrograms per kiolgram, SC, twice weekly). Zoledronic acid was administered starting immediately, early (from four weeks) or late (from eight weeks) after the induction of OA.

The MMT model is a useful model to interrogate the impact of cartilage and bone changes after mechanical injury. It demonstrates dynamic changes in cartilage and subchondral bone after injury and has been extensively used in testing new therapeutic interventions aimed at modulating cartilage and bone turnover during arthritis. The MMT model has also been used to test changes in pain behaviour, neuron phenotype and neuropeptide expression.

The study tested 154 animals. In the preliminary experiment, a total of 64 animals were used to observe the changes in cartilage and bone during OA progression. The animals were sacrificed at Week 2, 4, 8 and 12 after OA induction (n=8 at each time point). Another 40 animals were used to confirm the effect of zoledronic acid in the MMT model and to assess the effect of different dosings on subchondral bone. Zoledronic acid from Novartis Pharma Stein was administered subcutaneously twice weekly at low dose 10 micrograms per kilogram body weight and also at high dose 100 micrograms per kilogram body weight. The same volume of normal saline was given to sham animals. The animals (n=10 per group) were sacrificed at 12 weeks following the induction of OA. In evaluating pain behaviour, Yu et al., [19] measured weight-bearing asymmetry between the OA-induced (right) and contralateral (left) limb using an incapacitance meter. The authors found a marked reduction in limb weight-bearing one week post-OA induction, which was almost completely resolved by two weeks in all of the groups. Compared with MMT/NS controls at any time point tested, rats that received early zoledronic acid therapy showed less weight-bearing asymmetry that gradually become worse in a time-dependent manner. Interestingly, delayed administration of zoledronic acid at eight weeks after the induction of the MMT did not yield a statistically significant difference in weight-bearing.

With respect to other features of tissue damage after MMT in their study, Yu et al., [19] reported after 12 weeks, toluidine blue staining of cartilage degradation was widespread and profound with significant chondrocyte loss observed. However, this loss was significantly reduced by zoledronic acid administration. In results of experiments using micro-CT from animals in this study, MMT resulted in in increased bone accretion and cyst formation, whereas zoledronic acid treatment reversed these changes in a stage-dependent manner. In addition, there was evidence of osteosclerosis at the tibial metaphysis in animals treated with zoledronic acid, which occurred as a result of zoledronic acid inhibiting osteoclasts in active growth plates.

Yu et al., [19] also used Nissl staining for quantification of sensory nerves was similar in all five groups. The authors used fluorogold (FG) labelling to qauntifiy the number of CGRP positive neurons in MMT rats. They found that the percentage of CGRP-positive neurons in MMT/NS rats (48.9% +/- 3%) was increased compared with that observed in sham/NS rats (40.7% +/- 3%, $p< 0.01$). This ratio was significantly reduced by immediate and early zoledronic acid treatment i.e. at zero and four weeks, but not at advanced stages of the model at eight weeks.

The study outlined above suggests that bisphosphonates have a protective effect on cartilage and bone changes related to OA in a dose-dependent manner. Early treatment with zoledronic acid improved microstructural parameters, decreased the cartilage degeneration core and reduced weight-bearing asymmetry and CGRP expression. Late administration demonstrated no statistically significant efficacy ($p>0.05$). A CGRP is a marker of sensory neurons and was used by the investigators to identify the effects of zoledronic acid on joint pain. The expression of CGRP in Dorsal root ganglion (DRG) neurons innervating the joint was measured. Osteoarthritis has been shown to activate the nociceptive system and CGRP is elevated in DRGs [20].The study from [19] showed that the percentage of CGRP-positive neurons was markedly increased at advanced stages in the MMT model, whereas zoledronic acid treatment initiated at early stages reduced the expression of CGRP. These findings, combined with the results of pain behaviour studies, indicate that zoledronic acid treatment initiated at an early stage could relieve joint pain. The authors also demonstrated that early zoledronic acid treatment, but not later stages, delays cartilage degeneration and subchondral bone remodelling. Sensory nerves are also observed within vascular channels at the osteochondral junction in OA [21]. It is therefore possible that subchondral nerves may be exposed to painful stimuli in OA, which would lead to weight-bearing pain. An agent such as zoledronic acid could improve cartilage and bone integrity and thereby inhibit subchondral neovascular invasion.

A further study by Agnello et al., [22] has interrogated the effect of zoledronic acid in another mechanical model of OA: the cruciate transection model of OA in dogs. In their study, 21 adult dogs were allocated to 3 groups: control group, low-dose zoledronate [10 microg/kg, SC, for 12 months] and high-dose zoledronate [25 microg/kg, SC, for 12 months]. Serum osteocalcin (OC), serum bone-specific alkaline phosphatase (BAP), and urine pyridinoline and deoxypyridinoline concentrations were measured at Month 0, 1, 3, 6, 9, and 12 post-surgery. Bone mineral density (BMD) was determined in the distal portion of the femur and proximal portion of the tibia via computed tomography at each time point. The authors reported that zoledronic acid inhibited the production of osteocalcin in the high-dose zoledronic acid group at Month 9 and 12 and at 12 months in the low-dose group, compared with the control group. High-dose zoledronate decreased bone alkaline phosphatase BAP concentrations three and nine months after surgery. In the control group, BMD was decreased in the femoral condyle and caudal tibial plateau. Zoledronate prevented significant BMD decreases starting one month after transection, compared with control dogs. In the caudomedial aspect of the tibial plateau, both zoledronate groups had significant increases in BMD after three months, compared with control dogs. The same group also recently reported that collagenase cleavage was also inhibited in this model using zoledronic acid [23]. The authors concluded that zoledronic acid may reduce subchondral bone loss and effect markers of bone metabolism in dogs with experimentally induced instability of the stifle joint and subsequent development of osteoarthritis.

Investigation of Zoledronic Acid Using the Chymopapain Model

Muehlman et al., [24] used the chymopapain model in a model of cartilage matrix turnover. They investigated the effect of inhibition of bone remodeling, through the use of the bisphosphonate, zoledronic acid, on cartilage matrix damage in an animal model of cartilage matrix damage. New Zealand white rabbits were divided into four groups for treatment purposes: [1] untreated controls; [2] injected into one knee joint with the cartilage matrix degradation enzyme, chymopapain; [3] injected into one knee joint with chymopapain and also given subcutaneous injections of the bisphosphonate, zoledronic acid, three times per week until sacrifice at either day 28 or 56 post-chymopapain-injection; [4] received only the zoledronic acid injections. At sacrifice, the knee joints were examined grossly and histologically, and biochemically for proteoglycan content.

Urine samples were analysed, at intervals, for levels of collagen cross-links which are biochemical markers of cartilage and bone. Animals receiving both intra-articular chymopapain injections and subcutaneous zoledronic acid injections displayed a significantly lower degree of grossly and histologically detectable cartilage degeneration on the tibial articular surfaces (the articular surface displaying the greatest degree of degeneration) than did animals only receiving the chymopapain injections. In addition, urinary levels of collagen cross-links for bone and cartilage were significantly higher in those animals only receiving chymopapain injections. The bone resorption observed after chymopapain injection into the rabbit knee joint was inhibited through the use of the bisphosphonate, zoledronic acid. Interestingly, zoledronic acid did not increase the level of cartilage degeneration and had some chondroprotective effects in this model.

Clinical Trials of Zoledronic Acid in People with OA

The results of the literature search strategy identified a total of 116 studies (Figure 1). A total of four papers were deemed eligible. One further evaluation, two of these reported the same study, with two citations being conference abstracts (Laslett et al., 2011a; Laslett et al., 2011b) [25, 26] for the final definitive report (Laslett et al., 2012) [9].

Use of Zoledronic Acid as Non-Operative Treatment for Knee Osteoarthritis

In this study by Laslett et al., [9], a double-blind, randomised controlled trial design was adopted.

The researchers recruited 59 people, age range from 50 to 80 years, with ACR satisfying a diagnosis of OA knee who reported a minimum VAS pain score of 40mm or more and one or more bone marrow lesion on MRI.

Participants were randomised to receive either a single in-fusion of zoledronic acid (5mg/100ml; n=31) or a placebo medication (n=28). Outcomes were assessed at six and 12 months. They reported significant difference in VAS pain with improved outcomes in the zoledronic acid group compare to the placebo at six months (-14.5 mm, 95% CI -28.1 to -0.9).

However, this was not statistically significantly different between the groups at three or 12 months. Change in the Knee Injury and Osteoarthritis Outcome Score (KOOS) was not significant at any time point in this study ($p>0.05$). There was a statistically significant difference in favour of the zoledronic acid group compared to the placebo for reduction in total BML area at six months (-175.7 $mm^{2;}$ 95% CI: -327.2 to -24.3), with this trend continuing, but to a non-staitstically significant level, at 12 months (-146.5 $mm^{2;}$ 95% CI: -307.5 to 14.5).

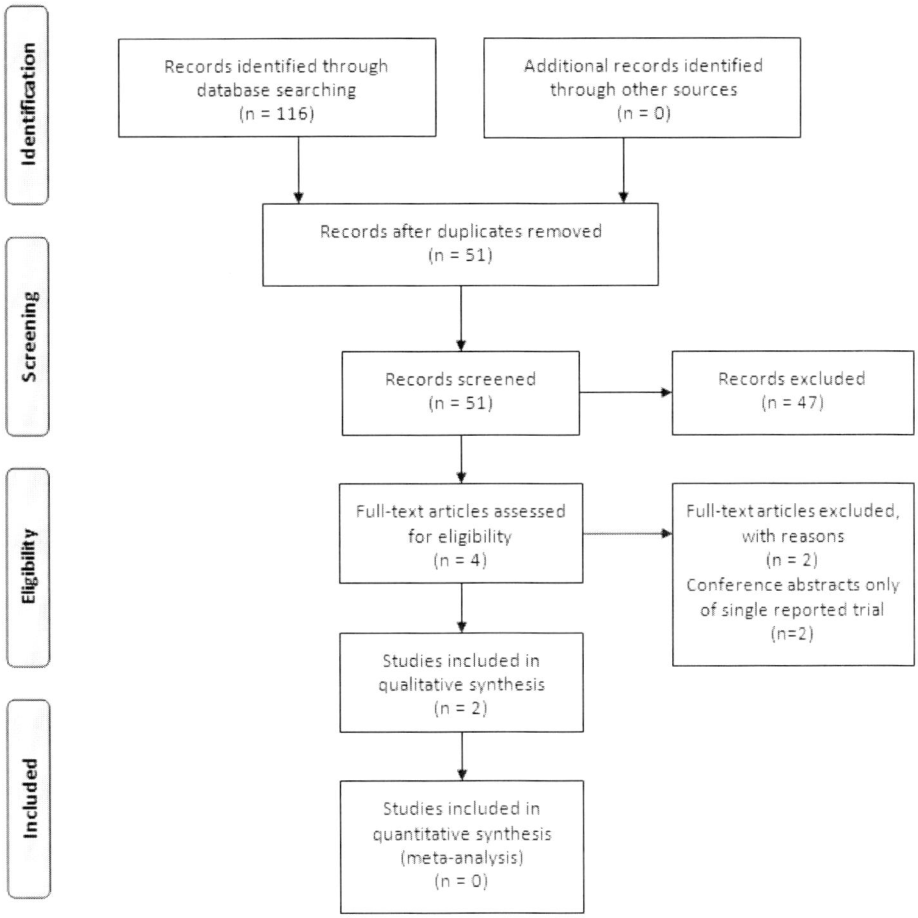

Figure 1. PRISMA flow diagram utilised for systematic review.

Furthermore, there was a greater proportion of participants in the zoledronic acid group who achieved a clinically significant reduction in BML size at six months compared to the placebo group (39% versus 18%, $p=0.044$). For adverse outcome measurements, the prevalence of adverse events in the zoledronate group was 90%. Of these adverse events, the most common was cold or flu symptoms, which was 78% of the 90% total.

Use of Zoledronic Acid Pre-Operatively in Knee Osteoarthritis

Harding et al., have shown [27] that bisphosphonates have been shown to reduce osteoclastic activity and enhance pin fixation in both experimental and clinical studies. In this prospective, randomised study of high tibial osteotomy using the hemicallotasis (HCO) technique, the authors evaluated whether treatment by one single infusion of zoledronic acid can enhance the pin fixation.

A total of 46 consecutive people (age range 35 to 65 years) were operated on for knee osteoarthritis by the HCO technique. After the osteotomy, two hydroxyapatite-coated pins were inserted in the metaphyseal bone and two non-coated pins in the diaphyseal bone. The insertion torque was measured by a torque force screw driver. Four weeks postoperatively, the patients were randomised to either one infusion of zoledronic acid or sodium chloride intravenously. At time for removal of the pins, the extraction torque forces of the pins were measured. All osteotomies healed and no difference was found in time to healing. The mean extraction torque force in the non-coated pins in the diaphyseal bone was doubled in the zoledronic treated group (4.5 Nm, Standard Deviation (SD) 2.1) compared to the placebo group (2.4 Nm: SD 1.0, $p<0.0001$).

The mean extraction torque forces of the hydroxyapatite-coated pins in the metaphyseal bone were similar in the zoledronic acid group (4.7 Nm, SD 1.3) and in the placebo group (4.0 Nm, SD 1.3). A single infusion of zoledronic acid improved twofold the fixation of non-coated pins in diaphyseal bone. Bisphosphonates might be an alternative to hydroxyapatite-coated pins in nonosteoporotic bone.

Potential Side-Effects

Bisphosphonates in general are known to have significant side-effects including renal failure, osteonecrosis of the jaw and atypical femoral fractures especially after long-term use. A further side-effect described in OA specifically has been flare-up of OA of the hand after zoledronic acid infusion [28]. Consideration of the side-effect profile of bisphosphonates is an important consideration in a condition which is chronic and any potential drug use needs to be considered carefully with its effect monitored over time.

Conclusion

In summary, this chapter outlines emerging data on the use of the bisphosphonate drug zoledronic acid in OA. There was been a body of animal model data suggesting potentially positive findings from these investigations. The minimal clinical trial data published to date have shown an improvement in OA pain in the short term, coupled with an effect on the size of bone marrow lesions following infusion of zoledronic acid. Therefore, it is possible that treatment with bisphosphonate drugs at earlier stages of the condition, as suggested by animal models of OA, may have a greater impact on modulating disease activity in this chronic, common arthritic disease.

ACKNOWLEDGMENT

We would like to thank Alison Davies (AD) for her assistance in earlier study identification, data extraction and critical appraisal.

REFERENCES

[1] Lems W. F., Geusens P. Established and forthcoming drugs for the treatment of osteoporosis. *Curr. Opin. Rheumatol.*, 2014 May; 26(3): 245-51.

[2] Viereck V., Emons G, Lauck V., Frosch K. H., Blaschke S., Grundker C., et al. Bisphosphonates pamidronate and zoledronic acid stimulate osteoprotegerin production by primary human osteoblasts. *Biochem. Biophys. Res. Commun.*, 2002 Mar 1;291(3):680-6.

[3] Eriksen E. F., Diez-Perez A., Boonen S. Update on long-term treatment with bisphosphonates for postmenopausal osteoporosis: A systematic review. *Bone*, 2014 Jan.;58:126-35.

[4] Pozzi S., Raje N. The role of bisphosphonates in multiple myeloma: Mechanisms, side effects, and the future. *Oncologist,* 2011;16(5): 651-62.

[5] Sofat N., Ejindu V., Kiely P. What makes osteoarthritis painful? the evidence for local and central pain processing. *Rheumatology (Oxford),* 2011 Dec.;50(12):2157-65.

[6] Hochberg M. C. Osteoarthritis year 2012 in review: Clinical. *Osteoarthritis Cartilage*, 2012 Dec.; 20(12):1465-9.

[7] Moher D., Liberati A., Tetzlaff J., Altman D. G., PRISMA Group. Preferred reporting items for systematic reviews and meta-analyses: The PRISMA statement. *PLoS Med.,* 2009 Jul. 21;6(7):e1000097.

[8] Jensen M. C., Brant-Zawadzki M. N., Obuchowski N., Modic M. T., Malkasian D., Ross J. S. Magnetic resonance imaging of the lumbar spine in people without back pain. *N. Engl. J. Med.,* 1994 Jul, 14; 331(2): 69-73.

[9] Laslett L. L., Dore D. A., Quinn S. J., Boon P., Ryan E., Winzenberg T. M., et al. Zoledronic acid reduces knee pain and bone marrow lesions over 1 year: A randomised controlled trial. *Ann. Rheum. Dis.*, 2012 Aug.;71(8):1322-8.

[10] Thakur M., Rahman W., Hobbs C., Dickenson A. H., Bennett D. L. Characterisation of a peripheral neuropathic component of the rat monoiodoacetate model of osteoarthritis. *PLoS One*, 2012;7(3):e33730.

[11] Strassle B. W., Mark L., Leventhal L., Piesla M. J., Jian Li X., Kennedy J. D., et al. Inhibition of osteoclasts prevents cartilage loss and pain in a rat model of degenerative joint disease. *Osteoarthritis Cartilage*, 2010 Oct.;18(10):1319-28.

[12] Yu D., Liu F., Liu M., Zhao X., Wang X., Li Y., et al. The inhibition of subchondral bone lesions significantly reversed the weight-bearing deficit and the overexpression of CGRP in DRG neurons, GFAP and iba-1 in the spinal dorsal horn in the monosodium iodoacetate induced model of osteoarthritis pain. *PLoS One,* 2013 Oct 30;8(10):e77824.

[13] Mach D. B., Rogers S. D., Sabino M. C., Luger N. M., Schwei M. J., Pomonis J. D., et al. Origins of skeletal pain: Sensory and sympathetic innervation of the mouse femur. *Neuroscience*, 2002;113(1):155-66.

[14] Whiteside G. T., Boulet J. M., Sellers R., Bunton T. E., Walker K. Neuropathy-induced osteopenia in rats is not due to a reduction in weight born on the affected limb. *Bone*, 2006 Mar.;38(3):387-93.

[15] Walsh D. A., McWilliams D. F., Turley M. J., Dixon M. R., Franses R. E., Mapp P. I., et al. Angiogenesis and nerve growth factor at the osteochondral junction in rheumatoid arthritis and osteoarthritis. *Rheumatology (Oxford)*, 2010 Oct.;49(10):1852-61.

[16] Bailey A. J., Mansell J. P., Sims T. J., Banse X. Biochemical and mechanical properties of subchondral bone in osteoarthritis. *Biorheology*, 2004;41(3-4):349-58.

[17] Burr D. B. Anatomy and physiology of the mineralized tissues: Role in the pathogenesis of osteoarthrosis. *Osteoarthritis Cartilage*, 2004;12 Suppl. A:S20-30.

[18] Bendele A. M. Animal models of osteoarthritis. *J. Musculoskelet. Neuronal. Interact.*, 2001 Jun.;1(4):363-76.

[19] Yu D. G., Yu B., Mao Y. Q., Zhao X., Wang X. Q., Ding H. F., et al. Efficacy of zoledronic acid in treatment of osteoarthritis is dependent on the disease progression stage in rat medial meniscal tear model. *Acta Pharmacol. Sin.*, 2012 Jul.;33(7):924-34.

[20] Bove S. E., Laemont K. D., Brooker R. M., Osborn M. N., Sanchez B. M., Guzman R. E., et al. Surgically induced osteoarthritis in the rat results in the development of both osteoarthritis-like joint pain and secondary hyperalgesia. *Osteoarthritis Cartilage*, 2006 Oct.;14(10): 1041-8.

[21] Suri S., Gill S. E., Massena de Camin S., Wilson D., McWilliams D. F., Walsh D. A. Neurovascular invasion at the osteochondral junction and in osteophytes in osteoarthritis. *Ann. Rheum. Dis.*, 2007 Nov.; 66 (11): 1423-8.

[22] Agnello K. A., Trumble T. N., Chambers J. N., Seewald W., Budsberg S. C. Effects of zoledronate on markers of bone metabolism and subchondral bone mineral density in dogs with experimentally induced cruciate-deficient osteoarthritis. *Am. J. Vet. Res.*, 2005 Sep.; 66(9): 1487-95.

[23] Dearmin M. G., Trumble T. N., Garcia A., Chambers J. N., Budsberg S. C. Chondroprotective effects of zoledronic acid on articular cartilage in dogs with experimentally induced osteoarthritis. *Am. J. Vet. Res.*, 2014 Apr.; 75 (4): 329-37.

[24] Muehleman C., Green J., Williams J. M., Kuettner K. E., Thonar E. J., Sumner D. R. The effect of bone remodeling inhibition by zoledronic acid in an animal model of cartilage matrix damage. *Osteoarthritis Cartilage*, 2002 Mar.;10(3):226-33.

[25] Laslett L., Dore D., Quinn S., Winzenberg T., Boon P., Jones G. Zoledronic acid reduces bone marrow lesions and improves knee pain over one year. *Intern. Med. J.*, May 2011a;41(34).

[26] Laslett L., Dore D. A., Quinn S. J., Winzenberg T. M., Boon P., Bavage E., et al. Zoledronic acid reduces bone marrow lesions and knee pain over one year. *Osteop. Intern.*, September 2011b;22(S596).

[27] Harding A. K., Toksvig-Larsen S., Tagil M., W-Dahl A. A single dose zoledronic acid enhances pin fixation in high tibial osteotomy using the hemicallotasis technique. A double-blind placebo controlled randomized study in 46 patients. *Bone*, 2010 Mar;46(3):649-54.

[28] Werner de Castro G. R., Neves F. S., de Magalhaes Souza Fialho S. C., Pereira I. A., Ribeiro G., Zimmermann A. F. Flare-up of hand osteoarthritis caused by zoledronic acid infusion. *Osteoporos. Int.*, 2010 Sep.; 21(9):1617-9.

In: Zoledronic Acid
Editor: Ronald Carman

ISBN: 978-1-63321-525-2

Chapter 4

TREATMENT WITH ZOLEDRONIC ACID IN PAGET'S DISEASE OF BONE

Javier Bachiller-Corral and Walter Alberto Sifuentes-Giraldo*
Department of Rheumatology, University Hospital Ramón y Cajal, Madrid, Spain

ABSTRACT

Paget's disease of bone (PDB) is characterized by an increase in bone turnover located at one or more foci of the skeleton. The initial pathophysiological mechanism is the increase in osteoclastic bone resorption and bisphosphonates are the most commonly used treatments for PDB. The new bisphosphonates with greater potency and binding affinity to hydroxyapatite, like zoledronic acid, are very useful for short and long-term control of disease activity. Zoledronic acid is indicated for PDB in Europe and America at dose of 5 mg given intravenously. In 2005, a risedronate-controlled trial, showed that zoledronic acid, administered as a single 15 minute infusion is highly effective in controlling metabolic activity in PDB after 6 months of administration. Therapeutic response occurred in 96% of patients (normalization of alkaline phosphatase in 89% and a 75% reduction in 7% of patients), which is significantly superior to the results obtained by the other bisphosphonates, including risedronate, and also improved physical function and overall evaluation (measured by the SF-36 questionnaire). Other studies have demostrated similar results in terms of effectiveness of bone turnover control with a single 5 mg infusion of zoledronic acid. This drug has also proven effective in patients with active PDB that had not responded to other bisphosphonates in the previous 6 months. Regarding duration of response, zoledronic acid was still effective 75 months after a single infusion in most of the patients during the follow-up, with loss of therapeutic response in only 12.5% of patients. Recently it has been reported that patients who had a relapse after a first dose of zoledronic acid may respond to a new 5 mg intravenous infusion. All these results make zoledronic acid the most effective therapy for the treatment of PDB to date, and the treatment of choice due to its efficiency, adherence and duration of response. The accepted indications for treatment of PDB include bone pain and neurological compression syndromes. Treatment before bone surgery is also recommended to prevent excess bleeding or hypercalcemia. Patients with high metabolic activity (alkaline phosphatase level more than twice the upper limit of

* Corresponding author's email: albertosifuentesg@gmail.com (Walter Alberto Sifuentes-Giraldo.

normal) should also be treated. A controversial indication is treatment with bisphosphonates in asymptomatic PDB patients to prevent progression or complications. Zoledronic acid has changed the management of PDB. Currently, a 15-minute intravenous zoledronic acid infusion is able to maintain biochemical control of the disease for at least 6.5 years. This has important practical implications in the clinical management of PDB patients. Long-term control of metabolic activity will probably reduce the risk of complications such as deformity, fracture, deafness and degenerative joint disease.

INTRODUCTION

Paget's disease of bone (PDB) is the second most common metabolic bone disease after osteoporosis. The most widely used treatments for PDB over the last 4 decades have been the bisphosphonates, which have allowed a metabolic disease control. However, the efficacy and duration of the response achieved with the first bisphosphonates were not optimal. In 2006, zoledronic acid, a potent amino bisphosphonate, was approved in Europe and America for use in patients with PDB at a single dose of 5 mg given intravenously. Over these last 10 years, results from several clinical trials and other research studies with zoledronic acid have been published. These results have placed this drug in the first-line therapy and have revolutionized the management of PDB, allowing new goals to be achieved. This chapter summarizes the disease characteristics and treatment indications, and reviews the evidence on the efficacy and safety of the use of zoledronic acid in this disease.

PAGET'S DISEASE OF BONE

PDB is a common bone disorder first described more than a century ago by the English surgeon James Paget [1]. It is a focal skeletal disorder characterized by a marked increase in bone remodeling. There is an initial accelerated bone resorption followed by a disorganized increase in bone formation. This increased bone remodeling leads to the development of a pathologic bone with tendency towards overgrowth, deformity and fractures [2]. Despite advances in recent decades in the knowledge of this disease, its etiology remains unknown. The most widely accepted etiological hypothesis is the simultaneous action of two factors, a genetic predisposition and an environmental factor (possibly a viral infection) that act synergistically [3]. The genetic factor has not been well characterized, but there is an association between PDB and polymorphisms in the TNFRSF11 gene on chromosome 18, as well as mutations in the sequestosome 1 gene (SQSTM1). Environmental factors that have been associated with PDB are the paramyxovirus, primarily measles, respiratory syncytial virus and canine distemper virus. Other possible external associated factors are trauma and toxic factors.

PDB mainly affects adults over 55 years old and the prevalence is slightly higher in males. It is extremely rare under age 40. The prevalence of the disease varies in different parts of the world, but there is a clear relationship with the people from northwest Europe, mainly of British origin [4]. So in England, North America and Australia the prevalence in adults over age 55 is between 1% and 5%, while the disease is very rare in Japan, the Middle East,

Africa and South America. Family aggregation has been described in 15-40% of patients [5], and in these cases the disease is transmitted in an autosomal dominant pattern with variable penetrance. Some regions or geographical areas in which the prevalence is higher than in surrounding regions have been reported [6, 7], without a known reason. In the past 15 years, several studies in different countries, have shown a decrease in both prevalence and severity of the disease [8, 9]. The reasons for this decline are unknown, but it may be related to migration and changes in the environmental factors.

The main pathophysiological mechanism of PDB is activation of osteoclasts, with an increase in size (up to 10-fold increase compared to the original size) and number of nuclei (between 50 and 100 nuclei), and a high osteoclastic activity, leading to an intense focal bone resorption within the affected bone. This initial mechanism is followed by an equally accelerated osteoblastic reaction in an attempt to maintain bone metabolic balance. But this osteoblastic reaction is disorganized and chaotic, and produces a coarse plexiform bone, with changes in the fibrillar pattern, resulting in a decreased mechanical strength [2]. This chronic disorder of bone remodeling results in a progressive replacement of the normal bone by a disorganized bone without the usual characteristics of flexibility and hardness. Bone growth also occurs mainly at the expense of cortical bone, which becomes evident after several years of evolution. A characteristic of this disease is the focal involvement; it affects one or more bones of the skeleton, while the remodeling in the remaining bones is apparently normal.

PDB most commonly involves several sites (poliostotic), but in up to 40% of cases the disease is located in only one affected site (monostotic PDB). The most commonly affected bones are the pelvis, femur, lumbar vertebrae, skull and tibia [2, 4], but any bone may be affected. It is very uncommon the involvement of new bones throughout the course of the disease. Most PDB patients are asymptomatic. The suspected diagnosis is established by elevated alkaline phosphatase (AP) on routine lab tests or an incidental finding on radiography. Due to the mild clinical symptoms this disease remains underdiagnosed. It is estimated that more than half of the patients are unaware of their disease. The most common clinical manifestations are pain and bone deformity [2, 4]. The pain may have different causes, such as increased bone remodeling, the occurrence of pseudofractures, compression of nerve structures due to bone growth, or the development of secondary arthropathy. Complications that may occur over time due to chronic changes are fractures, compressive deafness and malignant transformation. PBD is still considered to be an important cause of morbidity in elderly patients.

Assessment and monitoring of PDB activity is carried out using different biochemical markers that reflect bone resorption and formation. These markers usually have a high sensitivity to determine the metabolic activity of PDB and its therapeutic response. The most widely used markers are serum AP (bone formation marker) and 24-hour urine hydroxyproline (a marker of resorption). Serum AP is the gold standard due to its sensitivity, cost and availability in almost all medical settings [10]. Usually it is elevated in patients with PDB who have not received treatment. Serum AP may be normal in cases of low activity or monostotic involvement. In these cases, other biochemical markers such as bone AP, N-terminal propeptide of type I collagen and α-carboxytelopeptide of type I collagen may be useful.

The radiological changes are quite typical and specific, and have a characteristic pattern of cortical bone thickening, deformation, and alteration of the trabecular pattern with lytic and blastic areas. In cases of polyostotic PDB, there are often one or more foci with these radiological features and the diagnosis is usually straightforward. Technetium bone scan is useful in assessing the extent of disease and should be part of the initial evaluation in all patients with PDB. Computed tomography and magnetic resonance imaging may also be used to study the bone features and make a differential diagnosis with other processes.

The diagnosis of PDB is mainly based on clinical manifestations, radiological abnormalities and elevated bone markers. On a few occasions it is necessary to perform bone biopsy for histopathological diagnosis.

Treatment of Paget's Disease of Bone: Objectives and Indications

Currently there is no curative treatment of PDB, so the therapeutic goals have been focused on finding drugs to improve the symptoms and to control the metabolic activity, and secondly to reduce the development of long-term complications. To achieve these goals it is required correcting the primary pathogenic alteration, i.e. normalize the intense remodeling activity that exists in pagetic bone lesions. In order to achieve this control, drugs such as calcitonin and bisphosphonates have been used since the late 70s. The mechanism of action of both types of drugs is the reduction of the resorptive activity of osteoclast cells and the bone remodeling rate. Research on bisphosphonates has allowed the development of drugs with a progressively higher adherence to hydroxyapatite and greater antiresorptive potency. Pamidronate, clodronate and tiludronate in the 80s, as well as alendronate and risedronate in the 90s, led to a significant improvement in the treatment of PDB, in both potency and duration of the antiresorptive effect. The development of zoledronic acid in the new century has allowed for the dosage to be reduced, treatment times to be shortened, and the potency and duration of effect to be increased.

All the bisphosphonates are drugs with the ability to decrease the rate of bone turnover and reduce the activity of osteoclasts, primary pathogenetic core of PDB. In general, they have high tropism for minerals and high adherence to the bone. Tolerance is quite good, with few side effects. The oral absorption is poor and is influenced by multiple factors, which requires making fasting, be taken only with water and not eat until elapses at least 1 hour after taking. Intravenous administration avoids the digestive track and ensures the required dose of the drug. But until recently, hospital admission for 2 or 3 days was required for intravenous administration. Currently, due to the potency of the new bisphosphonates, primarily zoledronic acid, the necessary dosage has been reduced and, therefore, the infusion time has been considerably shortened. The intravenous aminobisphosphonates may produce fever and a flu-like syndrome after the infusion, which resolve within 72 hours. Sometimes may occur a transient leukopenia at the expense of reducing the number of lymphocytes. Other bisphosphonates as neridronate, ibandronate and olpadronate, have also proved efficacy in the control of metabolic activity in PDB, but there is currently no indication for their use.

In order to minimize the progressive long-term complications of the pagetic bone, it is necessary that the normalization of remodeling rate may be maintained over time. Although this aspect is still controversial due to the difficulty in studying it, new drugs such as zoledronic acid can achieve a real long-lasting control of the disease and reduce these complications.

Absolute indications for treatment are the presence of primary bone pain or neurological involvement due to compressive syndromes. In these cases, the disappearance of clinical depends directly on reducing the metabolism of pagetic bone. Other indications include the development of high-output heart failure, or the presence of hypercalcemia, especially in patients who need absolute rest [10, 11]. In patients who are to undergo surgery on pagetic bones, antiresorptive treatment is recommended during the weeks prior to surgery in order to reduce surgical bleeding. It may also be effective to treat patients who have cortical fissures or large deformities in the weigh-bearing bones (primarily the femur and tibia) in order to avoid the development of fractures. Finally, patients with high metabolic activity (AP level more than twice the upper limit of normal) should be treated, primarily young patients who have lesions settle in bones that could lead to evolutionary complications. Patients with painless lesions that involve bones that are not susceptible to progressive changes or complications do not require treatment [12].

Dosage Regimen and Treatment Recommendations with Zoledronic Acid in Paget's Disease of Bone

Zoledronic acid is used in PDB at a dosage of 5 mg as a single intravenous infusion over 15 minutes [13]. Usually only one infusion is sufficient. The administration needs to be repeated only if there is a relapse in the biochemical control after 6 months. It is recommended that patients be hydrated prior to treatment, especially those on diuretic treatment. The potent locking of the antiresorptive mechanism can cause a decrease in calcium serum levels, especially in patients with a deficiency of calcium and vitamin D. Before infusion of zoledronic acid is essential to rule out hypocalcemia and secondary hyperparathyroidism. All patients should receive calcium and vitamin D supplementation prior to, and for at least 10 days after administration of zoledronic acid. No dosage adjustment is necessary in patients with renal insufficiency with creatinine clearance above 30 ml/min, or in patients with liver disorders or advanced age. Use is not recommended in patients with severe renal impairment. Zoledronic acid must only be used by a doctor who has experience in the treatment of PDB

In order to relieve the flu-like illness associated with aminobisphosphonates, acetaminophen 1 g orally may be administered every 8 hours for 2-3 days following the infusion. Cautions should be taken in patients who are going to undergo dental procedures in order to prevent osteonecrosis of the jaw, which has been associated with new and potent bisphosphonates, especially with intravenous infusions [14].

Efficacy of Treatment with Zoledronic Acid in the Control of Short-Term Bone Metabolism

The powerful clinical effects of use of zoledronic acid in bone metastases and tumoral hypercalcemia were reported in the early years of this century. Studies were later designed to determine its usefulness in other diseases that share osteoclast activation, such as osteoporosis and PDB.

In 2005, Reid et al. [15] published a study that led to a breakthrough in the understanding of the efficacy of zoledronic acid on PDB. The results of this clinical trial shortly after opened the doors to its commercial authorization by American and European drug agencies. It was a multicenter, prospective, randomized, double-blind, phase III clinical trial controlled with risedronate. More than 350 patients from Europe, North America, Australia and South Africa with PDB were included with a mean age of 70 years. All subjects had elevated bone metabolic activity with serum AP level more than twice the normal upper limit (mean AP 2.6 times the upper limit of normal). Half of the patients were treated with zoledronic acid 5 mg as a single intravenous infusion, and the other half with oral risedronate 30 mg daily for 2 months. At month 6 after treatment, therapeutic response (normalization of AP, or a reduction of at least 75% in the AP excess) was obtained in 96% of patients treated with zoledronic acid (89% had a normalized AP and 7% had a 75% reduction). These results were significantly higher than those obtained in the risedronate group (74% achieved therapeutic response), and also clearly superior to the response rates previously reported with other bisphosphonates used for PDB (etidronate, tiludronate, pamidronate, clodronate and alendronate). The reduction of AP levels was faster in the zoledronic acid group with significant differences since the first month after treatment. In the extension phase of this clinical trial [16], 98% of patients with initially response maintained the AP normalization to the month 24 of follow-up.

The efficacy results of zoledronic acid use on PDB do not seem to depend on the duration of disease, the age or gender of the patient, nor previous treatment with other bisphosphonates. Although it has been previously reported that the location of the pagetic foci (specifically the cranial involvement) is associated with poor response or relapse with other bisphosphonates, this did not occurred with zoledronic acid.

In 2007 the results of an open-label study on the efficacy at the month 6 treatment with zoledronic acid versus pamidronate were published [17]. Patients treated with zoledronic acid received 4 mg intravenously as a single infusion and 97% achieved therapeutic response, much higher than results achieved with pamidronate. The most interesting finding in this study was that 18 patients who did not achieved therapeutic response with pamidronate were immediately treated with zoledronic acid, obtaining normalization of AP in all but one case. There have been other cases of PDB patients with resistance to pamidronate and other bisphosphonates which had a quick and satisfactory reduction of AP levels following administration of 5 mg of zoledronic acid [18-20].

A descriptive study on the use of zoledronic acid in patients with PDB in daily clinical practice has recently been published [21]. The efficacy results were similar to the clinical trial with a response rate of 91.6% during 3 years. The relapse rate was higher than figures previously reported, reaching 21% to the year 3 of follow-up. This study is the first in describing the efficacy of zoledronic acid in a large group of patients with PDB in the real world outside of the clinical trials.

In another observational study, 9 patients with active PDB (mean serum AP 322 IU/L) were treated with zoledronic acid. Normalization of AP was achieved to the month 3 in 8 cases and this response was maintained during 1 year [22]. In addition, a satisfactory reduction in scintigraphy activity was achieved to the month 3 in all cases.

EFFICACY IN LONG-TERM BONE METABOLISM CONTROL

In any chronic illness, convenient dosage is essential to their acceptance and adherence to treatment by patients. In order to improve PDB, effective and easily administered treatments are necessary to increase therapeutic compliance and, therefore, maintain a normalized bone remodeling.

Until the use of zoledronic acid, patients with PDB treated with other bisphosphonates had temporal responses during 1 or 2 years. However, relapses were common and new cycles of treatment were required to control the clinical manifestations and biochemical activity. Oral bisphosphonates require prolonged courses of treatment, with frequent digestive discomfort. Moreover, previous intravenously administered bisphosphonates obliged to a 3-day admission at hospital. The results obtained with zoledronic acid have allowed for a change in this situation.

The phase III clinical trial was continued for an extension phase to measure the long-term effect of a single infusion of zoledronic acid in the PDB. The results of this extension trial were published in 2011 after 72 months of follow-up of patients who had initial response [23]. Of the 152 patients treated with zoledronic acid and included in the follow-up, only 1 had relapse criteria (return of serum total AP activity to within 20% of the pretreatment value) and this occurred after 5 years follow-up. Another 19 cases (12.5%) had loss of response (response defined as normalization of AP). The remaining patients, who entered the follow-up period, had maintained AP levels within normal range. The relative risks for relapse and loss of response were 0.02 and 0.12, respectively, in the zoledronic acid-treated group. These efficacy results are the longest known to date in PDB and represent a milestone on the road to chronic normalization of bone remodeling and the possible cure of this disease. Loss of response to treatment was not associated with age, gender, weight or creatinine clearance, but there was an association with previous bisphosphonate treatments. Furthermore, patients who less reduced AP levels (and other markers of bone remodeling) after 6 months of treatment were those with higher rate of response loss. This relationship between nadir levels and duration of response, also described with other bisphosphonates, adjust scheduled medical visits during follow-up.

EFFICACY IN CONTROLLING CLINICAL MANIFESTATIONS

There are few studies assessing the efficacy of zoledronic acid use on the clinical manifestations of PDB. Symptoms directly related to increase bone remodeling, such as pain, neurological manifestations, and heart failure may improve with treatment.

In the pivotal study, patients in the zoledronic acid group had an improvement in health-related quality of life, both in the short term [15] and after 6.5 years of follow-up [23]. The assessment was made using the SF-36 health questionnaire which includes the pain and functional capacity. Patients treated with zoledronic acid had a greater increase in some areas, primarily in physical functioning and general health. However, changes in scores were small and probably not clinically significant. Conversely, in a series of 9 patients treated with zoledronic acid and monitored for 1 year, improvement in Paget related bone pain was described in 5 of the 6 cases who had pain at baseline. The pain control was rapid (between

10 days and 1 month) and was maintained for 1 year, except in one case in which the pain reappeared after 3 months of treatment [22]. Pain control is associated with a reduction in AP. However, there are reports of improvement in pain in patients with advanced PBD, which did not have elevation of biochemical markers of bone remodeling [24, 25]. Some isolated cases of response of neurological manifestations (compressive paralysis of the VI cranial nerve [26], normotensive hydrocephalus [27] and spinal cord compression [28]) in patients with marked increases in bone metabolism who were treated with an infusion of zoledronic acid have been also reported.

Several bisphosphonates have demonstrated efficacy in reducing bone pain and some neurological manifestations. Other clinical manifestations such as pain associated with pagetic arthropathy may also improve [29]. There are not enough data about the efficacy of control of bone metabolism to reduce long-term complications. In theory, when bone remodeling is controlled chronically, the newly-formed bone has a normal lamellar structure with its mechanical properties preserved. In this way, bone growth and deformation would be lower and the manifestations which depend directly on them, such as fractures, secondary arthropathy and deafness may be reduced. This hypothesis was tested in a study of a large group of English authors [30]. Over 1300 patients with PDB were randomized into 2 groups: the first received symptomatic treatment for pain, and if there was no response they were treated with bisphosphonates. The second group of patients received intense antiresorptive treatment with the objective of normalizing AP levels. After a mean follow-up period of 3 years, no differences in the occurrence of fractures, orthopedic surgery, pain or deafness were found between both groups. The study was probably too short in time to determine the differences in occurrence of long-term manifestations. In addition, zoledronic acid was not among the bisphosphonates administered to the intensive treatment group. Long-term studies with patients diagnosed in the initial phases of the disease are needed in order to test whether maintained normalization of AP is capable of reducing progressive changes and complications. Zoledronic acid is currently the drug of choice for studying this fundamental aspect of the disease.

Retreatment with Zoledronic Acid

Due to the power and duration of treatment with zoledronic acid, is now rare the need of retreatment for PDB. This regard, a recently published article studied the efficacy of a second treatment cycle with zoledronic acid in a small group of patients. They were all patients from the initial clinical trial who had relapsed after a response to the first cycle [31]. Only 6 patients with PDB were included, with a mean AP level of 200 IU/l. The mean time between the first and second cycle of zoledronic acid was 6.5 years. All patients responded to the month 3 after retreatment (all normalized AP levels) and achieved nadir levels similar to those achieved after the first dose. The authors found no cases of treatment resistance or side effects. Unfortunately, the duration of the treatment response in this group of patients was not studied. Another clinical study [21] reported 9 patients who required retreatment with zoledronic acid but precise data on their response are not available. There are also no data on the clinical response of a second treatment cycle with zoledronic acid in patients with pain. Presumably control of metabolic activity, would once again improve associated symptoms.

Although evidence is limited, if retreatment is required in patients who initially achieved response, zoledronic acid appears to be the best therapeutic option.

SAFETY

In the risedronate-controled trial the number of patients who suffered adverse effects was similar in both groups[15]. The most common adverse effects were flu-like syndrome (12%), fever (7%), headache (6%) and arthralgia (6%), with a similar frequency to other previous studies [32]. These symptoms appeared during the first days after infusion and usually resolved within one week. In the extension phase of the clinical trial after 6.5 years of treatment, the rate of serious adverse events was similar in the risedronate and zoledronic acid groups [23] (the rate was 0.085 per patient-year of observation). In the followed patients no cases of osteonecrosis of the jaw, nor an increase in the occurrence of atrial fibrillation or uveitis were reported. In clinical practice there have been isolated reports of patients with PDB who developed intracranial hypertension [33], hepatotoxicity [34], orbital inflammation [35], myocarditis [36] and acute tubular necrosis [37] after zoledronic acid infusion. A case of osteonecrosis of the hip has also been described as a possible side effect of zoledronic acid treatment [23].

CONCLUSION

Zoledronic acid has emerged as a powerful and safe treatment alternative for PDB. After nearly 10 years of clinical experience, it has become the first therapeutic option due to its efficacy, adherence and response duration. Clinicians now have a powerful tool that has allowed a reassessment of therapeutic goals and a change in clinical management. Early and sustained remission over time is now a realistic goal, which can be achieved in the majority of patients with a comfortable dosing regimen and minimal side effects. It is yet to demonstrate that zoledronic acid is able to restore normal lamellar bone in pagetic lesions and prevent long-term complications. The clinical results of this strategy of tight control of the disease will be evaluated in the next years.

REFERENCES

[1] Paget J. On a form of chronic inflammation of bone (osteitis deformans). *Med Chir Trans.* 1877;60:37-64.

[2] Siris ES, Roodman GD. Paget's disease of bone. In: Rosen C, ed. *Primer on the metabolic bone diseases and disorders of mineral metabolism.* Hoboken, NJ: Wiley, 2012:335-43.

[3] Ralston SH, Layfield R. Pathogenesis of Paget disease of bone. *Calcif Tissue Int.* 2012;91:97-113.

[4] Kanis JA. *Pathophysiology and treatment of Paget's disease of bone.* London: Martin Dunitz; 1998.

[5] Morales Piga A, Rey Rey J, Garcia Sagredo JM, Lopez.Abente G. Frecuency and characteristics of the familial aggregation in Paget´s disease of bone. *J Bone Miner Res.* 1995;10:1-8.

[6] Barker DJP, Chamberlain AT, Guyer PB, Gardner MJ. Paget´s disease of bone; the Lancashire focu. *Br Med J.* 1980;280:1105-7.

[7] Morales Piga A, Lopez-Abente G, Garcia Vadillo A, Elena Ibañez A, Gonzalez-Lanza M. Caracteristicas de la enfermedad de paget del hueso en un foco de elevada prevalencia. *Med Clin (Barc).* 1990;95:169-74.

[8] Cooper C, Schafheutle K, Dennison E, Kellingray S, Guyer P, Barker D. The epidemiology of Paget's disease in Britain: is the prevalence decreasing? *J Bone Miner Res.* 1999;14:192-7.

[9] Poór G, Donath J, Fornet B, Cooper C. Epidemiology of Paget's disease in Europe: the prevalence is decreasing. *J Bone Miner Res.* 2006;21:1545-9.

[10] Selby PL, Davie MWJ, Ralston SH, Stone MD. Guidelines on the management of Paget´s disease of bone. *Bone.* 2002;31:366-73.

[11] Ralston SH, Langston AL, Reid IR. Pathogenesis and management of Paget's disease of bone. *Lancet.* 2008;372:155-163.

[12] FR Singer. Paget disease: when to treat and when not to treat. *Nat Rev Rheumatol.* 2009;5:483-9.

[13] European Medicines Agency (EMA). Aclasta® Product information (European Public Assessment Report). Cited 2014 April 25th. Available from: http://www.ema.europa.eu/ema/index.jsp?curl=pages/medicines/ human/medicines/000595/human_med_000622.jsp&mid=WC0b01ac058001d124

[14] Wong PK, Borromeo GL, Wark JD. Bisphosphonate-related osteonecrosis of the jaw in non-malignant bone disease. *Rheumatol Int.* 2013;33:2189-98.

[15] Reid IR, Miller P, Lyles K, Fraser W, Brown JP, Saidi Y, Mesenbrink P, Su GQ, Pak J, Zelenakas K, Luchi M, Richardson P, Hosking D. Comparison of a single infusion of zoledronic acid with risedronate for Paget's disease. *N Engl J Med.* 2005; 353:898-908.

[16] Hosking D, Lyles K, Brown JP, Fraser WD, Miller P, Curiel MD, Devogelaer JP, Hooper M, Su G, Zelenakas K, Pak J, Fashola T, Saidi Y, Eriksen EF, Reid IR. Long-term control of bone turnover in Paget's disease with zoledronic acid and risedronate. *J Bone Miner Res.* 2007;22:142-8.

[17] Merlotti D, Gennari L, Martini G, Valleggi F, De Paola V, Avanzati A, Nuti R. Comparison of different intravenous bisphosphonate regimens for Paget's disease of bone. *J Bone Miner Res.* 2007;22:1510-7.

[18] Chung G, Keen RW. Zoledronate treatment in active Paget's disease. *Ann Rheum Dis.* 2003;62:275-6.

[19] Tucci JR. Therapy with zoledronic acid, 5 mg, for a patient with Paget disease of bone. *Endocr Pract.* 2008;14:607-10.

[20] Saban M, Fidalgo S, Díaz CA, Lutfi RJ. Effect of a single dose of zoledronic acid in a case of Paget bone disease. *Medicina (B Aires).* 2010;70:445-8.

[21] Devogelaer JP, Geusens P, Daci E, Gielen E, Denhaerynck K, Macdonald K, Hermans C, Vancayzeele S, Abraham I, Boonen S. Remission over 3 years in patients with Paget disease of bone treated with a single intravenous infusion of 5 mg zoledronic acid. *Calcif Tissue* Int. 2014;94:311-8.

[22] Avramidis A, Polyzos SA, Moralidis E, Arsos G, Efstathiadou Z, Karakatsanis K, Grollios G, Kita M. Scintigraphic, biochemical, and clinical response to zoledronic acid treatment in patients with Paget's disease of bone. *J Bone Miner Metab.* 2008;26:635-41.
[23] Reid IR, Lyles K, Su GQ, Brown JP, Walsh JP, del Pino-Montes J, Miller PD, Fraser WD, Cafoncelli S, Bucci-Rechtweg C, Hosking DJ. A single infusion of zoledronic acid produces sustained remissions in Paget disease: data to 6.5 years. *J Bone Miner Res.* 2011;26:2261-70.
[24] Polyzos SA, Anastasilakis AD, Anagnostis P, Kita M, Arsos G, Moralidis E, Papatheodorou A, Terpos E. Normal bone turnover markers in a patient with active Paget's disease of bone: response to treatment with zoledronic acid. *Endokrynol Pol.* 2012;63:312-5.
[25] Gkouva L, Andrikoula M, Kontogeorgakos V, Papachristou DJ, Tsatsoulis A. Active Paget's disease of bone with normal biomarkers of bone metabolism: a case report and review of the literature. *Clin Rheumatol.* 2011;30:139-44.
[26] Pane A. Paget disease manifesting with compressive sixth-nerve palsy that resolved with intravenous zoledronic acid therapy. *Arch Ophthalmol.* 2007;125:1440-1.
[27] Morton A. Pagetic hydrocephalus treated with zoledronate. *Ann Rheum Dis.* 2005;64:1386.
[28] Oikonomou A, Birbilis T, Gymnopoulou E, Prassopoulos P. Paget disease of the spine manifested by thoracic and lumbar epidural lipomatosis: magnetic resonance imaging findings. *Spine.* 2007;32:789-92.
[29] Siris ES, Lyles KW, Singer FR, Meunier PJ. Medical management of Paget's disease of bone: indications for treatment and review of current therapies. *J Bone Miner Res.* 2006;21:94-98.
[30] Langston AL, Campbell MK, Fraser WD, MacLennan GS, Selby PL, Ralston SH Randomized trial of intensive bisphosphonate treatment versus symptomatic management in Paget's disease of bone. *J Bone Miner Res.* 2010;25:20-31.
[31] Reid IR, Brown J, Levitt D, Ivorra J, Bachiller-Corral J, Su G, Antunez-Flores O, Aftring RP. Re-treatment of relapsed Paget's disease of the bone with zoledronic acid: results from an open-label study. *Bonekey Rep.* 2013;2:442.
[32] Reid IR, Gamble GD, Mesenbrink P, Lakatos P, Black DM. Characterization of and risk factors for the acute-phase response after zoledronic acid. *J Clin Endocrinol Metab.* 2010;95:4380-7.
[33] Ferraz-de-Souza B, Martin RM, Correa HPS. Symptomatic intracranial hypertension and prolonged hypocalcemia following treatment of Paget's disease of the skull with zoledronic acid. *J Bone Miner Metab.* 2013;31:360-5.
[34] Polyzos SA, Kountouras J, Anastasilakis AD, Litsas I, Kita M, Arsos G, Moralidis E, Terpos E. Zoledronic acid-induced transient hepatotoxicity in a patient effectively treated for Paget's disease of bone. *Osteoporos Int.* 2011;22:363-7.
[35] Ortiz-Perez S, Fernandez E, Molina JJ, Sanchez-Dalmau B, Navarro M, Corretger X, Olver JM. Two cases of drug-induced orbital inflammatory disease. *Orbit.* 2011;30:37-9.
[36] Watts MR, Ellims AH, Eccleston DS. Acute myopericarditis following intravenous zoledronic acid for the treatment of Paget's disease. *Med J Aust.* 2014;200:150.

[37] Markowitz GS, Fine PL, Stack JI, Kunis CL, Radhakrishnan J, Palecki W, Park J, Nasr SH, Hoh S, Siegel DS, D'Agati VD. Toxic acute tubular necrosis following treatment with zoledronate (Zometa). *Kidney Int.* 2003;64:281-9.

In: Zoledronic Acid
Editor: Ronald Carman

ISBN: 978-1-63321-525-2

Chapter 5

BISPHOSPHONATES: PHARMACOKINETICS, CLINICAL USES AND SAFETY

***Raquel Cobos*[1*] *and Gorka Orive*[2,3]**
[1]Health Research Unit of Alava, Basque Health Service, Vitoria-Gasteiz, Álava, Spain
[2]NanoBioCel Group, Laboratory of Pharmaceutics,
University of the Basque Country, School of Pharmacy
[3]Biomedical Research Networking Center in Bioengineering,
Biomaterials and Nanomedicine (CIBER-BBN), Vitoria, Spain

ABSTRACT

Since their introduction to clinical practice more than 3 decades ago, bisphosphonates have been increasingly used for a wide range of skeletal disorders and other conditions including heritable skeletal disorders in children, postmenopausal and glucocorticoid- induced osteoporosis (GIO), and bone metastases in patients with malignancies. Bisphosphonates of first generation have side chains minimally modified (clodronate or etidronate) or a chlorophenyl group (tiludronate). Bisphosphonates of second generation (alendronate or pamidronate) have a nitrogen group in the side chain and their power is 10 to 100 times greater than the first generation compounds. Finally, among third-generation of bisphosphonates (ibandronate, risedronate and zoledronate), the two last with the N atom included in a heterocyclic ring, are 10,000 times more potent than first generation agents. Their main therapeutic use is as antiosteolitic agent in patients with pathologies that possess increased bone resorption including Paget disease, osteoporosis and tumoral osteolysis and as inhibitors of ectopic calcifications and ossifications. Although bisphosphonates are generally well tolerated, the adverse effects are not rare, and they often produce the interruption of treatment. The adverse effects on the upper gastrointestinal tract are common with oral bisphosphonates, especially if taken incorrectly, so benefits and risk should be weighed. Oral absorption of bisphosphonates is very poor, as they are only absorbed between 1-3%, being higher when administered fasting. Between 20-80% of the absorbed dose is taken up by the bone tissue, and the

* Corresponding Author: Raquel Cobos; Health Research Unit of Alava, Basque Health Service, José Achótegui s/n, 01009, Vitoria-Gasteiz, Álava, Spain. E-mail: RAQUEL.COBOSCAMPOS@osakidetza.net; r.cobos@hotmail.es.

remaining dose is eliminated unchanged by the kidney. Protein plasma binding is variable between bisphosphonates (50-90%). This chapter describes and discusses the most important therapeutic effects together with the most relevant side-effects associated to the use of bisphosphonates.

1. INTRODUCTION

Since their introduction to clinical practice more than 3 decades ago, bisphosphonates have been increasingly used for a wide range of skeletal disorders. Bisphosphonates are now used to treat an increasing number of conditions including heritable skeletal disorders in children, postmenopausal and glucocorticoid- induced osteoporosis (GIO), and bone metastases in patients with malignancies [1]. Bisphosphonates can offer substantial clinical benefit in conditions in which an imbalance between osteoblast-mediated bone formation and osteoclast-mediated bone resorption underlies disease pathology [1].

1.1. Chemical Structure and Mechanism of Action

Bisphosphonates are analogues of pyrophosphate molecule where oxygen atom has been replaced with the carbon atom, and the two free valences of the carbon atom have been replaced by R1 and R2 radicals [2]. Bisphosphonates are characterized by their high affinity to hydroxyapatite crystals (calcium phosphate), and their main role is to inhibit the formation, aggregation and the dissolution of these crystals. The affinity of the different bisphosphonates depends on their side chain R2, being greater for zoledronate> alendronate> ibandronate = risedronate [3]. Bisphosphonates can bind hydroxyapatite in two ways: bidentate (an oxygen atom of each phosphonate binds calcium hydroxyapatite) and tridentate (besides the two above, are also joined by the hydroxyl group of the central carbon (radical R1) (Figures 1-3).

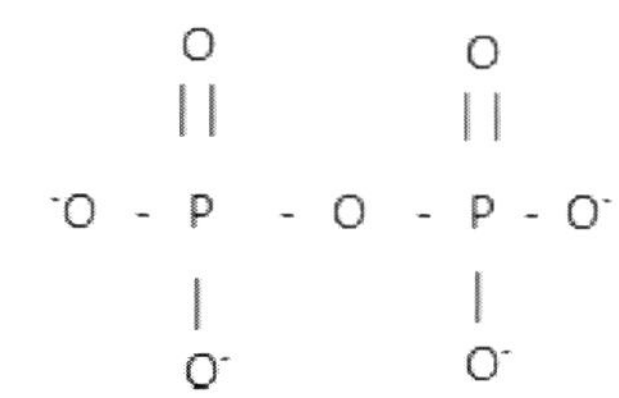

Figure 1. Inorganic pyrophosphate.

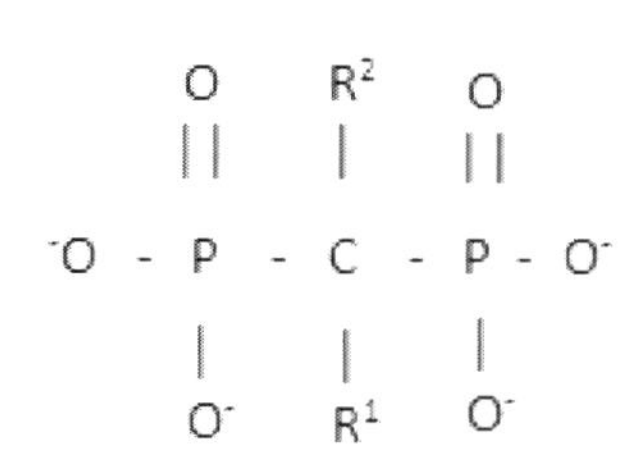

Figure 2. Biphosphonate.

Bisphosphonates	R1	R2
Etidronate	-OH	-CH3
Clodronate	-Cl	-Cl
Tiludronate	-H	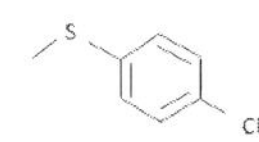
Alendronate	-OH	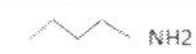
Pamidronate	-OH	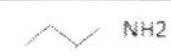
Ibandronate	-OH	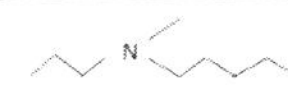
Risedronate	-OH	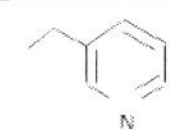
Zoledronate	-OH	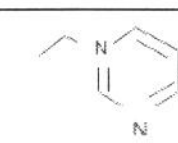

Figure 3. Side chain of radicals R1 and R2 of bisphosphonates.

The last binding is stronger and this could explain the difference potency of bisphosphonates to inhibit bone resorption [1, 2]. The presence of an amino group increases the antiresorptive potency of the bisphosphonates by 10 or 1000 versus the first non-nitrogen containing bisphosphonates. This is probably due to the fact that the nitrogen groups in the side chain R2 inhibit farnesyl pyrophosphate synthase (FPP) [6], an enzyme involved in the pathway of mevalonic acid required for the synthesis of cholesterol and isoprenoids lipids [7, 8]. Activity is dramatically increased when the amino group is contained in the aliphatic carbon chain. For example, alendronate, an aminobisphosphonate, is approximately 700-fold more potent than etidronate, both in vitro and in vivo [9].

Furthermore, it might be a correlation between the ability of nitrogenous biphosphonates to inhibit FPP synthase *in vitro* and the ability to inhibit bone resorption *in vivo* [8]. Assuming this, it has been observed that the less powerful drug is the etidronate whereas zoledronate is the most potent of the bisphosphonates family [1, 2, 6]. The main target of bisphosphonates is the osteoclasts. It has been observed that there are four mechanisms to explain the mechanism of action of this drug family [3]: i) inhibition of the formation / recruitment of osteoclasts by a mechanism that prevents their differentiation, ii) decrease of the adhesion of osteoclasts to bone matrix, reducing life osteoclasts by an increase of apoptosis, iii) inhibition of the activity of osteoclasts by penetrating inside and alteration of biochemical processes that produce disruption of the cytoskeleton and iv), morphological alterations, decrease of acid secretion, and alteration of enzymatic activity.

1.2. Pharmacokinetics

There are some important issues related to the biopharmacy and pharmacokinetics of the bisphosphonates that need to be addressed to understand their therapeutic activity and potential side-effects:

Absorption: Oral absorption of bisphosphonates is very poor, as they are only absorbed between 1-3% [2, 4, 5], being higher when administered fasting [5]. Oral bioavailability decreases in the presence of food. In particular foods containing calcium and other multivalent cations (aluminum, magnesium, iron), including milk can interfere with its absorption. Bisphosphonates should be administered only with water and the patient should remain without eating anything until at least half an hour later. Medications such as antacids, calcium and other multivalent cations also impede the absorption of bisphosphonates. There is very little difference in absorption between bisphosphonates. One particular aspect is that absorption of nitrogenous bisphosphonates (ibandronate, risedronate, pamidranato) is lower, being around 0.7%.

Distribution and elimination: Between 20-80% of the absorbed dose is taken up by the bone tissue (depends on the drug [2]) and remains there for months or years (2) depending on the individual affinity of each drug to the bone. The remaining dose is eliminated unchanged by the kidney (half-life of 0.5-2 hours [2, 5], and only a small amount is excreted in the bile [4]. The relative contribution of these two processes to overall plasma elimination differs significantly among bisphosphonates. To date, all bisphosphonates studied show no evidence of metabolism. Renal excretion is the only route of elimination, thus attention should be given with a impaired renal function. Once incorporated into the bone, the drug remains metabolically inactive until it is released by the activity of osteoclasts.

Bisphosphonates bind preferentially to bones which have high turnover rates, and their distribution in bone is not homogeneous. After bone uptake, the bisphosphonates are liberated again only when the bone in which they are deposited is resorbed. Thus, the half-life of bisphosphonates in bone is very long, ranging among different species from 1 to 10 years, depending largely on the rate of bone turnover.

Regarding drug distribution through blood, it has been observed that plasma protein binding is variable in the bisphosphonate family, being 87% for ibandronate, 56% for zoledronate and 54% pamidronate [10].

Renal function with binding to plasma proteins has been postulated as a possible determinant of renal toxicity of some bisphosphonates [11].

2. Therapeutic Activity and Clinical Uses

Bisphosphonates promote the apoptosis of osteoclasts actively engaged in the degradation of mineral on the bone surface. Accordingly, bisphosphonates have become the primary therapy for managing skeletal conditions characterized by increased osteoclast mediated bone resorption such us osteoporosis, Paget disease of bone, osteogenesis imperfecta (OI), hypercalcemia, and malignancy metastatic to bone [1]. Their main therapeutic use is as antiosteolitic agent in patients with pathologies with increased bone resorption including Paget disease, osteoporosis and tumoral osteolysis and as inhibitors of ectopic calcifications and ossifications [2].

2.1 Osteoporosis: Osteoporosis mainly affects postmenopausal women or subjects taking oral corticosteroids for long periods. *Postmenopausal osteoporosis* is characterized by an imbalance between osteoclast-mediated bone resorption and bone formation mediated by osteoblasts. As a consequence bone resorption is increased, bone mass is reduced, bone microstructure is altered and the risk of bone fracture enhanced [1, 2].

Bisphosphonates are effective in both prevention and treatment of postmenopausal osteoporosis. The primary choice is generally the alendronate or risedronate [12]. Alendronate and risedronate have conclusively shown that they reduce the number of vertebral fractures (Relative Risk-RR of Alendronate 0.53 -0.56 [13-15], RR of risedronate 2.5mg 0.54, and RR of risedronate 5mg 0.38 [16]) and hip fracture (RR of Alendronate 0.61 [15] and RR of risedronate 0.6 [15, 17]), and for many years have been used in the treatment of postmenopausal osteoporosis daily dosing regimens [3]. Later they were commercialized on a weekly basis [3]. Ibandronate only reduces the risk of vertebral fractures (RR 0.38) [18] and is available in a monthly regimen [3]. Zoledronic acid is available to be administered intravenously once a year [3]. Zoledronic acid also reduces the risk of vertebral fractures (RR 0.30-0.38) [15, 19] and hip fractures (0.62) [15].

Osteoporosis associated with glucocorticoids: While bisphosphonate therapy has become the treatment of choice in postmenopausal osteoporosis, few recognize that therapy with glucocorticoids lead to bone loss. However, glucocorticoids can reduce bone formation and promote bone resorption, leading to an imbalance in the process of bone turnover. This will produce a rapid loss of bone mass in addition to an alteration of the quality of the bone [20, 21].

In a case-control study conducted in the UK, it was revealed that the fracture rate is related to the administered oral corticosteroid dose, and the rate of vertebral fractures increases from 1.55 to 5.18 comparing the group of patients with low dose oral prednisolone (below 2.5 mg) and the group with high doses (up to 7.5 mg daily). The rate was increased during the first three months [22]. A recent study has shown that in patients taking at least one dose of 7.5 mg of prednisone, alendronate prevents bone loss more effectively than vitamin D3 [23].

Furthermore, in patients with glucocorticoid treatment, and high risk of fracture, the therapy with bisphosphonates is cost-effective (with the use of 5 mg glucocorticoids daily, the cost per one QALY (Quality-adjusted life year) gained with bisphosphonates was £41k in women aged <60, £17k in women aged 60–79, and £5k in women aged 80+ [24]). Patients having low bone mineral density and/or vertebral fractures and requiring treatment for long time with glucocorticoids, should be informed about existing therapies available to reduce the fracture risk, and they should receive drugs during glucocorticoid treatment [25].

2.2 Paget disease: Paget's disease of bone generates an overactive metabolism. There is a first phase called osteolitic phase where osteoclasts induce an extreme bone resorption, and a second phase known as osteoblastic phase characterized by an uncoordinated bone remodeling process. The prevalence is about 3% of the population above 40 years [26, 4]. Etidronate, the first bisphosphonate used in the clinical setting, demonstrated a reduction in bone turnover greater than calcitonin, that was the antiresorptive agent used until that moment. However, the presence of alterations in bone mineralization secondary to the use of etidronate limited the dose and duration of treatment (not exceeding 6 months). In addition, some patients showed early reactivation of the disease and the development of resistance [26].

2.3 Bone metastases: Bisphosphonates have been tested in patients with bone metastases and their use has been associated to reduced skeletal complications, bone pain, fractures, and improved life quality [1, 2, 4]. Bone is the most common site of metastatic disease, with up to 90% of patients with advanced cancer skeletal lesions [1].

2.4 Tumoral hipercalcemia: Hypercalcemia is deffined as an elevation of plasma calcium figures above 10.5mg/dl. In general, severe hypercalcemia (> 135mg/dl) is related to neoplastic processes. It usually occurs in around 30% of cancer patients and it is caused by an increase of bone release due to osteoclast activity [2, 4]. Treatment involves rehydrating the patient with saline serum, and furosemide can be administered as adjuvant therapy. If there is no improvement in reducing serum calcium, calcitonin can be administered.

In the last few years, a wide range of drugs have been designed and evaluate to treat this disease, being one the most recent ones intravenous bisphosphonate therapy. Bisphosphonates safely and effectively decrease serum calcium levels by interfering with osteoclast activity and by stimulating osteoclast apoptosis. Zoledronic acid is the most recent bisphosphonate approved by the US Food and Drug Administration for treatment of this disorder and is significantly more effective in reducing serum calcium levels than previously used bisphosphonates [27].

2.5 Therapy for children: The use of bisphosphonates is mainly associated with aging. However, it is also frequently used off-label to treat bone diseases in children incluing osteogenesis imperfect [28-30]. The last is caused by genetic defects in type 1 collagen production leading to brittleness of the bones. Pamidronate was successfully used in a study including 6 children with osteogenesis imperfecta; the treatment led to increased bone mineral density. The mean annual increase in lumbar spine area BMD (Bone Mineral Density) was 48% [28]. Furthermore, the treatment decreased fractures with minimal trauma, improved mobility and quality of life, and decreased bone pain [76]. Pamidronate (i.v.) is thus the drug of choice for the treatment of osteogenesis imperfecta in children [29], even though oral alendronate proved to be equally effective in milder forms [30].

3. Safety of Bishosphonates

Bishosphonates are generally considered safe drugs, with clinical benefits overcoming the risks associated with the treatment. Due to their widespread use in many patients suffering from different diseases, several adverse effects have been reported, but the relationship between the drug and adverse events is often difficult to establish because clear correlations are often missing due to co-medications or co-morbidities [4].

Gastrointestinal adverse effects: Although not observed in clinical trials, gastrointestinal intolerance, esophageal irritation, or erosion have been reported with the oral bisphosphonate use, especially if taken incorrectly [31]. Isolated cases of serious esophageal complications or upper gastrointestinal hemorrhage have been reported. Intravenous pamidronate may be used in patients with severe osteoporosis who have experienced fractures and cannot tolerate oral bisphosphonates [31].

Currently the appearance of major gastrointestinal adverse effects is questioned, particularly esophagus neoplasm. In 2007, it was reported the risk of the existence of an increased risk of this cancer in patients treated with oral bisphosphonates for a period of 5 years [32].

An observational study published at BMJ journal suggested that oral bisphosphonates could duplicate the risk of esophagus neoplasm versus people who didn't take them. In patients with a therapy longer than 3 years, the RR was 2.24 (confidence interval-CI 95%; 1.74-3.43), and there were not differences between bisphosphonates [33]. However, later studies found no association between the use of bisphosphonates and esophagus neoplasm

[34-36]. Since evidence is not conclusive, physicians should be aware that patients receiving bisphosphonate therapy for osteoporosis may constitute a patient group that could be at elevated risk of esophageal cancer and they should conduct appropriate examinations if patients develop pain, dysphagia or other symptoms suggestive of esophageal neoplasm [11]. Patients with known esophageal disease (e.g., achalasia, stricture, Barrett's esophagus, severe reflux and scleroderma) should avoid taking oral bisphosphonates [31].

Osteonecrosis of the Jaw (ONJ): One of most severe adverse events of bisphosphonates is osteonecrosis of the jaw, defined as an area of exposed bone in the maxillofacial region that persists for at least 8 week [37, 38]. It is extremely prevalent, as it appears in the 94% of patients who receive bisphosphonates intravenously (mainly zoledronic acid and pamidronate [39]), for cancer treatment.

The risk of ONJ in patients with cancer treated with high doses of intravenous bisphosphonates is higher, in the range of 1-10 per 100 patients (depending on duration of therapy). The risk of ONJ associated with oral bisphosphonate therapy for osteoporosis seems to be low, estimated between 1 in 10,000 and < 1 in 100,000 [40] patient-treatment years.

In relation to the specific location at jawbone, it has been proposed that periodontal inflammation, tooth abscesses and dental treatments increase the rate of bone turnover in the jaw, causing a larger deposit of bisphosphonates at this level, which would alter the response of bone against aggression [41].

The osteonecrosis of jaw induced by bisphosphonates, usually appears between 4 months and 6 years from the beginning of treatment. In case of oral bisphosphonates, halftime consumer is about 5.6 years, when intravenous administration, exposure time is lower than 1 year [42].

Hypocalcemia: It is mainly produced by intravenous bisphosphonates [1]. Bisphosphonates reduce calcium efflux from bone, resulting in a small and transient decrease in serum calcium (43, 44). Risk factors for symptomatic hypocalcemia include vitamin D deficiency, hypoparathyroidism, and impaired renal function [31].

Ocular inflammation: Nitrogenous bisphosphonates, especially, pamidronate, has been associated with the development of ocular inflammation in form of no specific conjunctivitis, uveitis, iritis, episcleritis, with an incidence between 0.046 and 1% [45, 46]. Most of the cases are related to pamidronate, but there are also some reports related to risedronate [47, 48] clodronate [49] and ibandronate [50].

These drugs can induce pro-inflammatory cytokine release including tumor necrosis factor and interleukin 1 and 6. These cytokines can induce inflammation and contribute to a immunological reaction at the uvea region [51, 52].

However, non-nitrogen containing bisphosphonates, as clodronate and etidronate, have also been implicated. In case of clodronate, ocular reactions might be due to an idiosyncratic reaction, rather than a process mediated by citokines [53].

Occurring within 6 to 48 h after infusion, these symptoms are most frequently reported after the first or second infusion, although they may appear as late as after the 6th infusion [54].

Acute inflammatory response: About 10-30% of patients who receive the first infusion of nitrogenous bisphosphonates, undergo an acute reaction characterized by pyrexia, myalgia, joint pain, headache, and flu-like symptoms [1, 11]. These symptoms appear during the first 72 hours after infusion and resolve in 3 days [11]. They can also occur after high oral doses of bisphosphonates [31].

Muscle, bone and joint pain: The FDA on January 7, 2008 published an alert regarding oral bisphosphonates, indicating that patients who are in treatment with oral bisphosphonates for osteoporosis may develop severe bone, joint or muscle pain. Pain can appear days or months after the beginning of the treatment (from the same day to 52 months). After discontinuation of treatment, some patients experienced complete relief of symptoms and others slow or incomplete resolution. Furthermore, this pain is different from that produced in the acute phase reactions [1, 10]. However, until now there is no a scientific explanation to justify this phenomenon.

Atrial fibrillation: In HORIZON Pivotal Fracture Trial, the number of patients who had arrhythmia in the zoledronic-acid group (266 patients, or 6.9%) was significantly higher than that in the placebo group (203 patients, or 5.3%; P = 0.003) [55]. By contrast, in the Fracture Intervention Trial (FIT), it was observed an increase of fibrillation risk in patients in treatment with bisphosphonates, though it was not a statistically significant increase (relative hazard, 1.14, 95% CI, 0.83 to 1.57, P = 0.42) [56].

In a recent meta-analysis evaluating 4 clinical trials, it was observed that the exposure to bisphosphonates was significantly associated with risk of serious atrial fibrillation (OR 1.47; 95% CI 1.01, 2.14; p = 0.04) [57].

However, there is a great uncertainty in relation to overall evidence. We can't make definitive conclusions, mainly due to the paucity of studies and heterogeneity of these.

Atypical femur fractures: There are an increasing number of studies showing that the long-term use of bisphosphonates is associated to an increased risk of low-energy or stress fractures [2, 13-16]. Generally these fractures appeared in older women treated for years with alendronate for osteoporosis. Fractures may occur spontaneously or after minimal trauma, and appeared in the proximal shaft or subtrochanteric area of the femur. They can be bilateral and are often preceded by pain in the affected area. Since bisphosphonates decrease bone resorption, in some patients chronic treatment might alter mineralization and lead to a brittle and fragile bone, despite the increase in bone mineral density [41]. Other studies, however, have found no such an association [58]. Although it has not been established a causal relationship, there is a consensus on the need to discontinue treatment in patients who develop these fractures [41].

Nephrotoxicity: Zoledronate and pamidronate have been associated with acute and chronic renal disease, being more frequent to date with zoledronate [5]. Ibandronate nephrotoxicity has been less observed, with a rate comparable to that produced by placebo in clinical trials [60, 61]. This might be due to a bigger plasma protein binding, which limits the free drug exposure to the kidney, and a short half-life in the renal tissue. Although acute renal failure may be clinically reversible, in some situation it may persist and lead to chronic renal failure. Renal failure is directly related to the dose and infusion time [62].

Toxicity pattern of pamidronate is the focal and segmental glomerulosclieriosis associated with tubular degenerative changes, in contrast with zoledronate that is primarily associated with tubular damage [63].

The American Society of Clinical Oncology 2007 recommends that pamidronate and zoledronate can be employed for patients with normal kidney function. In patients with mild-to-moderate kidney disease (estimated CrCl 30-60 cc/min), the dose of zoledronate should be reduced and the initial of pamidronate. For more severe kidney disease (estimated CrCl <30cc/min), zoledronate is not recommended and the time of infusion of pamidronate should be increased.

Conclusion

The administration of bisphophonates has grown steadily, with de introduction of simpler dosing regimens, the availability of lower-priced generics, and growing concerns about the safety of hormone replacement therapy in long term.

Bisphosphonates inhibit osteoclasts-mediated bone resorption and thus they have a hypocalcemic effect. Bisphosphonates are characterized by their high affinity to hydroxyapatite crystals (calcium phosphate), and their main role is to inhibit the formation, aggregation and the dissolution of these crystals, interfering with bone mineralization.

Their main therapeutic use is as antiosteolitic agent in patients with pathologies with increased bone resorption including Paget disease, osteoporosis and tumoral osteolysis and as inhibitors of ectopic calcifications and ossifications.

Although bisphosphonates are generally well tolerated, the adverse effects are not rare, and they often produce the interruption of treatment. The adverse effects on the upper gastrointestinal tract are common with oral bisphosphonates, especially if taken incorrectly.

On the other hand, the most prevalent adverse effect of intravenous bisphosphonates is an acute reaction characterized by pyrexia, myalgia, joint pain, headache, and flu-like symptoms due to the release of pro-inflammatory cytokines.

Despite, the considerable increase in the use of these drugs has shown that their consumption long term can lead to a number of major adverse events among which are: osteonecrosis of the jaw, atypical fractures, musculoskeletal pain, atrial fibrillation and renal toxicity. Although to a lower incidence, bisphosphonates may also induce ocular inflammatory disorders: conjunctivitis, episcleritis and uveitis.

References

[1] Matthew T. Drake, Bart L. Clarke, and Sundeep Khosla. Bisphosphonates: Mechanism of Action and Role in Clinical. *Practice. Mayo Clin. Proc.* 2008; 83(9): 1032–1045.

[2] Revisión clínica de la utilización de los bifosfonatos. Adrover Rigo M, Juste Díez de Pinos JL, Tuset Creus M, Codina Jané C, Ribas Sala J. *Farm. Hosp. 2000*; 24(2):74-82.

[3] Oliver Bock and Dieter Felsenberg. Bisphosphonates in the management of ostmenopausal osteoporosis – optimizing efficacy in clinical practice. *Clin. Interv. Aging*. 2008; 3(2): 279–297.

[4] Elisabeth V. Giger, Bastien Castagner, Jean-Christophe Leroux . Biomedical applications of bisphosphonates. *Journal of Controlled Release* 167 (2013) 175–188.

[5] Harold N Rosen. Pharmacology of bisphosphonates. Uptodate, last revision 2013 July 13.

[6] Russell RGG. Determinants of structure-function relationships among bisphosphonates. *Bone* 2007;40(suppl 2):S21-S25.

[7] Kavanagh KL, Guo K, Dunford JE, et al. The molecular mechanism of nitrogen-containing bisphosphonates as antiosteoporosis drugs. *Proc. Natl. Acad. Sci. USA* 2006 May 16;103(20):7829–7834.

[8] Dunford JE, Thompson K, Coxon FP, et al. Structure-activity relationships for inhibition of farnesyl diphosphate synthase in vitro and inhibition of bone resorption in

vivo by nitrogen-containing biphophonates. *J. Pharmacol. Exp. Ther.* 2001; 296:235-42.

[9] Lin JH. Bisphosphonates: a review of their pharmacokinetic properties. *Bone* 1996;18 (2):75-85.

[10] Mark A. Perazella, Glen S. Markowitz. Bisphosphonate Nephrotoxicity. *Kidney Int.* 2008; 74(11):1385-1393.

[11] Michael Pazianas, Bo Abrahamsen. Safety of bisphosphonates. *Bone* 2011; 49:103-110.

[12] Bifosfonatos. Guía de prescripción terapéutica. Available in: http://www.imedicinas.com/GPTage/Search.php?text=bifosfonatos.

[13] Black DM, Cummings SR, Karpf DB, et al. Fracture Intervention Trial Research Group. Randomised trial of effect of alendronate on risk of fracture in women with existing vertebral fractures. *Lancet* 1996;348(9041):1535–41.

[14] Cummings SR, Black DM, Thompson DE, et al. Effect of alendronate on risk of fracture in women with low bone density but without vertebral fractures: results from the Fracture Intervention Trial. *JAMA* 1998;280(24):2077–82.

[15] Serrano AJ,Begoña L, Anitua E, Cobos R, Orive G. Systematic review amd ,eta-analysis of the efficacy and safety of alendronate and zoledronate for the treatment of postmenospausal osteoporosis. *Gynecol. Endocrinol.* 2013; 29(12):1005-14.

[16] Harris ST, Watts NB, Genant HK, McKeever CD, Hangartner T, Keller M, Chesnut CH 3rd, Brown J, Eriksen EF, Hoseyni MS, Axelrod DW, Miller PD. Effects of risedronate treatment on vertebral and nonvertebral fractures in women with postmenopausal osteoporosis: a randomized controlled trial. Vertebral Efficacy With Risedronate Therapy (VERT) Study Group. *JAMA* 1999; 282(14):1344-52.

[17] McClung MR, Geusens P, Miller PD, et al. Hip Intervention Program Study Group. Effect of risedronate on the risk of hip fracture in elderly women. *N. Engl. J. Med.* 2001;344(5):333–40.

[18] Chesnut III Ch, Christiansen C, et al. Effects of oral inbandronate administered daily or intermittently on fracture risk in postmenopausal osteoporosis. *J. Bone Miner. Res.* 2004; 19:1241-9.

[19] Canalis E, Giustina A. Glucocorticoids-induced osteoporosis: summary of a workshop. *J. clin. Endocrinol. Metab.* 2001; 86: 5681-85.

[20] Black DM, Rosen CJ. Is risedronate or alendronate more effective at preventing nonvertebral fractures in women with osteoporosis?. *Nat. Clin. Pract. Rheumatol.* 2007; 3:378-9.

[21] Canalis E, Giustina A. Glucocorticoids-induced osteoporosis: summary of a workshop. *J. clin. Endocrinol. Metab.* 2001; 86: 5681-85.

[22] Van Staa TP, Leufkens HG, Abenhaim L, Zhang B, Cooper C. Use of oral corticosteroids and risk of fractures. *J. Bone Miner Res.* 2000 ;15(6):993-1000.

[23] De Nijs RN, Jacobs JW, Lems WF, Laan RF, Algra A, Huisman AM, Buskens E, de Laet CE, Oostveen AC, Geusens PP, Bruyn GA, Dijkmans BA, Bijlsma JW; STOP Investigators. Alendronate or alfacalcidol in glucocorticoid-induced osteoporosis. *N. Engl. J. Med.* 2006;355(7):675-84.

[24] Van Staa TP, Geusens P, Zhang B, Leufkens HG, Boonen A, Cooper C. Individual fracture risk and the cost-effectiveness of bisphosphonates in patients using oral glucocorticoids. *Rheumatology* (Oxford) 2007 Mar;46(3):460–66.

[25] Robert S. Weinstein. Glucocorticoid-Induced Bone Disease. *N. Engl. J. Med.* 2011; 365 (1):62-70.

[26] Lojo Oliveira L, Torrijos Eslava A. Tratamiento de la enfermedad ósea de Paget. *Reumatol. Clin.* 2012. doi:10.1016/j.reuma.2011.06.003

[27] Berenson JR. Treatment of hypercalcemia of malignancy with bisphosphonates. *Semin. Oncol.* 2002; (6 Suppl 21):12-8.

[28] Falk MJ, Heeger S, Lynch KA, DeCaro KR, Bohach D, Gibson KS, Warman ML. Intravenous bisphosphonate therapy in children with osteogenesis imperfecta. *Pediatrics.* 2003;111(3):573-8.

[29] N.J. Shaw, Management of osteoporosis in children, *Eur. J. Endocrinol.* 2008; 159: S33–S39.

[30] L.A. DiMeglio, M. Peacock, Two-year clinical trial of oral alendronate versus intravenous pamidronate in children with osteogenesis imperfect. *J. Bone Miner Res.* 2006; 21:.132–140.

[31] Michael McClung, Steven T. Harris, Paul D. Miller, Douglas C. Bauer, K. Shawn Davison, Larry Dian, David A. Hanley, David L. Kendler, Chui Kin Yuen, E. Michael Lewiecki. Bisphosphonate Therapy for Osteoporosis: Benefits, Risks, and Drug Holiday. *A. J. Med.* 2013; 26:13-20.

[32] M. A. Vidal, C. Medina y L. M. Torres˙ Seguridad de los bifosfonatos Safety of bisphosphonates. *Rev. Soc. Esp. Dolor* 2011; 18 (1): 43-55.

[33] Green J, Czanner G, Reeves G, Wise L, Watson J, Wise L, et al. Oral bisphosphonates and risk of cancer of oesophagus, stomach, and colorectum: casecontrol analysis within a UK primary care cohort *BMJ* 2010; 341: c4444.

[34] Wysowski DK. Reports of esophageal cancer with oral bisphosphonate use. *N. Engl. J. Med.* 2009; 360: 89-90.

[35] Cardwell CR, Abnet CC, Cantwell MM, Murray LJ. Exposure to oral bisphosphonates and risk of esophageal cancer. *JAMA* 2010; 304: 657-63.

[36] Solomon DH, Patrick A, Brookhart MA. More on reports of esophageal cancer with oral bisphosphonate use. *N. Engl. J. Med.2009*; 360: 1789-90.

[37] R. Rizzoli, N. Burlet, D. Cahall, P.D. Delmas, E.F. Eriksen, D. Felsenberg, J. Grbic, M. Jontell, R. Landesberg, A. Laslop, M. Wollenhaupt, S. Papapoulos, O. Sezer, M. Sprafka, JY. Reginster, Osteonecrosis of the jaw and bisphosphonate treatment for osteoporosis, *Bone* 2008; 42: 841–847.

[38] S. Khosla, D. Burr, J. Cauley, D.W. Dempster, P.R. Ebeling, D. Felsenberg, R.F. Gagel, V. Gilsanz, T. Guise, S. Koka, L.K. McCauley, J. McGowan, M.D. McKee, S. Mohla, D.G. Pendrys, L.G. Raisz, S.L. Ruggiero, D.M. Shafer, L. Shum, S.L. Silverman, C.H. Van Poznak, N. Watts, SB. Woo, E. Shane. Bisphosphonateassociated osteonecrosis of the jaw: report of a task force of the American Society for Bone and Mineral Research. *J. Bone Miner Res.* 2007; 22: 1479–1491.

[39] Woo SB, Hellstein JW, Kalmar JR. Narrative [corrected] review: Bisphosphonates and osteonecrosis of the jaws. *Ann. Intern. Med.* 2006;144(10):753–761.

[40] Felsenberg D. Osteonecrosis of the jaw; a potencial adverse effect of bisphosphonate treatment. *Nat. Clin. Pract.* 2006; 2: 662-3.

[41] Escuela Andaluza de Salud Pública. Bol Ter Andal 2010; 26 (2). Available in: http://www.cadime.es/docs/bta/CADIME_BTA2010_ 26_2.pdf

[42] Junquera IM, Martin Granizo R. Diagnostico, prevención y tratamiento de la osteonecrosis de maxilares por bifosfonatos. Recomendaciones de la SociedadEspanola de Cirugia Oral y Maxilofacial (SECOM). *Rev. Esp. Cir. Oral. Maxilofac.* 2008; 30(3): 145-56.

[43] Chesnut CH III, McClung MR, Ensrud KE, et al. Alendronate treatment of the postmenopausal osteoporotic woman: effect of multiple dosages on bone mass and bone remodeling. *Am. J. Med.* 1995;99:144- 152.

[44] Papapoulos SE, Harinck HI, Bijvoet OL, Gleed JH, Fraher LJ, O'Riordan JL. Effects of decreasing serum calcium on circulating parathyroid hormone and vitamin D metabolites in normocalcaemic and hypercalcaemic patients treated with APD. *Bone Miner.* 1986;1:69-78.

[45] Macarol V, Fraunfelder FT. Pamidronate disodium and possible ocular dverse drug reactions. *Am. J. Ophthalmol.* 1994;118:220–4.

[46] French DD, Margo CE. Postmarketing surveillance rates of uveitis and scleritis with bisphosphonates among a national veteran cohort. *Retina* 2008;28(6):889–93.

[47] Siris ES. Bisphosphonates and iritis. Lancet 1993; 341: 436-7. Vi.as G, Oliv. A, Holgado S, Costa J. Epiescleritis secundaria a risedronato. *Med. Clin. (Barc)* 2002; 118: 598-9.

[48] Aurich-Barrera B, Wilton L, Harris S, Shakir SA. Ophthalmological events in patients receiving risedronate: summary of informacion Gwynedd through folgo-up in a prescripcion-event monitoriong study in England. *Drug Saf.* 2006; 29(2): 151-60.

[49] Fietta P, Manganelli P, Lodigiani L. Clodronate induced uveitis. *Ann. Rheum. Dis.* 2003; 62: 378.

[50] Anonimo. Ibandronate (Boniva): a new oral bisphosphonate. *Med. Lett. Drugs Ther.* 2005; 47: 35.

[51] Moorthy RS, Valluri S, Jampol LM. Drug-induced uveitis. *Surv. Ophthalmol.* 1998; 42: 557-70.

[52] Malik AR, Campbell SH, Toma NM. Bilateral acute anterior uveitis after alendronate. *Br. J. Ophthalmol.* 2002; 86: 1443.

[53] Fietta P, Manganelli P, Lodigiani L. Clodronate induced uveitis. *Ann. Rheum. Dis.* 2003; 62: 378.

[54] Macarol V, Fraunfelder FT. Pamidronate disodium and possible ocular adverse drug reactions. *Am. J. Ophthalmol.* 1994; 118(2): 220–224.

[55] Black DM, Delmas PD, Eastell R, Reid IR, Boonen S, Cauley JA, et al. HORIZON pivotal Fracture Trial. *N. Engl. J. Med.* 2007; 356: 1809-22.

[56] Cummings SR. Schwartz AV. Black DM. Alendronate and atrial fibrillation. *NEJM* 2007; 356(18):1895-6.

[57] Loke YK, Jeevanantham V, Singh S. Bisphosphonates and atrial fibrillation: systematic review and meta-analysis. *Drug Saf.* 2009;32(3):219-28.

[58] Black DM, Reiss TF, Nevitt MC, Cauley J, Karpf D, Cummings SR. Biphosphonates and fractures of the subtrochanteric or diaphyseal femur. *N. Engl. J. Med.* 2010; 362(19): 1761-71.

[59] Tanvetyanon T, Stiff PJ. Management of the adverse effects associated with the intravenous bisphosphonates. *Ann. Oncol.* 2006; 17: 897-907.

[60] Body JJ, Diel IJ, Lichinitser MR et al. Intravenous ibandronate reduces the incidence of skeletal complications in patients with breast cancer and bone metastases. *Ann. Oncol. 2003*; 14(9): 1399–1405.

[61] Diel IJ, Bergstorm B, Barrett M. Long-term renal safety of intravenous ibandronate in patients with breast cancer and bone metastases: phase III data. *Ann. Oncol. 2005*; 16 (suppl 2): ii271–ii325.

[62] Perezella MA, Markowitz GS. Bisphosphonateg nephrotoxicity. Kidney international 2008; 74: 1385-1393.

[63] Kyle RA, Yee GC, Somerfield MR, Flynn PJ, Halabi S, Jagannth S, et al. American Society of Clinical Oncology 2007 Clinical Practice Guideline Update on the Role of Bisphosphonates in Multiple Myeloma. *Journal of clinical oncology* 2007; 25 (17):2464-72.

In: Zoledronic Acid
Editor: Ronald Carman

ISBN: 978-1-63321-525-2

Chapter 6

Clinical Role of Zoledronic Acid in Adjuvant and Metastatic Breast Cancer

Banys Malgorzata,[1,2] Natalia Krawczyk[1] and Tanja Fehm[1]
[1]Department of Obstetrics and Gynecology,
University of Duesseldorf, Duesseldorf, Germany
[2]Department of Gynecology and Obstetrics,
Marienkrankenhaus Hamburg, Hamburg, Germany

Abstract

In the recent decades, evidence has been accumulating concerning *in vivo* and *in vitro* anti-cancer activity of bisphosphonates. These effects are achieved through microevironmental changes, inhibition of tumor cell adhesion, invasion, neoangiogenesis and apoptosis induction. Zoledronic acid is known for its high potency with regard to antitumoral activity and has been to date studied in numerous clinical trials. In the adjuvant setting, postmenopausal patients benefit from zoledronate treatment; in the metastatic situation, zoledronate improves progression-free interval in patients with bone metastasis. Several authors hypothesized that bisphosphonates exhibit their oncologic effects through changes of bone marrow microenvironment making it less suitable for disseminated tumor cells; the presence of such cells in secondary sites is associated with higher risk of relapse and impaired prognosis. In the present review, we discuss experimental activity of bisphosphonates and review current data on the use of zoledronate acid in breast cancer patients.

Keywords: Breast cancer, zoledronic acid, bisphosphonates, disseminated tumor cell, apoptosis

Abbreviations

ABCSG	Austrian Breast and Colorectal Cancer Study Group
AZURE	Adjuvant Zoledronic Acid to Reduce Recurrence

BP	bisphosphonates
DFS	disease-free survival
DTC	disseminated tumor cell(s)
OS	overall survival
SRE	skeletal related events
ZICE	Zoledronate versus ibandronate comparative evaluation trial
ZO-FAST	Zometa-Femara Adjuvant Synergy Trials
ZOL	zoledronate

1. Introduction

Breast cancer is the most common malignancy in women, with more than 1.3 million new cases diagnosed yearly. Breast cancer-related mortality is in nearly all cases attributed to distant metastases and not the primary tumor. Despite successful surgery and adjuvant treatment, up to 30% of patients develop distant metastases in course of their disease. These recurrences may occur more than 10-15 years after completion of primary therapy, resulting in a phenomenon described as 'tumor dormancy' [1].

Breast cancer metastasizes typically to sites such as bone, lung, liver and brain. Bisphosphonates (BP), potent therapeutic agents used in the treatment of bone metastasis, has been recently reported to prolong survival in the adjuvant setting [2-4]. Possibly, anticancer activity of bisphosphonates may be associated with isolated tumor cells already present at secondary sites, called disseminated tumor cells (DTCs), and their elimination through microevironmental changes and apoptosis induction.

In the following review, we will discuss the current clinical value of zoledronic acid (ZOL) in adjuvant and metastatic setting.

2. Role of Zoledronic Acid in Metastatic Breast Cancer

Bisphosphonates are integral in the current therapy of breast cancer patients with metastases to the bones in order to prevent or reduce the incidence of skeletal related events (SRE), such as pathologic fractures, spinal cord compression or need for surgical/radiotherapeutic interventions. Moreover, BP can improve bone pain and are highly effective treatment for cancer-related hypercalcemia [5, 6]. Efficacy of different BP in metastatic breast cancer has been to date demonstrated by several studies; data from 19 randomized clinical trials with 6,646 patients have been evaluated in a Cochrane systemic review and meta-analysis [6].

In nine studies with 2,806 breast cancer patients with bone metastases different bisphosphonates (intravenous zoledronate, pamidronate and ibandronate and oral clodronate) versus placebo or no bisphosphonates have been analyzed. All BP, regardless of the substance, reduced the risk of SRE (excluding hypercalcemia) by overall 15% versus control (RR 0.85; 95% CI 0.77 to 0.94; P = 0.001). However, this effect was most prominent for intravenous zoledronic acid; ZOL reduced the risk of SRE by 41% versus control (RR 0.59; 95% CI 0.42 to 0.82; P = 0.001).

There are only a few studies to date performing direct comparison between different bisphosphonates. In a large multicenter randomized double-blind trial, Rosen et al. compared ZOL (4-8 mg i.v. every 3-4 weeks) versus pamidronate (90 mg i.v. every 3-4 weeks) for 12 months in 1,130 breast cancer patients with at least one bone metastasis [7, 8]. The multiple events analysis demonstrated a 20% additional reduction in the risk of SRE for patients in the ZOL arm compared with the pamidronate group; in women with osteolytic lesions, the benefit of ZOL was even greater. Within the osteolytic subgroup, ZOL significantly prolonged the time to first SRE compared with pamidronate (median, 310 days vs. 174 days, respectively; P = 0.013).

Recently, *the ZICE (Zoledronate versus ibandronate comparative evaluation) trial*, a multicenter randomized phase III study, compared intravenous ZOL and oral ibandronate in 1,404 breast cancer patients with bone metastases (NCT00326820) [9].

This open-label study was designed as a non-inferiority trial with SRE as primary endpoint. Annual SRE rates were 0.499 (95% CI 0.454—0.549) for oral ibandronate and 0.435 (0.393—0.480) for ZOL. Therefore, the null hypothesis that ibandronate was inferior to ZOL could not be rejected, confirming that zoledronic acid is preferable to ibandronate in the prevention of SRE in breast cancer patients with bone metastases.

3. Role of Zoledronic Acid in Early Breast Cancer

Beneficial effects of adding bisphosphonates to adjuvant treatment were demonstrated in a number of large clinical trials in non-metastatic breast cancer. So far, three prospective studies aimed at evaluating the impact of zoledronic acid on survival (Table 1) [3,4,10].

The Zometa-Femara Adjuvant Synergy Trials (ZO-FAST) initially investigated the bone-protective influence of ZOL; however, the survival analysis showed that ZOL may provide anticancer benefits in addition to the established bone-related effect ; (NCT00171340) [11]. Briefly, 1,065 postmenopausal women with hormone receptor positive breast cancer received letrozole 2.5 mg daily for 5 years in the adjuvant setting in this open-label, multicentre, randomized, phase III study [4]. After randomization, women in the "immediate arm" began treatment with zoledronic acid 4 mg every 6 months within one month after randomization and continued for 5 years; patients in the "delayed arm" received ZOL only upon a predetermined measure of bone loss (T-score below -2.0 or non-traumatic fracture). Patients in both arms received calcium and vitamin D orally. After 60 months of follow-up, a 34% relative reduction in the risk of disease recurrence or death were observed in the immediate ZOL-arm versus the delayed-ZOL-arm (hazard ratio [HR] = 0.66; $P = 0.0375$). These results could have been influenced by the initiation of ZOL in the delayed arm. Therefore, exploratory analyses of the delayed arm were conducted; patients who initiated ZOL due to bone loss or fracture had improved disease-free survival (DFS) compared to patients who received no ZOL treatment.

The Austrian Breast and Colorectal Cancer Study Group (ABCSG)-12 (NCT00295646), a randomized open-label phase III trial, investigated the impact of ZOL treatment in addition to adjuvant endocrine therapy [3]. In this four-arm study, 1,803 premenopausal women with hormone receptor positive early stage breast cancer were randomized to receive goserelin plus either tamoxifen or anastrozole, with or without ZOL 4 mg every 6 months for 3 years. This trial was aimed at evaluating the influence of ZOL on survival (primary end point: DFS).

Table 1. Studies evaluating anticancer activity of bisphosphonates in breast cancer

Study / clinical trial	N	Bisphospho-nate	Duration of therapy	Adjuvant therapy	Follow up	Survival benefit premenopausal	Survival benefit postmenopausal
Powles [28]	1069	Clodronate p.o.	2 years	CTX +/- Endocrine	66 months	Yes (OS, bone-metastasis free survival)	
Kristensen [29]	953	Pamidronate p.o.	4 years	CTX	n.d.	No	
Diel [30]	302	Clodronate p.o.	2 years	CTX +/- Endocrine	103 months	Yes (OS)	
Saarto [31]	299	Clodronate p.o.	3 years	CTX +/- Endocrine	120 months	No	
AZURE	3360	Zoledronate i.v.	5 years	CTX +/- Endocrine	60 months	No	Yes (DFS, OS)
NSABP-B34	3323	Clodronate p.o.	3 years	CTX +/- Endocrine	91 months	No	Yes (> 50 yrs. DFS, but not OS)
GAIN	3023	Ibandronate p.o.	2 years	Dose-dense dose-intense CTX	39 months	No	No (Trend > 60 yrs.)
ABCSG-12	1803	Zoledronate i.v.	3 years	Endocrine (Tam vs. AI +GnRH-Anal.)	84 months	Yes (DFS, OS)	-
ZO-FAST	1065	Zoledronate i.v.	5 years	Endocrine (AI)	60 months	-	Yes (DFS)

At a median follow-up of 62 months, addition of ZOL to adjuvant endocrine therapy improved DFS significantly (p=0.008). The reduction in events was reported for both local and distant recurrence in and outside the bone. Interestingly, younger women did not benefit from ZOL as much as older patients; in the subgroup analysis, ZOL did not reduce the risk for relapse in patients aged 40 or younger. In patients older than 40 years at study entry, the risk reduction was significant.

In contrast to the aforementioned trials, *the Adjuvant Zoledronic Acid to Reduce Recurrence (AZURE; BIG 01/04)* trial has been unable to demonstrate a significant benefit from adding ZOL to adjuvant therapy in the overall patient population (NCT00072020) [2]. This trial investigated the anticancer activity of ZOL combined with (neo)adjuvant chemotherapy as well as endocrine therapy in 3,360 pre- and postmenopausal axillary node-positive stage II/III breast cancer patients. Patients were randomly assigned to receive standard adjuvant systemic therapy either with or without ZOL (every 3-4 weeks for 6 doses and then every 3 to 6 months to complete 5 years of treatment). After 59 months of median follow-up, ZOL did not improve DFS in the overall population. However, a subgroup analysis revealed that patients who were more than 5 years postmenopausal benefitted significantly from ZOL treatment; in this study population, overall survival (OS) was better in the ZOL group by 29% (p = 0.017) and ZOL reduced DFS events in and outside the bone [2]. Interestingly, retrospective evaluation of the neoadjuvant subgroup (195 patients) showed that additional ZOL treatment reduced mean residual invasive tumor size by approximately 43% compared with neoadjuvant chemotherapy alone [10].

Interestingly, the survival improvement with ZOL in clinical trials was highest in patients older than 60 years or more than 5 years postmenopausal [2]. In the only large trial focusing on premenopausal patients (ABCSG-12), all women received GnRH agonist goserelin, thus inhibiting the production of estrogen in the ovary and creating low-estrogen environment as well ("fake menopause") [3]. Estrogen is an important player in the regulation of bone turnover through hormone receptors on bone cells; in estrogen-deprived or low-estrogen environment, bone resorption overweighs bone formation. Since one of the main mechanisms of action of bisphosphonates is the suppression of bone resorption, their antitumor potential might be particularly marked in estrogen-deprived microenvironment.

4. Antitumor Effects of Zoledronic Acid *In Vitro* and *In Vivo*

During the past two decades much more information has become available of the direct and indirect effects of bisphosphonates in vivo as well as in vitro (Figure 1). BP are known for their high affinity for bone and have been proven to inhibit bone resorption through several mechanisms such as the increase in osteoblast survival and impaired differentiation of osteoclasts [12]; these effects are useful in osteoporosis and bone metastasis treatment. Beyond these favorable bone health-related properties, both pre-clinical and clinical data confirm anti-metastatic and antitumoral properties of BP, including the inhibition of tumor cell invasiveness and adhesion, apoptosis induction and the inhibition of angiogenesis [13] [14, 15]. These findings support the currently discussed hypothesis that bisphosphonates prevent development of metastasis through microenvironmental changes and elimination of disseminated tumor cells.

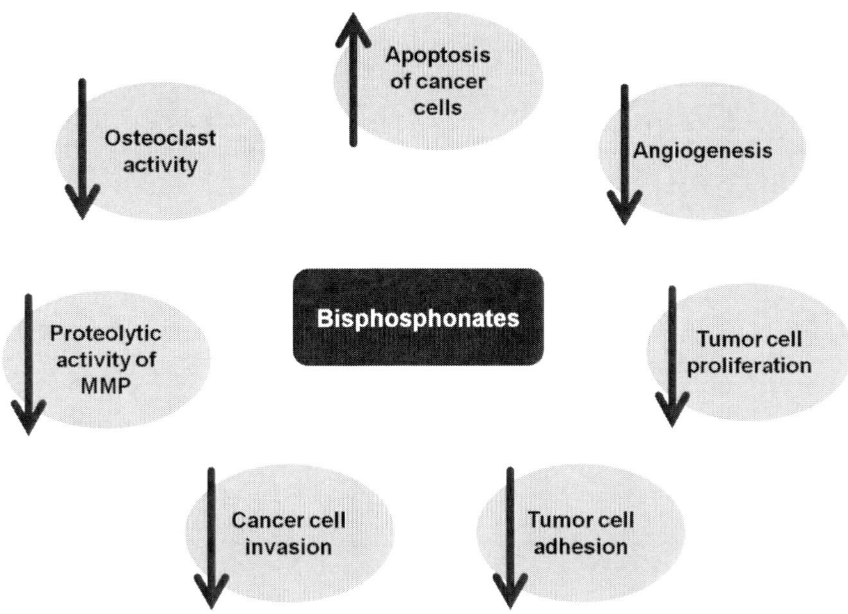

Figure 1. Effects of bisphosphonates contributing to their antitumoral activity.

The "seed and soil" hypothesis proposed by Stephen Paget in 1889 holds that secondary sites must provide a fertile "soil" for growth of the tumor "seed" in order to develop metastatic disease [16, 17]. The growth of distant disease recurrence could result from the ability of DTCs to stay dormant in the bone marrow, a stem-cell niche that possibly protects them from cytotoxic treatment [18, 19]. Results from large clinical trials, such as ZO-FAST, ABCSG-12 and AZURE, support the notion that ZOL may modify the microenvironment of the bone ("soil") in such a way as to make it less hospitable for the proliferation and survival of disseminated tumor cells ("seed").

Specifically, several studies showed that BP interplay with the components of bone microenvironment (e.g. matrix metalloproteinases) thus affecting the ability of bone marrow to host DTCs [20]; reduced proteolytic activity of matrix metalloproteinases seems to hinder tumor cells from digesting the basement membrane – a step necessary for further invasion [21]. In vitro, exposure of the bone to BP reduced breast cancer cell adhesion [13]; interestingly, tumor cells were more susceptible to BP exposure than normal bone cells [22].

We have previously reported that addition of ZOL to adjuvant treatment improves clearance of DTCs from bone marrow [23, 24]. In the open-label multicenter *ZOL-MRD-001 trial* (NCT00172068), 96 non-metastatic breast cancer patients with detectable DTCs in bone marrow at time of diagnosis, were randomized to receive intravenous ZOL 4 mg every 3-4 weeks plus adjuvant therapy or adjuvant therapy alone. DTC assessment per bone marrow biopsy was conducted after 12 and 24 months. After 24 months, 16% of patients in the control group had persistent DTCs whereas all women treated with ZOL became DTC negative ($P = 0.032$).

Another phase II study with focus on DTCs was conducted by Aft et al. (NCT00242203) [25]. 120 women with stage II-III breast cancer were enrolled before start of neoadjuvant chemotherapy; patients were randomized to receive 4 mg intravenous ZOL every 3 weeks for 1 year commencing with the first dose of cytotoxic treatment or no zoledronic acid. Bone marrow aspirations were performed at baseline (before start of chemotherapy), at surgery (three months after begin of study) and after 1 year. At 3 months, patients who were DTC-negative at baseline and were treated with ZOL were more likely to remain DTC free than patients in the control group ($P = 0.03$). Interestingly, patients with estrogen receptor-negative/HER2-negative cancer were more likely to achieve pathologic complete response with ZOL versus no ZOL.

Rack et al. examined 31 early breast cancer patients with DTCs in bone marrow who received ZOL 4 mg every 4 weeks for 6 months after completion of adjuvant surgery and performed matched-pair analysis with 141 DTC-positive patients who did not receive additional ZOL therapy [26]. At the second bone marrow aspiration, performed 8 months after enrollment in the ZOL group and after 12 months in the control group, 13% of patients treated with ZOL showed persistent DTCs compared to 27% in the control group ($P = 0.099$). Another study confirmed that ZOL treatment significantly decreased DTC levels versus baseline at 12 ($P < 0.001$) and 24 months ($P = 0.0026$) in DTC-positive breast cancer patients [27].

CONCLUSION

Zoledronic acid has long been used to reduce skeletal related complication in patients with bone metastasis. Recent clinical trials have shown that ZOL benefits patients with early breast cancer as well, improving disease-free and overall survival. These effects are particularly marked in low-estrogen environment following menopause. Possibly, these antitumor effects occur through alteration of bone marrow microenvironment making it less hospitable for persistence and proliferation of disseminated tumor cells.

REFERENCES

[1] Banys M, Hartkopf AD, Krawczyk N, et al. Dormancy in breast cancer. *Breast Cancer* (Dove Med Press) 2012; 4:183-191.

[2] Coleman RE, Marshall H, Cameron D, et al. Breast-cancer adjuvant therapy with zoledronic acid. *N. Engl. J. Med.* 2011; 365:1396-1405.

[3] Gnant M, Mlineritsch B, Stoeger H, et al. Adjuvant endocrine therapy plus zoledronic acid in premenopausal women with early-stage breast cancer: 62-month follow-up from the ABCSG-12 randomised trial. *Lancet Oncol.* 2011; 12:631-641.

[4] Eidtmann H, de Boer R, Bundred N, et al. Efficacy of zoledronic acid in postmenopausal women with early breast cancer receiving adjuvant letrozole: 36-month results of the ZO-FAST Study. *Ann. Oncol.* 2010; 21:2188-2194.

[5] Major P, Lortholary A, Hon J, et al. Zoledronic acid is superior to pamidronate in the treatment of hypercalcemia of malignancy: a pooled analysis of two randomized, controlled clinical trials. *J. Clin. Oncol.* 2001; 19:558-567.

[6] Wong MH, Stockler MR, Pavlakis N. Bisphosphonates and other bone agents for breast cancer. *Cochrane Database Syst. Rev.* 2012; 2:CD003474.

[7] Rosen LS, Gordon DH, Dugan W, Jr., et al. Zoledronic acid is superior to pamidronate for the treatment of bone metastases in breast carcinoma patients with at least one osteolytic lesion. *Cancer* 2004; 100:36-43.

[8] Rosen LS, Gordon D, Kaminski M, et al. Long-term efficacy and safety of zoledronic acid compared with pamidronate disodium in the treatment of skeletal complications in patients with advanced multiple myeloma or breast carcinoma: a randomized, double-blind, multicenter, comparative trial. *Cancer* 2003; 98:1735-1744.

[9] Barrett-Lee P, Casbard A, Abraham J, et al. Oral ibandronic acid versus intravenous zoledronic acid in treatment of bone metastases from breast cancer: a randomised, open label, non-inferiority phase 3 trial. *Lancet Oncol.* 2014; 15:114-122.

[10] Coleman RE, Winter MC, Cameron D, et al. The effects of adding zoledronic acid to neoadjuvant chemotherapy on tumour response: exploratory evidence for direct anti-tumour activity in breast cancer. *Br. J. Cancer* 2010; 102:1099-1105.

[11] Coleman R, de Boer R, Eidtmann H, et al. Zoledronic acid (zoledronate) for postmenopausal women with early breast cancer receiving adjuvant letrozole (ZO-FAST study): final 60-month results. *Ann. Oncol.* 2013; 24:398-405.

[12] Rodan GA. Mechanisms of action of bisphosphonates. *Annu. Rev. Pharmacol. Toxicol.* 1998; 38:375-388.

[13] van der Pluijm G, Vloedgraven H, van Beek E, van der Wee-Pals L, Lowik C, Papapoulos S. Bisphosphonates inhibit the adhesion of breast cancer cells to bone matrices in vitro. *J. Clin. Invest.* 1996; 98:698-705.

[14] Senaratne SG, Pirianov G, Mansi JL, Arnett TR, Colston KW. Bisphosphonates induce apoptosis in human breast cancer cell lines. *Br. J. Cancer* 2000; 82:1459-1468.

[15] Ory B, Heymann MF, Kamijo A, Gouin F, Heymann D, Redini F. Zoledronic acid suppresses lung metastases and prolongs overall survival of osteosarcoma-bearing mice. *Cancer* 2005; 104:2522-2529.

[16] Paget S. Distribution of secondary growths in cancer of the breast. *Lancet* 1889; 1:571.

[17] Langley RR, Fidler IJ. The seed and soil hypothesis revisited--the role of tumor-stroma interactions in metastasis to different organs. *Int. J. Cancer* 2011; 128:2527-2535.

[18] Meads MB, Hazlehurst LA, Dalton WS. The bone marrow microenvironment as a tumor sanctuary and contributor to drug resistance. *Clin. Cancer Res.* 2008; 14:2519-2526.

[19] Braun S, Vogl FD, Naume B, et al. A pooled analysis of bone marrow micrometastasis in breast cancer. *N. Engl. J. Med.* 2005; 353:793-802.

[20] Winter MC, Holen I, Coleman RE. Exploring the anti-tumour activity of bisphosphonates in early breast cancer. *Cancer Treat. Rev.* 2008; 34:453-475.

[21] Boissier S, Ferreras M, Peyruchaud O, et al. Bisphosphonates inhibit breast and prostate carcinoma cell invasion, an early event in the formation of bone metastases. *Cancer Res.* 2000; 60:2949-2954.

[22] Boissier S, Magnetto S, Frappart L, et al. Bisphosphonates inhibit prostate and breast carcinoma cell adhesion to unmineralized and mineralized bone extracellular matrices. *Cancer Res.* 1997; 57:3890-3894.

[23] Solomayer EF, Gebauer G, Hirnle P, et al. Influence of zoledronic acid on disseminated tumor cells in primary breast cancer patients. *Ann. Oncol.* 2012; 23:2271-2277.

[24] Banys M, Solomayer EF, Gebauer G, et al. Influence of zoledronic acid on disseminated tumor cells in bone marrow and survival: results of a prospective clinical trial. *BMC Cancer* 2013; 13:480.

[25] Aft R, Naughton M, Trinkaus K, et al. Effect of zoledronic acid on disseminated tumour cells in women with locally advanced breast cancer: an open label, randomised, phase 2 trial. *Lancet Oncol.* 2010; 11:421-428.

[26] Rack B, Juckstock J, Genss EM, et al. Effect of zoledronate on persisting isolated tumour cells in patients with early breast cancer. *Anticancer Res.* 2010; 30:1807-1813.

[27] Lin AY, Park JW, Scott J, et al. Zoledronic acid as adjuvant therapy for women with early stage breast cancer and disseminated tumor cells in bone marrow. *J. Clin. Oncol.* 2008; 26 (Suppl):20s (Abstract 559).

[28] Powles T, Paterson A, McCloskey E, et al. Reduction in bone relapse and improved survival with oral clodronate for adjuvant treatment of operable breast cancer [ISRCTN83688026]. *Breast Cancer Res.* 2006; 8:R13.

[29] Kristensen B, Ejlertsen B, Mouridsen HT, et al. Bisphosphonate treatment in primary breast cancer: results from a randomised comparison of oral pamidronate versus no pamidronate in patients with primary breast cancer. *Acta Oncol.* 2008; 47:740-746.

[30] Diel IJ, Jaschke A, Solomayer EF, et al. Adjuvant oral clodronate improves the overall survival of primary breast cancer patients with micrometastases to the bone marrow: a long-term follow-up. *Ann. Oncol.* 2008; 19:2007-2011.

[31] Saarto T, Vehmanen L, Virkkunen P, Blomqvist C. Ten-year follow-up of a randomized controlled trial of adjuvant clodronate treatment in node-positive breast cancer patients. *Acta Oncol.* 2004; 43:650-656.

In: Zoledronic Acid
Editor: Ronald Carman
ISBN: 978-1-63321-525-2

Chapter 7

ZOLEDRONIC ACID IN CHRONIC INFLAMMATORY RHEUMATIC DISEASES: A CRITICAL EVIDENCE OF ITS ANTIRESORPTIVE AND IMMUNOMODULATING EFFECTS

Laura Gonzalez-Lopez, M.D., M.Sc., Ph.D.[1,•],
Eva M. Olivas-Flores, M.D.[2],
David Bonilla-Lara, M.D.[3], ***Edsaul E. Perez-Guerrero, B.Sc.***[3],
Jessica D. Murillo-Vazquez, B.Sc.[3],
Tania M. Rodriguez Hernandez, M.D.[4]
and Jorge I. Gamez-Nava, M.D., M.Sc., Ph.D.[5]

[1]Department of Internal Medicine-Rheumatology,
Hospital General Regional 110, IMSS and Public Health Sciences Department,
Centro Universitario de Ciencias de la Salud Universidad de Guadalajara,
Guadalajara, Jal., Mexico
[2]Hospital General Regional 180, IMSS Tlajomulco, Jal., Mexico
[3]Programa de Doctorado en Farmacología,
Centro Universitario de Ciencias de la Salud (CUCS) Universidad de Guadalajara,
Guadalajara, Jal., Mexico
[4]Department of Internal Medicine-Rheumatology,
Hospital General Regional 110, IMSS, Guadalajara, Jal., Mexico
[5]Clinical Epidemiology Research Unit, Hospital de Especialidades,
Centro Médico Nacional de Occidente,
IMSS, and Public Health Sciences Department,
Centro Universitario de Ciencias de la Salud Universidad de Guadalajara,
Guadalajara, Mexico

• E-mail: dralauragonzalez@prodigy.net.mx.

ABSTRACT

Chronic inflammatory rheumatic diseases (CIRD) constitute a heterogeneous group of disorders that include rheumatoid arthritis (RA), systemic lupus erythematosus (SLE), ankylosing spondylitis (AS), psoriatic arthritis (PsA) and other diseases that affect a multiplicity of organs. Currently, it has been well recognized that a close link exists between the immune system and bone tissue, particularly in these disorders. CIRD have a high prevalence of osteoporosis (OP), observed between 25-59% in RA, 20-48% in SLE, 15-60% in AS and around 16% in PsA. Factors associated with OP in CIRD include the over-activation of osteoclasts by inflammatory cytokines, mainly tumor necrosis factor-alpha, and other interleukins (IL) including IL-1beta and IL-6, as well as other mechanisms such as impairment in joint function, and utilization of therapies that increase bone loss, mainly corticosteroids. OP is frequently underdiagnosed in CIRD; therefore, the onset of anti-osteoporotic therapy is delayed. Additionally, these patients have a high frequency of vertebral and non-vertebral fractures, with vertebral fractures being frequently asymptomatic or with non-severe symptoms leading to delays in treatment. Frequencies for vertebral fractures may vary; in RA around 21.7%, in SLE between 20-50%, in AS 19-65% and for PsA around 13%. According to the National Osteoporosis Foundation guidelines, adults with RA or any patient taking prednisone ≥5 mg/day or equivalent for ≥3 months should be evaluated for bone mineral density (BMD), and strategies to prevent fractures are required. Zoledronic acid (ZA) has been approved for the prevention and treatment of osteoporosis in patients expected to be on corticosteroid therapy for at least 12 months, as well as for the prevention of new clinical fractures. This review describes the current evidence of ZA to improve the BMD and as adjuvant therapy for controlling clinical inflammation in CIRD. In collagen-induced arthritis models, a combination of ZA plus methotrexate (MTX) prevents bone erosion, radiological damage and systemic bone loss, whereas clinical studies in patients with early RA suggest that this combination prevents bone erosions. On the other hand, the benefits of ZA in patients with established RA to prevent generalized bone loss are now recognized. Most of the evidence of ZA for OP is in postmenopausal women. Case reports in young patients and children with SLE describe how ZA decreases the incidence of bone fractures, although it is important to take into account the potential effects on growth. In animal models for AS, ZA prevents joint ankylosis; however, these preliminary data need to be evaluated in clinical studies. Patients with PsA treated with ZA have shown a decrease in the progression of bone edema, suggesting a suppression of osteitis that correlates with the improvement of disease activity in clinical measures. In tophaceous gout ZA increases BMD of the spine, neck of femur, total hip and total body, but does not influence bone erosions. In conclusion, ZA decreases generalized bone loss and focal bone damage, as well as improving some inflammatory parameters in some of the CIRD. The potential properties as immunomodulating need to be considered to define its possible role as adjuvant therapy directed against the mechanisms of inflammation in CIRD.

INTRODUCTION

Chronic inflammatory rheumatic diseases (CIRD) constitute a heterogeneous group of disorders that include rheumatoid arthritis (RA), systemic lupus erythematosus (SLE), spondyloarthropathies (SpA) (being the most representative ankylosing spondylitis (AS)), psoriatic arthritis (PsA) and other diseases such as systemic vasculitis, as well as diseases related to inflammatory myopathy and scleroderma. All of these disorders have the hallmark of a chronic inflammation mediated by autoimmunity mechanisms that may involve a multiplicity of organs frequently affecting the musculoskeletal system [1]. CIRD are associated with bone manifestations that include osteopenia and osteoporosis (OP) (defined as generalized bone loss and microarchitecture bone deterioration leading to a decrement in bone strength and consequently to an increase of fracture risk) deteriorating the functional capacities, quality of life and higher morbidity and mortality.

Epidemiology of Osteoporosis in Chronic Inflammatory Rheumatic Diseases

Currently, in most CIRD, it is well recognized that there is a close link between the immune system and bone, whereby the immune system participates in the pathogenesis of abnormalities in bone remodeling and loss of bone mass. CIRD are associated with a high prevalence of OP, with RA being probably the most evaluated and in which the frequency of OP ranges between 25 and 59% [2, 3]. Also in Bone Mass Density (BMD) evaluations in SLE many studies have found a frequency of OP between 20 and 48%. AS has a prevalence of OP between 15 and 60% [4] and OP is present in approximately 16% of PsA [5].

Risk Factors for Osteoporosis and Low Bone Mass Density in Chronic Inflammatory Rheumatic Diseases

OP in patients with CIRD had been related to a wide variety of risk factors. These can be classified as genetic, epidemiological, secondary to the inflammatory effects of the disease on bone, effects derived from complications (disability, poor mobility) or comorbidities associated with these diseases, and finally, secondary to the bone effects of the therapy used to treat these diseases. Most of the guidelines used to prevent or to treat patients with OP place an emphasis on the primary factors affecting bone mass such as corticosteroid therapy, chronic inflammation, the severity of the disease, disability-related immobilization and comorbid diseases that are often concurrent such as thyroid disease, diabetes mellitus and renal failure [6, 7]. These risk factors are summarized in Table 1. For physicians and researchers the acknowledgement of a wide variability in the prevalence and incidence of OP in CIRD findings across different studies is important. This variability is a consequence of many factors that include several differences in the inclusion criteria among the studies, types of study design, methodology for the assessment of OP, origin site of the included patients, the frequency of epidemiological factors related to OP that these patients may have (including ethnicity, old age, alcohol or tobacco abuse, female gender), genetic antecedents (such as a history of hip fracture in the family), or use and intensity of utilization of drugs affecting bone mass (such as corticosteroids). Some of these factors are considered in many studies as confounders leading to the exclusion of patients with one or more of these characteristics, making comparability across the studies difficult [8, 9].

Table 1. Risk Factors for Osteoporosis in CIRD

Factors	Associated Variables
Genetics	Family history of fractures
Epidemiological	Age >40
	Ethnicity (Caucasian)
	Alcohol or tobacco abuse
	Female gender
	Postmenopause
	Low body mass index
Disease or treatment associated	Persistent disease activity
	Corticosteroid therapy (≥ 7.5 mg/day Predictable or prevailing duration of > 3 months of corticosteroid therapy)
	Limited joint functioning
	Renal involvement
Comorbid diseases	Thyroid disease
	Diabetes mellitus
	Chronic Renal failure
Other	Lack of prevention with Vitamin D and calcium supplements

OSTEOIMMUNOLOGY AND CHRONIC INFLAMMATORY RHEUMATIC DISEASES

Currently the concept of osteoimmunology is referred to as an integrative scientific discipline of both the immune and musculoskeletal systems, which investigates the linkage between immune and skeletal cells, cytokines, ligands and receptors, with the aim of improving the understanding of the molecular regulation and joint destruction [10]. Osteoimmunology encompasses the concepts of the participation of the immune system in the regulation of bone degradation, the relationship between bone formation and inflammatory processes, and the participation of the bone marrow as a starting point for the recruitment of cells from bone marrow to the inflammatory sites [11].

A dysregulation in the bone-remodeling process that increases osteoclast resorption has been highlighted by many investigators as the central key to the development of pathological bone erosions in patients with some CIRD. A disruption in the receptor activator of nuclear factor κB (RANK) and the receptor activator of nuclear factor κB ligand (RANKL) system plays a relevant role in the differentiation and maturation of osteoclasts leading to an accelerated bone resorption and consequently to OP. Also, an overexpression of RANKL in swollen joints is associated with bone destruction [12]. A variety of immune system cells express RANKL, including osteoblast precursors and mature osteoblasts, as well as activated T cells [13, 14]. Several cytokines are involved in the upregulation of RANKL expression including interleukin-1 (IL-1), IL-6, IL-11, IL-17 and tumor necrosis factor-alpha (TNF-α) [13, 15]. Another molecule that plays an interesting role in the bone-remodeling process is the macrophage colony-stimulating factor (M-CSF); this cytokine also participates in the osteoclast activation [16]. A summary of several cytokines playing a role in the bone-remodeling process is shown in Table 2. Although cytokines do not constitute the unique actors in the genesis of secondary OP observed in CIRD. Several cells related to the immune response also participate. T cells play a significant role in bone mineral regulation, because under physiological conditions, T cells express interferon-gamma (INF-γ) which constitutes a cytokine with major effects on the inhibition of osteoclastogenesis, and the inhibition of RANKL signaling pathways [17]. In contrast, under pathological conditions of inflammation as observed in CIRD, the activated T cells stimulate an overproduction of RANKL and stimulate the secretion of TNF-α and IL-1 by macrophages, enhancing the osteoclastogenesis with the subsequent increase of bone resorption. Under these conditions the RANKL-osteoclastogenic signal can overcome the anti-osteoclastogenic effect induced by INF-γ, leading to an increase of bone resorption and osteoporosis [18]. Additionally, IL-17-producing T cells (Th17) participate in autoimmune inflammation and contribute considerably to bone destruction in some CIRD, particularly RA [19]. Th17 cells are found into the synovial tissue in RA; this tissue also characteristically produces lower quantities of INF-γ, contributing to local inflammation and the enhancement of RANKL production on synovial fibroblast [20].

Kotake et al. have reported that the concentration of IL-17 in synovial fluids of RA patients was higher compared to that in OA patients. They suggest that IL-17 indirectly mediates the osteoclastogenic effects of Th17 cells in a process related to prostaglandin (PG) E_2 [21]. The osteoclastogenic effect of the RANK/RANKL system is conterregulated by osteoprotegerin (OPG), a decoy receptor of the TNF receptor superfamily [22]. Additionally, under physiological conditions, after bone resorption induced by osteoclast there is a compensatory process of bone formation performed by activated osteoblasts to control the bone resorption. The factors involved in the differentiation and activity of osteoblasts include parathyroid hormone (PTH), wingless protein (Wnt) family and the bone morphogenic protein family including transforming growth factor beta (TGF-β) [23]. The Wnt pathway performs the pivotal role for osteoblastic differentiation from mesenchymal precursors [11].

Osteoimmunology in Osteoporosis Associated with Rheumatoid Arthritis

On the other side are some of the high levels of pro-inflammatory cytokines observed in CIRD, such as TNF-α which may promote the expression of inhibitory proteins for bone formation such as Dickkopf-1 (Dkk-1) and sclerostin, molecules that downregulate osteoblast differentiation and bone formation of the Wnt pathway [23]. Synovial fibroblasts obtained from synovial joints in arthritis produce Dkk-1, negatively affecting the bone formation [11]. Garnero et al., in a study of patients with RA, reported the association between elevated circulating Dkk-1 and a higher risk of progression of bone erosions observed in these patients [24].

Pro-inflammatory cytokines such as TNF-α, IL-1, IL-6 and IL-17 play a pivotal role in the pathogenesis of OP in RA through RANKL expression [21].

Table 2. Cytokines Involved in Osteoclastogenesis

Cytokine	Expressing cells	Function
IL-1	Macrophages, dendritic cells	Potent stimulator and activator of osteoclastogenesis.
IL-6	Macrophages, dendritic cells and synovial fibroblasts	Osteoclastogenic activity.
IL-8	Monocytes/macrophages, fibroblasts, chondrocytes, synoviocytes	Osteoclastogenic activity.
IL-11	Osteoblasts	Osteoclastogenic activity.
IL-17	Th17 cells	RANKL expression. Osteoclast activation by RANKL.
TNF-α	Macrophages and dendritic cells	Through RANKL osteoclastogenic activity.
IL-4	Th2 cells and mast cells	Anti-osteoclastogenic.
IL-10	Macrophages and Th2 cells	Anti-osteoclastogenic.
IL-13	Th1 and Th2 cells, CD8+ T cells, mast cells, basophils, eosinophils and NK cells	Anti-osteoclastogenic activity.
IL-18	Monocytes, synovial fibroblast and osteoblast	Anti-osteoclastogenic activity.
M-CSF	Osteoblast	Promotes osteoclast-precursor proliferation and RANK expression.
IFN-γ	Th1 cells and NK cells	Inhibits osteoclastogenesis.
TGF-β	Treg cells and dendritic cells	Inhibits osteoblast differentiation and osteoclastogenesis.

IL: Interleukin; TNF-α: Tumor necrosis factor alpha; IFN-γ: Interferon gamma; TGF-β: Transforming Growth Factor beta; RANKL: Ligand of Receptor Activator Nuclear Factor κB; NK: Natural killer; M-CSF: Macrophage-colony stimulating factor.

Xu et al. observed that RA patients had lower OPG plasma levels and greater RANKL plasma levels compared with those of the control group, being implicated in the pathogenesis of OP a decrement in the plasmatic OPG/RANKL ratio [25]. Chabaud et al. identified that the increase in IL-17 is involved in the enhancement of IL-6 production in the synovium tissue and upturn the degradation of type I collagen [26]. Kotake et al. observed that synovial fluids in RA patients had higher concentrations of IL-17 compared to the synovial fluids of osteoarthritis (OA) patients, thus inducing PGE_2-mediated osteoclast differentiation [21].

Osteoimmunology in Osteoporosis Associated with Systemic Lupus Erythematosus

SLE is characterized by an overactivation of T cells and polyclonal B lymphocytes, with an increase in auto-antibodies, and immune complexes production, leading to organ damage. Several studies have shown an imbalance of Th1/Th2 cytokines with an increase in the synthesis of pro-inflammatory cytokines, including IFN-γ, TNF-α, IL-10, IL-6, IL-12, IL-12-IL-23 and IL-1β [27, 28]. These pro-inflammatory cytokines have a relevant role in the pathogenesis of OP in SLE because of their leading performance to an accelerated osteoclastogenesis [29]. Osteoblasts are cells derived from human mesenchymal stem cells (MSCs).

Hess et al. found that TNF-α mediated Nuclear factor kappa-light-chain-enhancer of activated B cells (NF-kB) activation, supporting osteogenic differentiation and matrix mineralization by increasing bone morphogenetic protein-2 (BMP-2) expression [30]. BMPs promote a differentiation of MSCs into chondrocytes and osteoblasts, and also promote the differentiation of osteoprogenitor cells into osteoblast. The systemic inflammatory status in SLE may enhance bone resorption, decreasing osteoblast mediated bone formation [31]. In SLE an over-activation of T-cells by oxidized lipids leads to an increment of RANKL production and TNF enhancing the osteoclasts' activity and differentiation [32]. Bone formation may be negatively affected by oxidized LDL involved in a decrease in osteoblast differentiation [33]. Petri et al. reported in the Hopkins Lupus Cohort that low levels of the fraction of complement C4 constitute a risk factor for the development of low BMD in the spine [34].

Osteoimmunology in Osteoporosis Associated with Ankylosing Spondylitis

In AS there is often reduced bone mineral density that enhances bone fragility. Nevertheless, the diagnosis of OP in patients with AS represents a challenge due to the interference of syndesmophytes with bone bridges at lumbar spine that produce an overestimation of lumbar BMD. Ectopic bone formation, which eventually leads to ligament joint fusion, especially vertebrae fusion, has been considered the hallmark of AS. Cytokines with relevance in the pathogenesis of AS including both IL-6 and TNF-α, but Wnt and BMPs also participate [35, 36]. Gratacos et al. found increased serum IL-6 levels and TNF-α levels in patients with AS compared to patients with non-inflammatory lower back pain. They also observed a positive correlation between the increased serum IL-6 levels and disease activity [35]. Wnt is involved as a mediator in the formation of bony spurs and at the same time inhibits bone resorption through OPG induction [36]. Furthermore, BMPs are implicated in the pathway that leads to joint fusion [37]. Taylan et al. observed that serum levels of the Wnt pathway inhibitors, such as Dkk-1 and sclerostin, had no differences between patients with AS and control groups [38]. However, other authors have found different results. Appel et al. assessed the expression of sclerostin by immunohistochemistry in patients with AS; they observed a significant reduction of the expression of sclerostin [39].

Heiland et al. evaluated the relationship between the presence of syndesmophytes and the serum levels of Dkk-1 in patients with AS. They found that in patients with no syndesmophyte development the serum levels of Dkk-1 were significantly higher compared with patients with formation of syndesmophytes [40]. Inflammatory infiltrates formation in the bone marrow in AS is related to vertebral osteoporosis [36]. Appel et al. observed an increased quantity of T and B cells and persistent inflammation in zygapophyseal joints of patients with AS compared to non-AS controls, implying the role of these features in the pathophysiology of AS [41]. Unlike the pathogenesis of RA, in AS the bone-remodeling balance is in favor of bone formation instead of bone resorption, sustained by the upregulation of the Wnt pathway.

Osteoimmunology in Osteoporosis Associated with Psoriatic Arthritis

In psoriatic arthritis (PsA) there is a focal bone erosion mediated by osteoclasts at the bone–pannus junction [42]. This increased bone erosion is mediated by an increase of osteoclastogenic factors with increasing numbers of osteoclasts. Dalbeth et al. observed in a cross-sectional study that patients with PsA presented higher serum levels Dkk-1 and M-CSF compared with healthy controls and patients with psoriasis without arthritis [43]. These authors also observed a positive correlation of M-CSF and RANKL levels with bone erosions. On the other hand, Ritchlin et al. observed that in bone samples of PsA patients there is a large number of osteoclast resorption pits at the bone-pannus junction and subchondral bone. These authors also found a greater amount of osteoclast precursor cells in the blood samples of patients with PsA compared with healthy controls, being higher in those patients with erosive arthritis [44]. Colucci et al. observed in osteoclastogenesis models of PsA that osteoclastogenesis is regulated by an overexpression of RANKL, TNF-α and IL-7 of T cells [45].

Osteoimmunology in Osteoporosis Associated with Gout

It has been suggested by Chhana et al. that in patients with tophaceous gout there is an abnormality of the bone turnover on bone-tophus interface, with an increase of osteoclasts and decrease of osteoblasts, leading to severe bone resorption. They also reported that the addition of monosodium urate crystals (MSU) to osteoblast cultures reduces the osteoblast viability [46]. Lee et al. observed that the osteoblast inhibition by adding MSU could be explained through the induction of IL-1, IL-6 and TNF-α expression in infiltrated mononuclear cells; meanwhile, RANKL was expressed in T cells [47]. Dalbeth et al. reported that peripheral blood, synovial fluid and tophus had an increased quantity of osteoclasts. Therefore, there is a positive correlation between RANKL serum levels and severe erosive and tophaceous gout where there is presence of multinucleated cells with osteoclast markers at sites of bone erosion [48]. Lee et al. found that tartrate-resistant acid phosphatase (TRAP+) osteoclasts were present in tophi samples of patients with gout, suggesting their contribution to bone erosions [47].

Osteoimmunology in Osteoporosis Associated with Osteoarthritis

Although osteoarthritis (OA) does not constitute a CIRD, an evaluation of the mechanisms of bone resorption is relevant. An alteration in the metabolism and function of osteoblasts has been observed in OA (49). Hopwood et al. found abnormalities in genes encoding WNT and TGF-β1/BMP signaling pathway genes. They suggest that this alteration affecting the OA bone microenvironment causes an imbalance in bone remodeling [50]. Two different groups of OA osteoblasts have been distinguished in OA: low OA osteoblasts, associated with low levels of prostaglandin E2 (PGE2) and IL-6, similar to normal cells; and high OA osteoblasts associated with high levels of PGE2 and IL-6 [51]. In high OA osteoblasts extracted from subchondral bone there is an increase of OPG with a decrement of expression of RANKL and the OPG/RANKL ratio where there is higher osteoblast compared with normal and low osteoblast [49]. Moreover, Ephrin type-B receptor 4 (EphB4) is highly expressed in osteoclast extracted from subchondral bone and its activation by the specific ligand ephrin B2 inhibits the expression of IL-1β, IL-6 and RANKL, but not of OPG [52]. These data together could be the explanation for the abnormal metabolism in OA subchondral bone by inhibiting resorption factors and their activities and the presence of a higher bone mineral density in OA.

Zoledronic Acid in Animal Models for Chronic Inflammatory Rheumatic Diseases

A better understanding of the role of osteoclasts in the development of pathological bone erosion in several rheumatic disorders - particularly RA - has led to consideration of these cells as a therapeutic target to preserve the bone integrity in inflammatory arthritis. Currently, the most accepted drugs for the inhibition of osteoclast-mediated bone resorption are bisphosphonates [53]; of these ZA has the major antiresorptive potency [54]. Although in CIRD this bisphosphonate not only acts as antiresorptive, but ZA also has a suppressive effect of the bone resorption through the inhibition of the formation and survival of osteoclast contributing to the observed effectiveness for the prevention of bone mass loss. Table 3 summarizes the studies regarding the use of ZA in animal models. Le Goff et al., in a collagen-induced arthritis (CIA) model, evaluated the effect of ZA as monotherapy versus the combination of ZA plus methotrexate (MTX) for preventing bone erosions. They observed that the combination of ZA plus MTX prevents bone erosion and radiological damage, and decreases generalized bone loss, therefore increasing the BMD [55]. Sims et al. evaluated the effects of ZA on juxtaarticular bone in a CIA model through micro-computed tomography analysis. These authors observed an increment in the trabecular bone in those animals treated with ZA, decreasing the bone erosions with a correlation of this decrement with the utilized doses. Therefore, on the basis of these results, Sims et al. suggested that the anti-erosive effect of ZA is dose-dependent [56].

In another study, Herrak et al., evaluated the decrement in the rate of bone erosions in an inflammation model for systemic bone loss using human TNF-transgenic (hTNFtg) mice after application of a single-dose of ZA. They observed that ZA prevents the development of bone erosions, increasing total bone density by 30% and cortical thickness by 84%, measured by micro-CT scans of tibial bones. On the other hand, repeated application of ZA shows a 58% increment in total bone density and a 96% increment in cortical thickness.

A main reason for the gain in bone density influenced by ZA was essentially the consequence of an increase in trabecular bone density. In contrast, ZA had no influence on clinical and histologic sings of inflammation, regardless of whether the application was a single-dose or repeated-dose regimen [54]. In a medial meniscal tear (MMT) rat model Yu et al. evaluated the development and progression of OA in animals treated with ZA. Their results pointed out that ZA, administered in the early stages of OA animal models, improved the subchondral microstructural parameters substantially, decreasing the cartilage degeneration; nevertheless, in animals with a delay in treatment with ZA there were no significant effects on these parameters [57].

Table 3. Zoledronic Acid in Animal Models

Author	Year	Animal Model	Evaluation	Results
Herrak et al. [54]	2004	Systemic inflammatory bone loss model	Bone erosion after a single-dose of ZA	ZA block bone erosion and increase total bone density
Sims et al. [56]	2004	CIA model	Effect of ZA on juxtaarticular bone	Increment of trabecular bone and a dose-dependent anti-erosive effect of ZA
Lories et al. [60]	2008	AS model	Incidence and severity of arthritis and bone formation	No changes in bone formation
Le Goff et al. [55]	2009	CIA model	Effect of ZA (monotherapy) vs ZA plus MTX on bone erosion	ZA plus MTX prevents bone erosion and increases BMD
Strassle et al. [59]	2010	Painful degenerative joint disease model	Radiographic and histological change in BMD with ZA	ZA increases BMD and inhibits cartilage degeneration
Yu et al. [57]	2012	MMT model	The osteoarthritis progression with ZA	Administration of ZA at early stage improved subchondral microstructural parameters and mitigate cartilage degeneration
Cinar et al. [58]	2014	OA model	Effect of intra-articular ZA on synovial tissue and joint cartilage	Less inflammation and necrosis of synovial tissue

ZA: zoledronic acid; CIA: collagen-induced arthritis; AS: ankylosing spondylitis; MTX: methotrexate; BMD: bone mass density; MMT: medial meniscal tear; OA: osteoarthritis.

Cinar et al. evaluated the effects of intra-articular administration of ZA on synovial tissue and joint cartilage in a rat model for OA, observing that the histological inflammation, as well as the necrosis of synovial tissue, was significantly lower in the group receiving ZA compared with the control group. Nevertheless, they did not observe any substantial preventive effect of ZA on the joint cartilage [58]. Strassle et al. evaluated the modifications in BMD after ZA as monotherapy, in a model of painful degenerative joint disease in rats, based on the administration of monosodium iodoacetate (MIA). These authors observed that an early introduction of ZA significantly increases the BMD and inhibits cartilage degeneration, showing dose-dependent responses [59]. Several animal models for AS show that ZA has conflicting results regarding the protective effect of disease progression. Lories et al., in an animal model for AS using DBA/1 mice, evaluated the rate of bone formation associated with ankylosis after the administration of ZA. These authors did not observe a significant change in the bone formation after intensive treatment with ZA for 14 weeks [60]. These data regarding AS models remain controversial and further investigations are required.

RHEUMATOID ARTHRITIS, OSTEOPOROSIS AND ZOLEDRONIC ACID

Rheumatoid arthritis (RA) is a chronic inflammatory disease affecting synovial joints, characteristically developing bone erosions leading to diverse grades of disability. RA is considered the most frequent type of autoimmune inflammatory arthritis. Pelaez-Ballestas et al. described in a population-based study performed in Mexico that the prevalence of RA is 1.6% (95% CI 1.4-1.8%) [61]. In a Mexican study Morales-Romero et al. reported that RA constitutes the first cause for consultation in Rheumatology services [62]. Osteoporosis (OP) is highly prevalent in patients with RA. Several studies have documented a prevalence for OP of between 22% and 55% [2, 63, 64]. Our group observed that around 24% of 191 patients with a long duration of RA disease had osteoporosis [63]. RA is also associated with a high prevalence of fragility fractures. Ghazi et al., in a case-control study, reported that 21.7% of patients with RA had vertebral fractures [2]. Characteristics associated with OP in RA include epidemiological factors (aging, female gender, menopause, coexistence of other comorbidities), variables associated with the disease (longer disease duration, higher disease activity, positive rheumatoid factor or anti-CCP antibodies, elevated erythrocyte sedimentation rate, higher radiological damage and impairment in functioning) as well as some therapeutic variables (corticosteroids use, MTX utilization, low calcium intake, vitamin D deficiency) [64, 65]. Conversely, an adequate control of the disease is associated with lower prevalence of OP. Whereas, vertebral fractures in RA are closely related to lower spine or femoral T-scores observed in the bone mineral densitometry, as well as longer RA duration, and severe disease activity [3]. Non-vertebral osteoporotic fractures are also increased in RA; variables associated with these fractures include the antecedents of vertebral fractures [2]. In a nested case-control study Roussy et al. identified some factors associated with non–vertebral fractures in patients aged ≥50 years with RA [66]. These authors were unable to identify any substantial protective effect of biological disease-modifying antirheumatic drugs (DMARDs) for the development of non-vertebral fractures. Vis et al., in a 5-year prospective cohort study, evaluated the development of vertebral and non-vertebral fractures [67]. The incidence of new non-vertebral fractures at 5 years was 16% (annual incidence of 3.2 per 100 patients/year) whereas the 5-year incidence of new vertebral osteoporotic fractures was 19% (3.7% per 100 patients/year [67].

This evidence shows that patients with RA have a high risk of osteoporosis as well as vertebral and non-vertebral osteoporotic fractures. Therefore, RA is included in the guidelines of the National Osteoporosis Foundation (NOF) as a risk factor that requires prevention and management for osteoporosis [7]. These guidelines also describe how patients chronically receiving corticosteroids, such as a high proportion of patients with RA, would require prevention with antiresorptive drugs, calcium and vitamin D supplements. Nevertheless, several studies have shown that only a low proportion of patients with RA among those requiring osteoporosis treatment receive anti-osteoporotic therapy. Our group reported the results of a cross-sectional study evaluating 520 patients with RA, and identified that although 79% of the patients chronically received corticosteroids, only 13% had antiresorptive agents [68]. Also, Overman et al. described in a survey that only 28.4% of postmenopausal women and 9.7% of men aged ≥ 50 years self-reported anti-osteoporotic therapy, whereas 81.2% of postmenopausal women and 75.8% of men aged ≥50 were chronic corticosteroid users. These authors concluded that there is a significant gap between the patients truly treated and the patients that require treatment or prevention for corticosteroid-induced osteoporosis [69]. Another concern is that a high proportion of patients with RA are nonadherent to bisphosphonates. Richards et al. evaluated the adherence to bisphosphonates in a retrospective cohort study of 573 patients with RA. These authors observed that approximately half (52.7%) were nonadherent to bisphosphonates [70]. Factors associated with nonadherence in the multivariate analysis were longer disease duration of RA, a duration of bisphosphonate therapy >32 months, and non-Caucasian ethnicity. Additional factors that were associated with nonadherence only in the univariate analysis were lower education (<12 years) and a higher disease activity [70].

Zoledronic Acid in Rheumatoid Arthritis

A significant number of patients with RA have received ZA with the aim of preventing corticosteroid-induced osteoporosis. Reid et al. described the results of a one-year randomized, double dummy non-inferiority study comparing intravenous infusion of ZA versus daily oral risedronate and assessing the percentage change in BMD of the lumbar spine at the end of one year. These authors observed that ZA was more effective in increasing BMD in the lumbar spine, although the frequency of adverse effects was higher in the ZA group, mainly related to transient symptoms during the first 3 days after infusion [71].

Use of Zoledronic Acid as Adjuvant Therapy for Inflammation in Rheumatoid Arthritis

There is a lack of controlled studies evaluating the clinical effects of ZA on disease activity parameters in RA. In a 26-week randomized controlled trial Jarrett et al. evaluated the administration of ZA 5 mg versus placebo in combination with MTX in order to reduce the development of new erosions observed on magnetic resonance image (MRI). These authors found a significant difference in favor of ZA in a lower number of bone erosions in the hands and wrists. The proportion of patients with RA developing new MRI bone edema was lower in the group with ZA compared with the placebo group [72].

In conclusion, in patients with RA an annual administration of ZA (5 mg iv) can be considered an adequate therapeutic option directed to prevent or to treat osteoporosis. ZA should especially be considered in those patients with previous antecedents of osteoporotic fractures, prolonged utilization of corticosteroid therapy and use of polypharmacy. To date, there is not enough information to recommend ZA as an adjunctive therapy to help in the control of disease activity or bone erosions. Nevertheless, the data obtained by a clinical trial suggest that ZA may offer benefits not only in the increase of BMD, but also in reducing the progression of radiological damage. These data need to be reproduced by other studies, increasing the sample size, duration of treatment and assessment of other relevant clinical variables.

SYSTEMIC LUPUS ERYTHEMATOSUS, OSTEOPOROSIS AND ZOLEDRONIC ACID

SLE is a systemic chronic autoimmune disease characterized by persistent inflammation leading to damage to several organs, with the production of autoreactive cells, cytokines and auto-antibodies [73]. Pelaez-Ballestas et al., in their population-based study, identified a prevalence of SLE in Mexico of 0.06 (95%CI 0.03.0.10) [61]. Morales-Romero et al. found that SLE is the second most frequent rheumatic autoimmune disease seen in rheumatology services in Mexico [62]. In these patients the use of corticosteroids as a corner-stone for the treatment of this disease is highly frequent because these drugs are useful to treat some manifestations associated with the inflammation of organs which substantially increases the survival of these patients. Nevertheless, a significant number of adverse effects may result from corticosteroid utilization; some of these side effects can be considered dose and duration dependent [74]. Among these complications, whereas other effects are associated with individual susceptibility, one of the most relevant is the decrement in bone mass and OP, constituting a major health problem to be considered in patients with SLE [75]. In patients with SLE both OP and osteoporotic fractures are relevant complications caused by a multiplicity of factors [31]. The frequency of osteopenia in SLE varies from 24–74% [76, 77], whereas the frequency of OP varies from 1.4 to 68% [78, 79]. These differences across studies are dependent on several factors such as characteristics of the patients (height, age, sex, and ethnicity), variables associated with the disease (disease severity, complications, renal involvement) and factors related to the treatments (corticosteroids doses and other drugs associated with osteoporosis) [1]. Corticosteroid doses differ between patients with different organ involvement and severity of the disease, whereby those with an active disease may receive higher doses of corticosteroids. In a cohort study Boyanov et al. reported that the corticosteroid therapy enhanced bone loss. They observed that 68.7% of their patients treated with corticosteroids had osteoporosis [78]. Other risks factors for OP in SLE are similar to those observed in the general population such as aging, postmenopausal status, and low body weight or low body mass index (BMI). Liyanage has described that low lean body mass is also associated with low BMD in SLE [80]. Most of the studies performed on BMD in SLE exclusively include females; therefore, the frequency of OP in males has been described less frequently. Mok et al. observed a higher decrease in BMD in male patients with SLE compared with healthy controls [81]. Lakshminarayanan et al. observed that ethnicity influences the prevalence of OP in SLE, whereby white women have lower BMD [82]. Ethnicities other than Caucasian seem to play a protective role regarding OP in SLE. Li et al. identified a very low prevalence of OP in their Chinese patients with SLE (4 to 6%), suggesting that the effects of the disease on BMD in these Asian patients with SLE is lower than other populations, even if they receive corticosteroid therapy [83]. In Mexican patients with SLE the frequency observed for OP described by Mendoza-Pinto et al. is 17.7% and factors associated with the presence of vertebral fracture may include chronic disease damage, low BMI, and cumulative corticosteroid dose in pre-menopausal SLE patients [84]. Other epidemiological factors that have been investigated in OP associated with SLE include smoking and excessive alcohol use. Yeap et al. reported a lack of association between smoking and low BMD in SLE [85]. Mok reported that alcohol consumption was associated with bone loss in male lupus patients in Hong Kong [81]. On the other hand, there is an elevated frequency of osteoporotic fractures in SLE. Furukawa et al. reported a prevalence for vertebral fractures in around 50% of their patients with SLE [86]. Li et al. observed that 20.4% of their patients with SLE had asymptomatic vertebral fractures, although they relevantly identified that 30% of patients with vertebral fractures had normal BMD in densitometry [87]. Ekblom-Kullberg et al. observed that the risk of any symptomatic fracture in women with SLE is higher compared to controls [OR=1.8 95% CI 1.3 to 2.4%], but this difference is only observed in females [88]. Bultink et al. reported that corticosteroid use in SLE in the previous 6 months raised the risk of clinical fracture (adjusted RR= 1.27, 95% CI 1.02 to 1.58), other factors associated with clinical fractures being history of cerebrovascular events, seizures and previous OP fractures [89]. Garcia-Carrasco et al. identified that the presence of vertebral fractures is associated with a decreasing quality of life, whereby patients with vertebral fractures have worse physical function [90]. Factors related to the severity of the disease are also related to osteoporotic fractures. Zhu et al., in a five-year cohort study, reported that higher scores for organ damage are related to vertebral fractures, whereas corticosteroid therapy duration and OP at the lumbar spine were factors related to non-vertebral fractures [9]. In a population-based cohort Wang et al. identified an incidence rate for hip fractures in SLE of 8.60 per 10,000 person-years. This incidence was 3.17-fold higher in SLE compared with their controls [8]. Although the high frequency observed of OP in adults with SLE is recognized, in children with SLE there is also a deteriorated BMD. Compeyrot-Lacassagne et al. reported that the prevalence of OP in children with SLE is 20.3%, whereas the frequency of osteopenia is 37.5%. Variables associated with OP in children with SLE in this study were: age of the patients at the time of dual X-ray absorptiometry (DXA), disease duration, cumulative corticosteroid dose, azathioprine, mycophenolate mofetil, cyclophosphamide, history of nephritis, renal biopsy showing class III–IV lupus nephritis and damage [91].

Zoledronic Acid in Systemic Lupus Erythematosus

The NOF guidelines and Food and Drug Administration (FDA) approved ZA as a drug for the prevention and treatment of OP in men and women expected to be on corticosteroid therapy for at least 12 months. ZA is also indicated for the prevention of new clinical fractures in patients who have recently had a low-trauma hip fracture [7]. The American College of Rheumatology (ACR) in 2010 published recommendations for the prevention and treatment of corticosteroid-induced osteoporosis. Among their recommendations are weight-bearing activities, smoking cessation, and diagnostic methods like DXA, orientated to identify the Fracture Risk Assessment (FRAX) score.

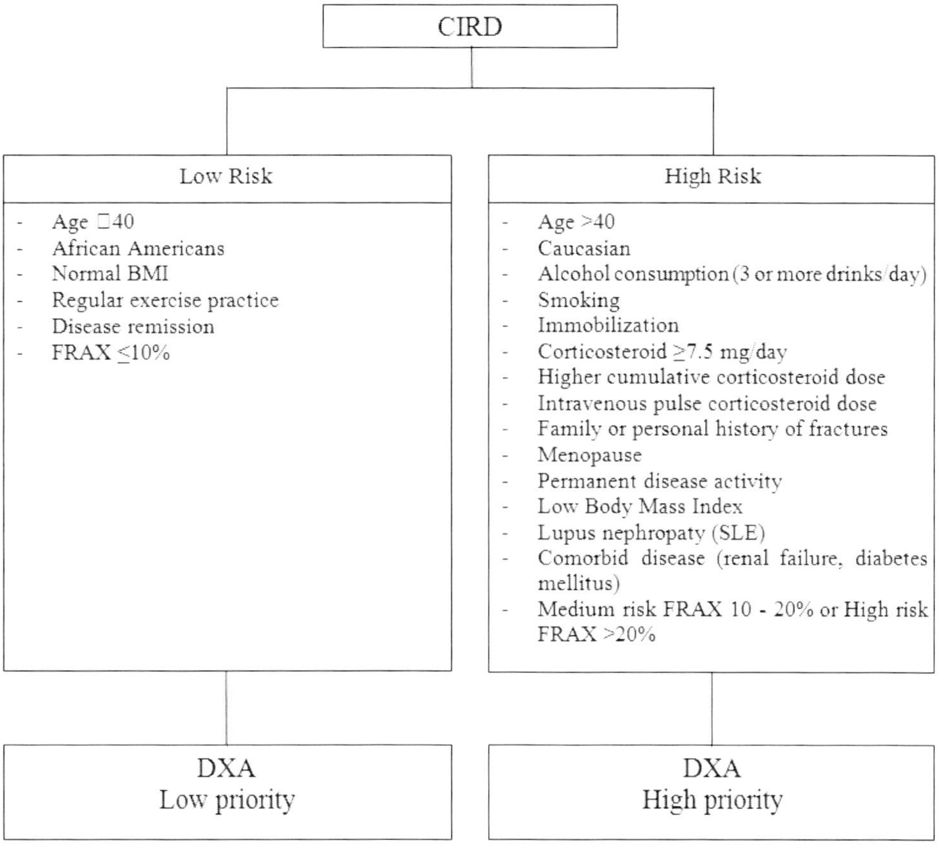

Flowchart 1. Clinical features to consider the evaluation of BMD with dual X-ray absorptiometry (DXA).

In patients considered at low risk, if corticosteroid doses are <7.5 mg/day, no pharmacological treatment is recommended, but in patients with >7.5 mg/day these guidelines recommend the use of bisphosphonates (alendronate, risedronate or ZA) [6]. Administration of ZA in SLE has special considerations and requires an adequate evaluation of the patient's characteristics; two of them are oriented to evaluate whether the patients may or may have not a renal or cardiovascular involvement. Lupus nephropathy (LN) is a frequent complication in SLE. Feldman et al. in the United States observed that the prevalence of LN was 30.9%; Pons-Estel et al. in a Latin American cohort observed the frequency of LN was 17.9% [92]. Active LN or a deteriorated creatinine clearance secondary to this nephritis, therefore, may contraindicate ZA administration. It is highly relevant to take into account in patients under ZA treatment that around one-third of the dose administrated IV is excreted by glomerular filtration; therefore, in patients with SLE, ZA must not be recommended in patients with a creatinine clearance lower than 35 mL/min [93]. Any patient with SLE candidate for ZA must be evaluated for renal function. Thus, it is recommended to avoid the administration of ZA in those patients with a diagnosis of moderate or severe nephropathy. Following the administration of ZA, some patients may also decrease creatinine clearance or increase the creatinine levels; therefore, these levels should be monitored [93]. On the other hand, cardiac manifestations are another relevant clinical feature in patients with SLE. Garcia et al. reported the prevalence of arrhythmia in SLE of 11.4 % of a Latin American cohort [94]. This feature should be considered as indicating among those patients a candidate to receive ZA, because this bisphosphonate is associated with the development of arrhythmias, particularly in oncology patients. Yazici et al. reported that the frequency of development of arrhythmias with ZA infusion in patients with bone metastasis is high, reaching 28.8% for supraventricular premature complexes and 26.9% for ventricular premature complexes during the infusion period [95]. Nevertheless, these data described by Yazici et al. cannot be extrapolated to SLE and ZA patients need to be assessed for arrhythmias. Studies reporting ZA in specific patients with juvenile SLE are rare. Souza et al. reported a case of a 13-year-old Caucasian girl with a diagnosis of SLE and vertebral fractures localized in the thoracic vertebrae (T2 and T5) with a DXA study showing low BMD in the spine, femoral neck and whole body. This girl received ZA (4 mg, once). The new BMD measurements after 6 months showed an increase in BMD of 52% in the spine; an increase of 12.8% in the femoral neck; and an increase of 11.2% for the whole body [96].

In conclusion, there is a lack of controlled-clinical trials evaluating the efficacy of ZA in the specific group of patients with SLE. This bisphosphonate administration should be considered to prevent or to treat osteoporosis, mainly during periods of inactive disease. This is an interesting research area that requires well-designed prospective cohorts as well as controlled-clinical trials. Nevertheless, this bisphosphonate is not recommended in patients with nephritis, myocarditis or arrhythmias, and patients' creatinine levels need to be supervised after the administration of this bisphosphonate.

Spondyloarthritis, Osteoporosis and Zoledronic Acid

Spondyloarthropathies constitute a group of inflammatory diseases affecting the spine, sacroiliac joints, and sites of enthesis, as well as peripheral joints and other periarticular structures. These diseases are usually linked with positivity for the human leucocyte antigen type B 27 (HLA-B27), and are usually negative rheumatoid factor. Among the most frequent spondyloarthropathies are ankylosing spondylitis (AS), Reiter's syndrome, psoriatic arthritis (PsA), arthritis related to inflammatory bowel diseases and undifferentiated spondyloarthropathy. In a community-based study Pelaez-Ballestas et al. have reported a prevalence of SpA in the Mexican population of 0.6% [97]. Our group observed that AS constituted one of the first five most frequent inflammatory joint disorders seen in rheumatology services in Mexico, with two-thirds of the affected patients being male [62]. Osteoporosis is highly prevalent in most of the series evaluating BMD in AS, although most of the studies included only male patients. These studies show that OP frequency varies largely from 19 to 62% [98, 99]. Although these studies differ substantially in the characteristics of the population being included, particularly in variables related to OP such as age or gender (some papers included males only, whereas other articles include patients of both sexes); also, there are differences across the studies in disease duration, disease severity, and treatments. Other relevant differences between these works are the study designs (retrospective, cross-sectional or cohorts) and the methods used to establish OP (dual energy x-ray absorptiometry, quantitative computed tomography). Some studies even differ in the anatomical regions being assessed by DXA (some articles included only the spine and hip, whereas others also evaluated the forearm). Some of these data are shown in a systematic review published by van der Weijden et al., assessing the studies of the prevalence of low-bone mineral density in patients with AS [100]. Vertebral fractures in AS are more prevalent than those observed in the general population. Muñoz-Ortego et al., in a case-control study based in a large population-based public health database in Spain, compared the frequency of vertebral and non-vertebral fractures in 6,474 patients with AS with 32,346 matched controls, identifying that the patients with AS had a higher frequency of vertebral fractures (0.86%) than the control group (0.41%). This increase in prevalence was also observed in non-vertebral fractures in the group with AS versus the controls (3.4% versus 2.7%, respectively). In the adjusted analysis these authors observed that AS is associated with a higher risk of vertebral fractures (hazard ratio 1.93, 95% CI 1.39 to 2.68, $p<0.001$) and also a higher risk of non-vertebral fractures (hazard ratio 1.19 95% CI 1.02 to 1.39, $p=0.03$) [101]. Nevertheless, due to most vertebral fractures being asymptomatic, the prevalence of vertebral fractures increases when they are systematically evaluated with a radiological method. Klingberg et al. identified that 12% of their 204 patients with AS had vertebral fractures; most of them had not been previously diagnosed [102]. Factors associated with vertebral fractures are aging, smoking, longer disease duration, higher scores of radiological damage, higher impairment in metrology index, major impact of the disease as perceived by the patients, postmenopausal status in women, and low BMD in the spine or femoral neck [102]. Spinal fractures in AS can be of three types: a) fractures of the vertebral body, b) fractures affecting the components of the dorsal arch and c) fractures of the syndesmophytes (calcified ligaments in AS) [99]. Bone turnover markers are not consistently increased in AS, reflecting the complexity of the disease and its bone repercussion. Taylan et al. described the utility of several biomarkers and cytokines related to bone turnover including OPG, serum band 5 tartrate-resistant acid phosphatase (TRAP-5), bone-specific alkaline phosphatase (BAP), cross-linked N-telopeptide of type I collagen (NTx), sRANKL, secreted frizzled-related protein 1 (sFRP-1), Dickkopf-related protein 1 (DKK-1), and sclerostin [38]. They found no significant statistical differences between patients with AS and controls; they only observed in AS patients lower serum OPG levels and a higher RANKL/OPG ratio compared to healthy controls [38]. Nevertheless, in another study Chen et al. identified that the serum levels of sRANKL and OPG were significantly higher in AS patients than in healthy controls [103].

On the other hand, Arends et al. examined the serum levels of markers for bone formation (procollagen type 1 N-terminal peptide (PINP) and osteocalcin (OC)), as well as markers for bone resorption (serum C-telopeptides of type I collagen (sCTX)). These authors adjusted the serum levels of these biomarkers by the Z-scores of BMD. According to their results, the sCTX Z-score and OC Z-score were independently related to low BMD in AS [104]. In another study, Arends et al. evaluated in a cohort study the effect of anti-TNF therapy on markers of bone turnover in AS [105]. These authors observe that the treatment with anti-TNF agents increased bone-specific alkaline phosphatase (bone formation biomarker); there was a decreased serum collagen-telopeptide (sCTX), (bone resorption biomarker) in concordance with an increasing BMD in the lumbar spine [105].

Zoledronic Acid in Spondyloarthritis

There is some evidence that the addition of bisphosphonates to the therapy increases the BMD in AS. Kang et al. suggested that the combination of bisphosphonates plus anti-TNF therapy may significantly increase the BMD in AS [106]. Bisphosphonates may also have anti-inflammatory properties in spondyloarthropathies.

CIRD

Consider treatment with bisphosphosnates if:

- History of any osteoporotic fracture
- T-score $\leq$ -2.5 at femoral neck or spine
- Low bone mass (T-score between -1.0 and -2.5 at femoral neck or spine) + Age > 50 + postmenopause
- Higher daily corticosteroid dose Prednisone $\geq$ 7.5 mg/day*
- Higher cumulative corticosteroid dose
- A significant decrease in BMD between 2 different measurements
- Higher levels of bone turnover markers

Bisphosphonates

Alendronate
Risedronate
Zoledronic Acid

*Predictable or prevailing duration of > 3 months of corticosteroid therapy.

Flowchart 2. Considerations to indicate treatment with bisphosphonates.

Toussirot et al. reviewed the evidence of pamidronate in AS, concluding that most of the evidence is based on open trials that observe an effect of pamidronate in the improvement of clinical symptoms of AS, particularly in axial disease, although it may also have an effect on peripheral arthritis [107]. Maksymowych et al. performed a six-month randomized, controlled, double-blind trial comparing two different doses of intravenous pamidronate (60 mg versus 10 mg) in the treatment of AS refractory to nonsteroidal anti-inflammatory drugs [108]. These authors observed a significant improvement in the clinical scales for disease activity (BASDAI), functioning (BASFI), and other clinical scales in favor of pamidronate 60-mg [108]. Supporting that, the anti-inflammatory effects of pamidronate are dose-pendent. Viapiana et al. evaluated the anti-inflammatory effects of neridronate (100 mg iv, monthly) versus infliximab (5 mg/kg) therapy in a 6-month open-label, single-center study on patients with active AS [109].

These authors observed an improvement in BASDAI, axial pain and BASFI at 3 months, and all of these parameters also improved in both arms over 6 months except for functioning, where the improvement was observed only in the neridronate arm. At the end of the study no significant differences were found between neridronate versus infliximab in the clinical parameters although the arms of the patients treated with neridronate had a significant increase in BMD at the lumbar spine [109]. Anti-TNF agents are currently considered the "gold standard" for the treatment of AS; nevertheless, there is a proportion of patients that have no response to these therapies. A therapeutic alternative is the application of adjuvant therapy to these agents. To date, there is a lack of controlled-clinical trials evaluating whether ZA may play a role as adjuvant therapy in the management of disease activity in patients with AS. However, recent information derived from a non-controlled study hallmarks the relevance of testing ZA in the treatment of spondyloarthropathies, particularly in AS. Clunie et al. evaluated in an open pilot trial the effects of ZA on osteitis lesions in AS using an MRI index [110]. These authors included 7 patients who had osteitis in MRI, observing an improvement in 4/7 patients after 3 months of the ZA 5 mg infusion. After 6 months of the infusion 6 of 7 patients achieved an improvement of the osteitis as well as in the symptomatology related to the inflammatory activity [110].

Although this is the first report observing that ZA may reduce spinal osteitis in AS. This evidence is relevant because osteitis is associated with syndesmophyte formation; the lack of a controlled parallel group makes it necessary to consider this study only as exploratory, and their results as preliminary, requiring validation by further randomized controlled-clinical trials. Therefore, this information generates important questions about the role of ZA in SpA which require the most intensive research.

In conclusion, to date there is some evidence derived from cohort studies that identifies the benefits of the administration of bisphosphonates in increasing BMD. ZA can be considered a therapeutic option in the prevention of osteoporotic fractures in AS and other spondyloarthropathies. A significant proportion of patients with AS or other spondyloarthritis have antecedents of uveitis. However, there is a lack of information about the development of uveitis flares secondary to ZA administration in SpA, including AS patients with uveitis associated to spondyloarthropathies. These patients should probably be excluded from ZA treatment.

This recommendation is based on the published information of uveitis development after ZA administration in postmenopausal patients [111]. An assessment of a comparison between ZA versus other bisphosphonates is required to evaluate the efficacy, tolerability, adherence and permanence of the effects in this group of patients.

PSORIATIC ARTHRITIS, OSTEOPOROSIS AND ZOLEDRONIC ACID

Psoriatic arthritis (PsA) is a chronic inflammatory musculoskeletal disease related to psoriasis and characterized by inflammation of the synovial joints, loss of function and a diminished quality of life, most of the time associated with negativity for rheumatoid factor. Setty et al., in a systematic review, reported a prevalence of PsA in different studies from 0.02% to 0.25% [112]. In Mexico there is a lack of data about the prevalence of the disease although PsA is considerably observed with lower frequency compared with other CIRD. Busquets et al. have estimated the prevalence of osteoporosis in PsA at around 16% and identified a frequency for osteoporotic fractures in these patients of about 13% [5]. Pedreira et al. estimated the prevalence of any osteoporotic fractures is 33.3% in postmenopausal PsA patients [113].

Zoledronic Acid in Psoriatic Arthritis

To date there is a lack of systematized studies evaluating the effects of ZA on PsA. Using PubMed with the key words "psoriatic arthritis", "treatment" AND "zoledronic acid" we were able to identify only one randomized controlled trial evaluating the efficacy of ZA in PsA. McQueen et al. evaluated the efficacy of the administration of ZA versus placebo on bone erosions in PsA using MRI. This trial shows that ZA decreased the findings of bone edema, although it did not improve bone erosions in these patients [114]. This study has two important limitations: firstly, a limited sample-size that might be associated with insufficient statistical power to identify significant differences between those treated with ZA and those not treated; and secondly, an insufficient length of follow-up that may decrease the probability of detecting significant changes in patients under treatment with ZA, especially on the erosion score of the MRI. Nonetheless, the results of the study encourage the performance of new controlled-clinical trials with a larger sample of patients with a longer follow-up time in order to put into place the possible protective effect of ZA on articular erosions of patients with PsA.

GOUT, OSTEOPOROSIS AND ZOLEDRONIC ACID

Gout is a chronic debilitating disorder caused by the deposition of monosodium urate crystals within joints after chronic hyperuricaemia [115, 116]. Acute gout is a painful form of arthritis, characterized by swelling, erythema and the abrupt onset of severe joint pain [117]. Prevalence of gout in the population varies from 0.26% to 3.7% [118]. In Mexico, Pelaez-Ballestas reported the prevalence of gout as 0.3% [61]. Tophaceous gout is a complication of gout whereby bone erosions can lead to joint damage, structural deformities and musculoskeletal disability [119]. The prevalence of these bone erosions in gout varies from 33.8 to 49.4% [120].

Zoledronic Acid in Gout

In a randomized controlled trial Dalbeth et al. evaluated the effect of a 5 mg annual administration of ZA versus placebo on the bone erosions of tophaceous gout during two-years' follow-up. Although these authors did not observe a significant improvement in bone erosions, administration of ZA was associated with an increase in BMD on the spine, neck of the femur, total hip and total body and with a significant decrement in some clinical variables such as the frequency of gout attacks, improvement in functioning, pain and patient global assessment [121]. Therefore, from these data we can conclude that additional controlled studies are required to determine the utility of ZA on bone erosions, decrement of gout attacks or other clinically relevant variables in patients with tophaceous gout. This important area of research should be explored by further studies.

Osteoarthritis, Osteoporosis and Zoledronic Acid

Although osteoarthritis (OA) is not considered in the spectrum of CRID, it is one of the most frequent rheumatic disorders diagnosed in the general population. OA is a chronic disease characterized by deterioration of articular cartilage of the joints with subchondral bone remodeling and associated symptoms including pain, aches, or stiffness in the affected joint [122, 123]. According to the study performed by Zhang et al., it is estimated that about 13.3% of men and 26.2% of women have at least one hand joint affected by symptomatic OA [124]. Felson et al., in a population-based study, observed that 11% of women and 7% of men had symptomatic OA in the knees [125]. In Mexico the prevalence of OA is 10.5% [61]. Therefore, OA constitutes one of the most frequent causes of consultation due to musculoskeletal disorders, especially at the primary care level. Several authors have suggested that there is an inverse relationship between OA and osteoporosis [126-129]; in fact, studies using DXA have shown an increase of BMD in OA. Nevertheless, there is controverted information regarding whether or not OA decreases fracture risk. Some have correlated the high BMD with increasing fracture risk [130, 131], whereas other groups have observed a decrement of the risk for osteoporotic fractures associated with an increase of BMD in OA [132, 133]. This discrepancy regarding the correlation of BMD with risk of fracture between studies on fractures in OA may be caused by many factors, including the type of OA, characteristics of the patients selected for the study, and the method of OA assessment which may differ between studies.

Zoledronic Acid in Osteoarthritis

Pain is the most prominent and disabling symptom of OA. Arthritic pain is associated with worse functioning outcomes and decrement in the scores of quality of life compared with other chronic conditions [134]. Among a multiplicity of hypotheses about the causes of pain in this disease, it has been suggested that in patients with OA there is a loss of the osteochondral integrity that may expose subchondral nerves to pro-inflammatory cytokines and other molecules that mediate pain, allowing the growth of sensory nerves in the cartilage and causing increased bone pain [135]. Furthermore, it has been suggested that osteoclast triggers the activation and sensitization of the nerves through a reduction in the pH level of the subchondral junction [136, 137]. Bisphosphonates have been evaluated in the treatment of pain in OA. Davis et al. reported in a systemic review the evidence related to the use of bisphosphonates in OA. After the review of 13 controlled trials, these authors concluded that there is strong evidence that the use of bisphosphonates decreases the pain related to OA in studies compared with placebo or non-treatment controls in OA [138]. In a randomized placebo controlled clinical trial, Laslett et al. compared the effects of a single infusion of ZA (5 mg) versus placebo on knee pain and bone marrow lesions (BML) [139]. This clinical trial shows significant improvement in pain at 6 months and BML evaluated by the Visual Analog Scale (VAS) and MRI, respectively. However, this difference did not remain at 12 months. Furthermore, there was no change in knee injury, OA outcome score or total bone marrow lesions.

Zoledronic Acid in Hypertrophic Osteoarthropathy (HOA)

Hypertrophic osteoarthropathy (HOA) is a syndrome characterized by a combination of digital clubbing, joint and bone pain, and proliferative periostitis [140]. The results of ZA administration have been described in some HOA case reports. There is a case report of a 62-year-old woman with pain and inflammatory polyarthritis who had treatment failure with low doses of prednisone, tramadol and pamidronate infusion. After administration of ZA the pain completely resolved without recurrence [141]. These results suggest the need for controlled studies that evaluate whether ZA can be considered in the management of bone and joint pain associated with HOA.

Autoimmune Diseases Associated with the Use of Zoledronic Acid

ZA produces adverse drug reactions including hypersensitivity reactions. The principal side effect of ZA is the induction of an acute phase reaction. The mechanism for this response seems to be related to a release of pro-inflammatory cytokines, particularly TNF-α and IL-6 [142]. Some case reports have described an association between ZA and the development of symptoms and signs of rheumatic diseases. One example is the development of dermatomyositis, an infrequent but severe CIRD characterized by inflammatory myopathy involving mainly striated muscles, which causes muscle weakness as well as cutaneous involvement with a typical skin rash with a heliotrope rash – of a purple or violet color - observed on the upper eyelids and a Gottron rash characterized by a violaceous rash or papules at the knuckles, predominantly in metacarpophalangeal or interphalangeal joints. A case series describes the development of dermatomyositis after the administration of a single dose of 5 mg of zoledronic acid in two patients diagnosed with osteoporosis. None of them had previous history of symptoms related to myositis [143, 144]. The time for development of dermatomyositis after ZA administration was different in both patients although the diagnosis of dermatomyositis in both was confirmed. Although case reports are unable to establish a definite causal relationship and usually the patients are taking other drugs related to autoimmune reactions, these aspects should alert the clinician to the need to evaluate these rare effects. On the other hand, there is one case report of an 82-year-old patient diagnosed with giant cell arteritis who developed vision loss following the administration of ZA [145]. Vision loss is a well-recognized complication in patients with giant cell arteritis [146]; however, in the case described by Metyas et al. there was vision loss shortly after ZA infusion. Therefore, the physician should be aware of this potential complication of ZA in patients with giant cell arteritis. A hypothesis for this worsening is that ZA administration may promote the impairment of arterial wall inflammation secondary to release of pro-inflammatory cytokines with a thickness of the intimal layer of the arterial wall that leads to vision loss. On the other hand, ZA infusion is associated with arthralgias, regional or diffuse musculoskeletal pain or infrequently with joint swelling [111]. Therefore, it may increase the symptoms in patients with a subjacent chronic rheumatic disease. There is a case report of one woman who developed a flare of symptoms related to hand osteoarthritis after ZA; this exacerbation probably resulted from a release of pro-inflammatory cytokines induced by this bisphosphonate [147].

SAPHO and Zoledronic Acid

SAPHO (synovitis, acne, pustulosis, hyperostosis, and osteitis) is a chronic disorder characterized by an inflammatory condition with skin and osteoarticular manifestations [148]. Due to the presence of osteitis and periostitis, bisphosphonates have been proposed in the treatment of SAPHO [148]. Kopterides et al. described a case report of a patient with SAPHO syndrome who received ZA in order to improve jaw pain due to SAPHO. After three consecutive years of administration of 4 mg of ZA, the patient had no episode of jaw pain and discontinued NSAIDs, and the bone scan revealed significant improvement [149].

Zoledronic Acid in Corticosteroid-Induced Osteoporosis

Chronic treatment with corticosteroids in CIRD is associated with bone mineral loss and increase in the rate of development of fractures. There is clinical evidence that ZA is useful to treat patients with OP secondary to long-term corticosteroid utilization. Devogelaer et al. compared in a study the effects of ZA versus oral risedronate on bone turnover markers in patients with corticosteroids induced OP [150].

These authors observed a significant difference favoring ZA in reducing β-C-terminal telopeptides of type 1 collagen (β-CTx), N-terminal telopeptide of type I collagen (NTx), procollagen type 1 N-terminal propeptide (P1NP) and bone-specific alkaline phosphatase (BSAP) levels in these patients independently of corticosteroid dose [150]. In another study Sambrook et al. compared the responses between ZA and risedronate in male patients with corticosteroid-induced osteoporosis [151].

Table 4. Prevalence of OP in Rheumatoid Arthritis

Author, Year, Country	Study	Patients	Control group	Osteoporosis (%)
Chen, 2014, China [154]	Cross sectional	110	110	33.6
Gonzalez-Lopez, 2012, Mexico [63]	Cross sectional	191	No	24.1
Mobini M, 2012, Iran [65]	Cross sectional	121	No	32.3
Lee SG, 2012, Korea [155]	Cross sectional	299	246	22.1
Ghazi, 2012, France [2]	Cross sectional	101	303	55.4
Dao, 2011, Vietnam [156]	Cross sectional	105	105	37
El Maghraoui, 2010, Morocco [157]	Cross sectional	172	No	44.2
Zhang J, 2010, USA [158]	Cross sectional	141	No	44.9
Haugen, 2007, Norway [159]	Cross sectional	194	122	19.4
Westhoff, 2007, Germany [160]	Cross sectional	967	No	11.3
Nolla, 2006, Spain [161]	Cross sectional	187	No	21
Ørstavik,2004, Norway [162]	Cross sectional	147	51	30.6
Lodder, 2004, Netherlands [163]	Cross sectional	373	No	12.6

The selected studies were included if they had a sample size $\geq$ 100 patients with RA, assessed by BMD.

Table 5. Prevalence of Vertebral and Non-vertebral Fracture in Rheumatoid Arthritis

Author, Year, Country	Type of study	Patients	Control group	Vertebral fracture (%)	Non-vertebral fracture (%)
Lee, 2014, Canada [164]	Cross sectional	100	No	47	-
Ghazi, 2012, France [2]	Cross sectional	101	303	21.7	-
El Maghraoui, 2010, Morocco [157]	Cross sectional	172	No	36	-
Nampei, 2008, Japan [165]	Cross sectional	209	No	11.5	-
Baskan, 2007, Turkey [166]	Cross sectional	100	56	30	-
Arai, 2006, Japan [167]	Cross sectional	117	62	21	-
Ørstavik,2004, Norway [162]	Cross sectional	147	51	22.1	17.3
Lodder, 2004, Netherlands [163]	Cross sectional	373	No	15.3	-

These authors observed that ZA was superior to risedronate in increasing the BMD of the lumbar spine at 12 months; also, they described a greater reduction in serum β-CTx and P1NP obtained with ZA compared with risedronate [151].

Similar data were reported previously by Reid et al. in a 1-year randomized, double-blind, double-dummy, non-inferiority study, observing that ZA was superior to risedronate for increasing the BMD of the lumbar spine in both the prevention and treatment groups of osteoporosis induced by corticosteroids [71]. Reid et al. identified a reduction in the risk of fractures with ZA compared with placebo even in those who received a single dose [152]. Zhang et al. identified in a meta-analysis of placebo-controlled trials that ZA reduces the rate of fracture compared with placebo [153].

Conclusion

Osteoporosis is highly prevalent in CIRD. Tables 4 and 5 show selected studies on the prevalence of OP and osteoporotic fractures in RA, respectively. Tables 6 and 7 describe the prevalence of OP in SLE and osteoporotic fractures in several cross-sectional studies from different countries. Tables 8 and 9 show the prevalence of OP and osteoporotic fractures in AS reported by some cross-sectional studies. Finally, Table 10 summarizes the prevalence of OP in PsA.

Table 6. Prevalence of Osteoporosis in Systemic Lupus Erythematosus

Author, Year, Country	Type of study	Patients	Control group	Osteoporosis (%)
Jacobs, 2013, Netherlands [75]	Cross sectional	126	No	6.3
Lee, 2012, Canada [168]	Cross sectional	271	No	14.6
Souto, 2012, Brazil [4]	Cross sectional	159	No	28
Mendoza-Pinto, 2009, Mexico [84]	Cross sectional	210	No	17.7
Almehed, 2007, Sweden [169]	Cross sectional	163	No	23
Lee, 2006, USA [170]	Cross sectional	307	No	6.9
Bultink,2005, Netherlands [171]	Cross sectional	107	No	4
Yee, 2005, *United Kingdom [172]*	Cross sectional	242	No	10.2
Pineau, 2004, Canada [173]	Cross sectional	205	No	18

The selected studies were included if they had a sample size of ≥ 100 patients with SLE, assessed by BMD.

These tables highlight the epidemiological relevance of OP in CIRD and therefore, treatments oriented to prevent or to treat osteoporotic fractures in these patients. Bisphosphonates plus calcium and vitamin D supplements constitute a well-validated therapeutic strategy for these patients. However, among the CIRD most of the patients treated with bisphosphonates reported in trials have RA. ZA has a well-recognized benefit in the prevention of glucocorticoid induced OP, in patients with established OP or oriented to prevent the decrement in bone mass. After examining the evidence of ZA in CIRD, we can conclude that this bisphosphonate constitutes a therapeutic option to prevent or treat osteoporosis in CIRD. In most of these diseases there is conclusive evidence of an increase in the rate of osteoporotic fractures (asymptomatic in a relevant proportion). Therefore, a structured evaluation of osteoporosis and fractures should be considered in patients with CIRD, mainly in those with severe or persistent disease activity, chronic use of corticosteroids, or those with other epidemiological risk factors for OP. ZA should be considered as a therapeutic option offering a demonstrated efficacy in reducing fracture risk in postmenopausal OP or in patients chronically receiving corticosteroids but this evidence needs to be confirmed by controlled studies in patients with specific CIRD. Some patients with CIRD may develop a worsening of articular symptoms or even develop a flare of the disease after ZA administration. To date, there has been some evidence of an additional effect of ZA in improving the symptoms of inflammatory joint diseases as well as some evidence observed in image studies, but this information is still inconclusive regarding clinical decisions oriented to the possible role of ZA as adjuvant therapy in CIRD.

Table 7. Prevalence of Vertebral and Non-vertebral Fracture in Systemic Lupus Erythematosus

Author, Year, Country	Type of study	Patients	Control Group	Vertebral fracture (%)	Non-vertebral fracture (%)
Zhu, 2014, China [9]	Cross sectional	127	No	0.94	1.26
Ekblom-Kullberg, 2013, Finland [88]	Cross sectional	222	720	-	42
Lee, 2012, Canada [168]	Cross sectional	271	No	-	9.4
Almehed, 2010, Sweden [169]	Cross sectional	150	No	29	-
Li, 2009, China [87]	Cross sectional	152	No	20.4	-
Mendoza-Pinto, 2009, Mexico [84]	Cross sectional	210	No	26.1	-
Bultink, 2005, Netherlands [171]	Cross sectional	107	No	20	-
Yee, 2005, *United Kingdom [172]*	Cross sectional	242	No	9.1	-

Table 8. Prevalence of osteoporosis in Ankylosing Spondylitis

Author, Year, Country	Type of study	Patients	Control group	Osteoporosis in spine (%)	Osteoporosis in hip (%)
Singh, 2013, India [174]	Cross sectional	100	150	22	9
Klingberg, 2013, Sweden [175]	Cross sectional	69	68	6	-
Klingberg, 2012, Sweden [102]	Cross sectional	151	No	10	5
Vasdev, 2011, India [176]	Cross sectional	80	160	28.7	11.5
Muntean, 2011, Romania [177]	Cross sectional	44	39	59.5	47.7
Ghozlani, 2009, Morocco [178]	Cross sectional	80	No	25	-

The selected studies were included if they had patients with AS, assessed by BMD last 10 years.

Table 9. Prevalence of Osteoporotic Fractures in Ankylosing Spondylitis

Author, Year, Country	Study	Patients	Control group	Vertebral fracture (%)
Klingberg, 2013, Sweden [175]	Cross sectional	69	No	12
Van der Weijden, 2012, Netherlands [179]	Cross sectional	113	No	15
Arends, 2011, Netherlands [104]	Cross sectional	128	No	39
Ghozlani, 2009, Morocco [178]	Cross sectional	80	No	18.8

Table 10. Prevalence of Osteoporosis in Psoriatic Arthritis

Author, Year, Country	Type of study	Patients	Control group	Osteoporosis spine (%)	Osteoporosis hip (%)
Busquets, 2014, Spain [5]	Cross sectional	155	No	7	11
Grazio, 2011, Croatia [180]	Cross sectional	69	No	7.2	1.4
Borman, 2008, Turkey [181]	Cross sectional	47	No	5	-
Hofbauer, 2006, Germany [182]	Cross sectional	116	No	6	-

The selected studies included have been conducted during the last 10 years.

Therefore, new information derived from double-blind controlled trials is required and constitutes an important target for further research.

ACKNOWLEDGMENT

This review was financed with a grant from the Instituto Mexicano del Seguro Social (Grant number FIS/IMSS/PROT/MD09/733).

REFERENCES

[1] Bultink I. E., Vis M., van der Horst-Bruinsma I. E., Lems W. F. Inflammatory rheumatic disorders and bone. *Current rheumatology reports,* 2012;14(3):224-30.

[2] Ghazi M., Kolta S., Briot K., Fechtenbaum J., Paternotte S., Roux C. Prevalence of vertebral fractures in patients with rheumatoid arthritis: revisiting the role of glucocorticoids. *Osteoporosis international: a journal established as result of cooperation between the European Foundation for Osteoporosis and the National Osteoporosis Foundation of the USA*, 2012;23(2):581-7.

[3] Mohammad A., Lohan D., Bergin D., Mooney S., Newell J., O'Donnell M., et al. The prevalence of vertebral fracture on vertebral fracture assessment imaging in a large cohort of patients with rheumatoid arthritis. *Rheumatology (Oxford, England)*, 2014;53(5):821-7.

[4] Souto M. I., Coelho A., Guo C., Mendonca L. M., Pinheiro M. F., Papi J. A., et al. The prevalence of low bone mineral density in Brazilian patients with systemic lupus erythematosus and its relationship with the disease damage index and other associated factors. *Journal of clinical densitometry : the official journal of the International Society for Clinical Densitometry,* 2012;15(3):320-7.

[5] Busquets N., Vaquero C. G., Moreno J. R., Vilaseca D. R., Narvaez J., Carmona L., et al. Bone mineral density status and frequency of osteoporosis and clinical fractures in 155 patients with psoriatic arthritis followed in a university hospital. *Reumatol. Clin.,* 2014;10(2):89-93.

[6] Grossman J. M., Gordon R., Ranganath V. K., Deal C., Caplan L., Chen W., et al. American College of Rheumatology 2010 recommendations for the prevention and treatment of glucocorticoid-induced osteoporosis. *Arthritis care and research,* 2010;62(11):1515-26.

[7] Watts N. B., Lewiecki E. M., Miller P. D., Baim S. National Osteoporosis Foundation 2008 Clinician's Guide to Prevention and Treatment of Osteoporosis and the World Health Organization Fracture Risk Assessment Tool (FRAX): what they mean to the bone densitometrist and bone technologist. *Journal of clinical densitometry : the official journal of the International Society for Clinical Densitometry,* 2008; 11(4): 473-7.

[8] Wang S. H., Chang Y. S., Liu C. J., Lai C. C., Chen W. S., Chen T. J., et al. Association of systemic lupus erythematosus with a higher risk of cervical but not trochanteric hip fracture: a nationwide population-based study. *Arthritis care and research,* 2013; 65 (10): 1674-81.

[9] Zhu T., Griffith J., Au S. K., Tang X. L., Kwok A., Leung P. C., et al. Incidence of and risk factors for non-vertebral and vertebral fracture in female Chinese patients with systemic lupus erythematosus: a five-year cohort study. *Lupus,* 2014.

[10] Arboleya L., Castaneda S. Osteoimmunology: the study of the relationship between the immune system and bone tissue. *Reumatol. Clin.*, 2013;9(5):303-15.
[11] Schett G. Osteoimmunology in rheumatic diseases. *Arthritis research and therapy,* 2009; 11(1):210.
[12] Gravallese E. M., Manning C., Tsay A., Naito A., Pan C., Amento E., et al. Synovial tissue in rheumatoid arthritis is a source of osteoclast differentiation factor. *Arthritis and rheumatism,* 2000;43(2):250-8.
[13] Lacey D. L., Timms E., Tan H. L., Kelley M. J., Dunstan C. R., Burgess T., et al. Osteoprotegerin ligand is a cytokine that regulates osteoclast differentiation and activation. *Cell,* 1998;93(2):165-76.
[14] Takayanagi H. Inflammatory bone destruction and osteoimmunology. *Journal of periodontal research,* 2005;40(4):287-93.
[15] Zhao R. Immune regulation of bone loss by Th17 cells in oestrogen-deficient osteoporosis. *European journal of clinical investigation,* 2013;43(11):1195-202.
[16] Takayanagi H. Osteoimmunology: shared mechanisms and crosstalk between the immune and bone systems. *Nature reviews Immunology*, 2007;7(4):292-304.
[17] Takayanagi H., Ogasawara K., Hida S., Chiba T., Murata S., Sato K., et al. T-cell-mediated regulation of osteoclastogenesis by signalling cross-talk between RANKL and IFN-gamma. *Nature,* 2000;408(6812):600-5.
[18] Gao Y., Grassi F., Ryan M. R., Terauchi M., Page K., Yang X., et al. IFN-gamma stimulates osteoclast formation and bone loss in vivo via antigen-driven T cell activation. *The Journal of clinical investigation,* 2007;117(1):122-32.
[19] Takayanagi H. Osteoimmunology and the effects of the immune system on bone. *Nature reviews Rheumatology,* 2009;5(12):667-76.
[20] Danks L., Takayanagi H. Immunology and bone. *Journal of biochemistry,* 2013; 154 (1):29-39.
[21] Kotake S., Udagawa N., Takahashi N., Matsuzaki K., Itoh K., Ishiyama S., et al. IL-17 in synovial fluids from patients with rheumatoid arthritis is a potent stimulator of osteoclastogenesis. *The Journal of clinical investigation,* 1999;103(9):1345-52.
[22] Simonet W. S., Lacey D. L., Dunstan C. R., Kelley M., Chang M. S., Luthy R., et al. Osteoprotegerin: a novel secreted protein involved in the regulation of bone density. *Cell,* 1997;89(2):309-19.
[23] Schett G., Saag K. G., Bijlsma J. W. From bone biology to clinical outcome: state of the art and future perspectives. *Annals of the rheumatic diseases*, 2010;69(8):1415-9.
[24] Garnero P., Tabassi N. C., Voorzanger-Rousselot N. Circulating dickkopf-1 and radiological progression in patients with early rheumatoid arthritis treated with etanercept. *The Journal of rheumatology,* 2008;35(12):2313-5.
[25] Xu S., Wang Y., Lu J., Xu J. Osteoprotegerin and RANKL in the pathogenesis of rheumatoid arthritis-induced osteoporosis. *Rheumatology international,* 2012;32(11): 3397-403.
[26] Chabaud M., Lubberts E., Joosten L., van Den Berg W., Miossec P. IL-17 derived from juxta-articular bone and synovium contributes to joint degradation in rheumatoid arthritis. *Arthritis research,* 2001;3(3):168-77.
[27] McCarthy E. M., Smith S., Lee R. Z., Cunnane G., Doran M. F., Donnelly S., et al. The association of cytokines with disease activity and damage scores in systemic lupus erythematosus patients. *Rheumatology (Oxford, England)*, 2014.

[28] Wong C. K., Lit L. C., Tam L. S., Li E. K., Wong P. T., Lam C. W. Hyperproduction of IL-23 and IL-17 in patients with systemic lupus erythematosus: implications for Th17-mediated inflammation in auto-immunity. *Clinical immunology,* 2008;127(3):385-93.
[29] Tang Y., Xie H., Chen J., Geng L., Chen H., Li X., et al. Activated NF-kappaB in bone marrow mesenchymal stem cells from systemic lupus erythematosus patients inhibits osteogenic differentiation through downregulating Smad signaling. *Stem cells and development,* 2013;22(4):668-78.
[30] Hess K., Ushmorov A., Fiedler J., Brenner R. E., Wirth T. TNFalpha promotes osteogenic differentiation of human mesenchymal stem cells by triggering the NF-kappaB signaling pathway. *Bone,* 2009;45(2):367-76.
[31] Bultink I. E. Osteoporosis and fractures in systemic lupus erythematosus. *Arthritis care and research,* 2012;64(1):2-8.
[32] Svenungsson E., Fei G. Z., Jensen-Urstad K., de Faire U., Hamsten A., Frostegard J. TNF-alpha: a link between hypertriglyceridaemia and inflammation in SLE patients with cardiovascular disease. *Lupus,* 2003;12(6):454-61.
[33] Moerman E. J., Teng K., Lipschitz D. A., Lecka-Czernik B. Aging activates adipogenic and suppresses osteogenic programs in mesenchymal marrow stroma/stem cells: the role of PPAR-gamma2 transcription factor and TGF-beta/BMP signaling pathways. *Aging cell,* 2004;3(6):379-89.
[34] Petri M. Musculoskeletal complications of systemic lupus erythematosus in the Hopkins Lupus Cohort: an update. *Arthritis care and research : the official journal of the Arthritis Health Professions Association,* 1995;8(3):137-45.
[35] Gratacos J., Collado A., Filella X., Sanmarti R., Canete J., Llena J., et al. Serum cytokines (IL-6, TNF-alpha, IL-1 beta and IFN-gamma) in ankylosing spondylitis: a close correlation between serum IL-6 and disease activity and severity. *British journal of rheumatology,* 1994;33(10):927-31.
[36] Schett G. Structural bone changes in spondyloarthritis: mechanisms, clinical impact and therapeutic considerations. *The American journal of the medical sciences,* 2011;341 (4): 269-71.
[37] Lories R. J., Derese I., Luyten F. P. Modulation of bone morphogenetic protein signaling inhibits the onset and progression of ankylosing enthesitis. *The Journal of clinical investigation,* 2005;115(6):1571-9.
[38] Taylan A., Sari I., Akinci B., Bilge S., Kozaci D., Akar S., et al. Biomarkers and cytokines of bone turnover: extensive evaluation in a cohort of patients with ankylosing spondylitis. *BMC musculoskeletal disorders*, 2012;13:191.
[39] Appel H., Ruiz-Heiland G., Listing J., Zwerina J., Herrmann M., Mueller R., et al. Altered skeletal expression of sclerostin and its link to radiographic progression in ankylosing spondylitis. *Arthritis and rheumatism,* 2009;60(11):3257-62.
[40] Heiland G. R., Appel H., Poddubnyy D., Zwerina J., Hueber A., Haibel H., et al. High level of functional dickkopf-1 predicts protection from syndesmophyte formation in patients with ankylosing spondylitis. *Annals of the rheumatic diseases*, 2012; 71 (4): 572-4.
[41] Appel H., Kuhne M., Spiekermann S., Ebhardt H., Grozdanovic Z., Kohler D., et al. Immunohistologic analysis of zygapophyseal joints in patients with ankylosing spondylitis. *Arthritis and rheumatism*, 2006;54(9):2845-51.

[42] Rahimi H., Ritchlin C. T. Altered bone biology in psoriatic arthritis. *Current rheumatology reports,* 2012;14(4):349-57.
[43] Dalbeth N., Pool B., Smith T., Callon K. E., Lobo M., Taylor W. J., et al. Circulating mediators of bone remodeling in psoriatic arthritis: implications for disordered osteoclastogenesis and bone erosion. *Arthritis research and therapy,* 2010;12(4):R164.
[44] Ritchlin C. T., Haas-Smith S. A., Li P., Hicks D. G., Schwarz E. M. Mechanisms of TNF-alpha- and RANKL-mediated osteoclastogenesis and bone resorption in psoriatic arthritis. *The Journal of clinical investigation,* 2003;111(6):821-31.
[45] Colucci S., Brunetti G., Cantatore F. P., Oranger A., Mori G., Quarta L., et al. Lymphocytes and synovial fluid fibroblasts support osteoclastogenesis through RANKL, TNFalpha, and IL-7 in an in vitro model derived from human psoriatic arthritis. *The Journal of pathology*, 2007;212(1):47-55.
[46] Chhana A., Callon K. E., Pool B., Naot D., Watson M., Gamble G. D., et al. Monosodium urate monohydrate crystals inhibit osteoblast viability and function: implications for development of bone erosion in gout. *Annals of the rheumatic diseases,* 2011;70(9):1684-91.
[47] Lee S. J., Nam K. I., Jin H. M., Cho Y. N., Lee S. E., Kim T. J., et al. Bone destruction by receptor activator of nuclear factor kappaB ligand-expressing T cells in chronic gouty arthritis. *Arthritis research and therapy,* 2011;13(5):R164.
[48] Dalbeth N., Smith T., Nicolson B., Clark B., Callon K., Naot D., et al. Enhanced osteoclastogenesis in patients with tophaceous gout: urate crystals promote osteoclast development through interactions with stromal cells. *Arthritis and rheumatism,* 2008;58(6):1854-65.
[49] Kwan Tat S., Pelletier J. P., Lajeunesse D., Fahmi H., Lavigne M., Martel-Pelletier J. The differential expression of osteoprotegerin (OPG) and receptor activator of nuclear factor kappaB ligand (RANKL) in human osteoarthritic subchondral bone osteoblasts is an indicator of the metabolic state of these disease cells. *Clinical and experimental rheumatology*, 2008;26(2):295-304.
[50] Hopwood B., Tsykin A., Findlay D. M., Fazzalari N. L. Microarray gene expression profiling of osteoarthritic bone suggests altered bone remodelling, WNT and transforming growth factor-beta/bone morphogenic protein signalling. *Arthritis research and therapy,* 2007;9(5):R100.
[51] Massicotte F., Lajeunesse D., Benderdour M., Pelletier J. P., Hilal G., Duval N., et al. Can altered production of interleukin-1beta, interleukin-6, transforming growth factor-beta and prostaglandin E(2) by isolated human subchondral osteoblasts identify two subgroups of osteoarthritic patients. *Osteoarthritis and cartilage / OARS, Osteoarthritis Research Society*, 2002;10(6):491-500.
[52] Kwan Tat S., Pelletier J. P., Amiable N., Boileau C., Lajeunesse D., Duval N., et al. Activation of the receptor EphB4 by its specific ligand ephrin B2 in human osteoarthritic subchondral bone osteoblasts. *Arthritis and rheumatism,* 2008;58 (12): 3820-30.
[53] Cranney A., Guyatt G., Griffith L., Wells G., Tugwell P., Rosen C. Meta-analyses of therapies for postmenopausal osteoporosis. IX: Summary of meta-analyses of therapies for postmenopausal osteoporosis. *Endocrine reviews,* 2002;23(4):570-8.

[54] Herrak P., Gortz B., Hayer S., Redlich K., Reiter E., Gasser J., et al. Zoledronic acid protects against local and systemic bone loss in tumor necrosis factor-mediated arthritis. *Arthritis and rheumatism*, 2004;50(7):2327-37.

[55] Le Goff B., Soltner E., Charrier C., Maugars Y., Redini F., Heymann D., et al. A combination of methotrexate and zoledronic acid prevents bone erosions and systemic bone mass loss in collagen induced arthritis. *Arthritis research and therapy*, 2009;11(6):R185.

[56] Sims N. A., Green J. R., Glatt M., Schlict S., Martin T. J., Gillespie M. T., et al. Targeting osteoclasts with zoledronic acid prevents bone destruction in collagen-induced arthritis. *Arthritis and Rheumatism*, 2004;50(7):2338-46.

[57] Yu D. G., Yu B., Mao Y. Q., Zhao X., Wang X. Q., Ding H. F., et al. Efficacy of zoledronic acid in treatment of teoarthritis is dependent on the disease progression stage in rat medial meniscal tear model. *Acta pharmacologica Sinica*, 2012;33(7):924-34.

[58] Cinar B. M., Ozkoc G., Bolat F., Karaeminogullari O., Sezgin N., Tandogan R. N. Intra-articular zoledronic acid in a rat osteoarthritis model: significant reduced synovitis may indicate chondroprotective effect. *Knee surgery, sports traumatology, arthroscopy : official journal of the ESSKA*, 2014.

[59] Strassle B. W., Mark L., Leventhal L., Piesla M. J., Jian Li X., Kennedy J. D., et al. Inhibition of osteoclasts prevents cartilage loss and pain in a rat model of degenerative joint disease. *Osteoarthritis and cartilage / OARS, Osteoarthritis Research Society*, 2010; 18(10):1319-28.

[60] Lories R. J., Derese I., Luyten F. P. Inhibition of osteoclasts does not prevent joint ankylosis in a mouse model of spondyloarthritis. *Rheumatology (Oxford, England)*, 2008;47(5):605-8.

[61] Pelaez-Ballestas I., Sanin L. H., Moreno-Montoya J., Alvarez-Nemegyei J., Burgos-Vargas R., Garza-Elizondo M., et al. Epidemiology of the rheumatic diseases in Mexico. A study of 5 regions based on the COPCORD methodology. *The Journal of rheumatology Supplement*, 2011;86:3-8.

[62] Morales-Romero J., Cázares-Méndez J. M., Gámez-Nava J. I., Triano-Páez M., Villa-Manzano A. I., López-Olivo M. A., et al. La atención médica en reumatología en un hospital de segundo nivel de atención. *Reumatología Clínica*, 2005;1(2):87-94.

[63] Gonzalez-Lopez L., Gamez-Nava J. I., Vega-Lopez A., Rodriguez-Jimenez N. A., Gonzalez-Montoya N., Aguilar-Chavez E., et al. Performance of risk indices for identifying low bone mineral density and osteoporosis in Mexican Mestizo women with rheumatoid arthritis. *The Journal of rheumatology*, 2012;39(2):247-53.

[64] Hauser B., Riches P. L., Wilson J. F., Horne A. E., Ralston S. H. Prevalence and clinical prediction of osteoporosis in a contemporary cohort of patients with rheumatoid arthritis. *Rheumatology (Oxford, England)*, 2014.

[65] Mobini M., Kashi Z., Ghobadifar A. Prevalence and associated factors of osteoporosis in female patients with rheumatoid arthritis. *Caspian journal of internal medicine*, 2012;3(3):447-50.

[66] Roussy J. P., Bessette L., Bernatsky S., Rahme E., Lachaine J. Biologic disease-modifying anti-rheumatic drugs and the risk of non-vertebral osteoporotic fractures in patients with rheumatoid arthritis aged 50 years and over. *Osteoporosis international: a journal established as result of cooperation between the European Foundation for*

Osteoporosis and the National Osteoporosis Foundation of the USA, 2013;24(9): 2483-92.

[67] Vis M., Haavardsholm E. A., Boyesen P., Haugeberg G., Uhlig T., Hoff M., et al. High incidence of vertebral and non-vertebral fractures in the OSTRA cohort study: a 5-year follow-up study in postmenopausal women with rheumatoid arthritis. *Osteoporosis international: a journal established as result of cooperation between the European Foundation for Osteoporosis and the National Osteoporosis Foundation of the USA*, 2011;22(9):2413-9.

[68] Gamez-Nava J. I., Zavaleta-Muniz S. A., Vazquez-Villegas M. L., Vega-Lopez A., Rodriguez-Jimenez N. A., Olivas-Flores E. M., et al. Prescription for antiresorptive therapy in Mexican patients with rheumatoid arthritis: is it time to reevaluate the strategies for osteoporosis prevention? *Rheumatology international*, 2013;33(1):145-50.

[69] Overman R. A., Toliver J. C., Yeh J. Y., Gourlay M. L., Deal C. L. U.S. adults meeting 2010 American College of Rheumatology criteria for treatment and prevention of glucocorticoid-induced osteoporosis. *Arthritis care and research*, 2014.

[70] Richards J. S., Cannon G. W., Hayden C. L., Amdur R. L., Lazaro D., Mikuls T. R., et al. Adherence with bisphosphonate therapy in US veterans with rheumatoid arthritis. *Arthritis care and research*, 2012;64(12):1864-70.

[71] Reid D. M., Devogelaer J. P., Saag K., Roux C., Lau C. S., Reginster J. Y., et al. Zoledronic acid and risedronate in the prevention and treatment of glucocorticoid-induced osteoporosis (HORIZON): a multicentre, double-blind, double-dummy, randomised controlled trial. *Lancet*, 2009;373(9671):1253-63.

[72] Jarrett S. J., Conaghan P. G., Sloan V. S., Papanastasiou P., Ortmann C. E., O'Connor P. J., et al. Preliminary evidence for a structural benefit of the new bisphosphonate zoledronic acid in early rheumatoid arthritis. *Arthritis and rheumatism*, 2006;54(5): 1410-4.

[73] Kiriakidou M., Cotton D., Taichman D., Williams S. Systemic lupus erythematosus. *Annals of internal medicine*, 2013;159(7):Itc4-1.

[74] Zonana-Nacach A., Barr S. G., Magder L. S., Petri M. Damage in systemic lupus erythematosus and its association with corticosteroids. *Arthritis and rheumatism*, 2000; 43(8):1801-8.

[75] Jacobs J., Korswagen L. A., Schilder A. M., van Tuyl L. H., Dijkmans B. A., Lems W. F., et al. Six-year follow-up study of bone mineral density in patients with systemic lupus erythematosus. *Osteoporosis international : a journal established as result of cooperation between the European Foundation for Osteoporosis and the National Osteoporosis Foundation of the USA*, 2013;24(6):1827-33.

[76] Mok C. C., Mak A., Ma K. M. Bone mineral density in postmenopausal Chinese patients with systemic lupus erythematosus. *Lupus*, 2005;14(2):106-12.

[77] Yeap S. S., Othman A. Z., Zain A. A., Chan S. P. Vitamin D levels: its relationship to bone mineral density response and disease activity in premenopausal Malaysian systemic lupus erythematosus patients on corticosteroids. *International journal of rheumatic diseases*, 2012;15(1):17-24.

[78] Boyanov M., Robeva R., Popivanov P. Bone mineral density changes in women with systemic lupus erythematosus. *Clinical rheumatology*, 2003;22(4-5):318-23.

[79] Uaratanawong S., Deesomchoke U., Lertmaharit S., Uaratanawong S. Bone mineral density in premenopausal women with systemic lupus erythematosus. *The Journal of rheumatology,* 2003;30(11):2365-8.

[80] Liyanage A., Lekamwasam S., Dissanayake S. P., Munidasa D. Factors that determine body composition of female systemic lupus erythematosus (SLE) patients in Sri Lanka: a comparative study using dual-energy x-ray absorptiometry. *Lupus,* 2013;22(9):972-6.

[81] Mok C. C., Ying S. K., To C. H., Ma K. M. Bone mineral density and body composition in men with systemic lupus erythematosus: a case control study. *Bone,* 2008;43(2):327-31.

[82] Lakshminarayanan S., Walsh S., Mohanraj M., Rothfield N. Factors associated with low bone mineral density in female patients with systemic lupus erythematosus. *The Journal of rheumatology,* 2001;28(1):102-8.

[83] Li E. K., Tam L. S., Young R. P., Ko G. T., Li M., Lau E. M. Loss of bone mineral density in Chinese pre-menopausal women with systemic lupus erythematosus treated with corticosteroids. *British journal of rheumatology,* 1998;37(4):405-10.

[84] Mendoza-Pinto C., Garcia-Carrasco M., Sandoval-Cruz H., Munoz-Guarneros M., Escarcega R. O., Jimenez-Hernandez M., et al. Risk factors of vertebral fractures in women with systemic lupus erythematosus. *Clinical rheumatology,* 2009;28(5):579-85.

[85] Yeap S. S., Fauzi A. R., Kong N. C., Halim A. G., Soehardy Z., Rahimah S., et al. Influences on bone mineral density in Malaysian premenopausal systemic lupus erythematosus patients on corticosteroids. *Lupus,* 2009;18(2):178-81.

[86] Furukawa M., Kiyohara C., Horiuchi T., Tsukamoto H., Mitoma H., Kimoto Y., et al. Prevalence and risk factors of vertebral fracture in female Japanese patients with systemic lupus erythematosus. *Modern rheumatology / the Japan Rheumatism Association,* 2013;23(4):765-73.

[87] Li E. K., Tam L. S., Griffith J. F., Zhu T. Y., Li T. K., Li M., et al. High prevalence of asymptomatic vertebral fractures in Chinese women with systemic lupus erythematosus. *The Journal of rheumatology,* 2009;36(8):1646-52.

[88] Ekblom-Kullberg S., Kautiainen H., Alha P., Leirisalo-Repo M., Julkunen H. Frequency of and risk factors for symptomatic bone fractures in patients with systemic lupus erythematosus. *Scandinavian journal of rheumatology,* 2013;42(5):390-3.

[89] Bultink I. E., Harvey N. C., Lalmohamed A., Cooper C., Lems W. F., van Staa T. P., et al. Elevated risk of clinical fractures and associated risk factors in patients with systemic lupus erythematosus versus matched controls: a population-based study in the United Kingdom. *Osteoporosis international : a journal established as result of cooperation between the European Foundation for Osteoporosis and the National Osteoporosis Foundation of the USA,* 2014;25(4):1275-83.

[90] Garcia-Carrasco M., Mendoza-Pinto C., Riebeling C., Sandoval-Cruz M., Nava A., Etchegaray-Morales I., et al. Influence of prevalent vertebral fractures on the quality of life of patients with systemic lupus erythematosus. *The Israel Medical Association journal : IMAJ,* 2011;13(6):333-7.

[91] Compeyrot-Lacassagne S., Tyrrell P. N., Atenafu E., Doria A. S., Stephens D., Gilday D., et al. Prevalence and etiology of low bone mineral density in juvenile systemic lupus erythematosus. *Arthritis and rheumatism,* 2007;56(6):1966-73.

[92] Pons-Estel G. J., Alarcon G. S., Burgos P. I., Hachuel L., Boggio G., Wojdyla D., et al. Mestizos with systemic lupus erythematosus develop renal disease early while

antimalarials retard its appearance: data from a Latin American cohort. *Lupus,* 2013; 22(9):899-907.

[93] Boonen S., Sellmeyer D. E., Lippuner K., Orlov-Morozov A., Abrams K., Mesenbrink P., et al. Renal safety of annual zoledronic acid infusions in osteoporotic postmenopausal women. *Kidney international,* 2008;74(5):641-8.

[94] Garcia M. A., Alarcon G. S., Boggio G., Hachuel L., Marcos A. I., Marcos J. C., et al. Primary cardiac disease in systemic lupus erythematosus patients: protective and risk factors--data from a multi-ethnic Latin American cohort. *Rheumatology (Oxford, England),* 2014.

[95] Yazici O., Aksoy S., Ucar O., Ozdemir N., Demir M., Sendur M. A., et al. Arrhythmias during and after zoledronic acid infusion patients with bone metastasis. *Medical oncology (Northwood, London, England),* 2013;30(3):609.

[96] Souza S. C., Borges C. T., Jorgetti V., Pereira R. M. The effect of intravenous zoledronic acid on glucocorticoid-induced multiple vertebral fractures in juvenile systemic lupus erythematosus. *Revista do Hospital das Clinicas,* 2004;59(5):302-5.

[97] Pelaez-Ballestas I., Navarro-Zarza J. E., Julian B., Lopez A., Flores-Camacho R., Casasola-Vargas J. C., et al. A community-based study on the prevalence of spondyloarthritis and inflammatory back pain in Mexicans. *Journal of clinical rheumatology : practical reports on rheumatic and musculoskeletal diseases,* 2013; 19 (2): 57-61.

[98] Bessant R., Keat A. How should clinicians manage osteoporosis in ankylosing spondylitis? *The Journal of rheumatology,* 2002;29(7):1511-9.

[99] Vosse D., de Vlam K. Osteoporosis in rheumatoid arthritis and ankylosing spondylitis. *Clinical and experimental rheumatology,* 2009;27(4 Suppl. 55):S62-7.

[100] van der Weijden M. A., Claushuis T. A., Nazari T., Lems W. F., Dijkmans B. A., van der Horst-Bruinsma I. E. High prevalence of low bone mineral density in patients within 10 years of onset of ankylosing spondylitis: a systematic review. *Clinical rheumatology,* 2012;31(11):1529-35.

[101] Munoz-Ortego J., Vestergaard P., Rubio J. B., Wordsworth P., Judge A., Javaid M. K., et al. Ankylosing Spondylitis is Associated with an Increased Risk of Vertebral and Non-Vertebral Clinical Fractures: A Population-Based Cohort Study. *Journal of bone and mineral research: the official journal of the American Society for Bone and Mineral Research,* 2014.

[102] Klingberg E., Geijer M., Gothlin J., Mellstrom D., Lorentzon M., Hilme E., et al. Vertebral fractures in ankylosing spondylitis are associated with lower bone mineral density in both central and peripheral skeleton. *The Journal of rheumatology,* 2012;39(10):1987-95.

[103] Chen C. H., Chen H. A., Liao H. T., Liu C. H., Tsai C. Y., Chou C. T. Soluble receptor activator of nuclear factor-kappaB ligand (RANKL) and osteoprotegerin in ankylosing spondylitis: OPG is associated with poor physical mobility and reflects systemic inflammation. *Clinical rheumatology,* 2010;29(10):1155-61.

[104] Arends S., Spoorenberg A., Bruyn G. A., Houtman P. M., Leijsma M. K., Kallenberg C. G., et al. The relation between bone mineral density, bone turnover markers, and vitamin D status in ankylosing spondylitis patients with active disease: a cross-sectional analysis. *Osteoporosis international: a journal established as result of cooperation*

between the European Foundation for Osteoporosis and the National Osteoporosis Foundation of the USA, 2011;22(5):1431-9.

[105] Arends S., Spoorenberg A., Houtman P. M., Leijsma M. K., Bos R., Kallenberg C. G., et al. The effect of three years of TNFalpha blocking therapy on markers of bone turnover and their predictive value for treatment discontinuation in patients with ankylosing spondylitis: a prospective longitudinal observational cohort study. *Arthritis research and therapy*, 2012;14(2):R98.

[106] Kang K. Y., Lee K. Y., Kwok S. K., Ju J. H., Park K. S., Hong Y. S., et al. The change of bone mineral density according to treatment agents in patients with ankylosing spondylitis. *Joint, bone, spine : revue du rhumatisme,* 2011;78(2):188-93.

[107] Toussirot E., Wendling D. Antiinflammatory treatment with bisphosphonates in ankylosing spondylitis. *Current opinion in rheumatology,* 2007;19(4):340-5.

[108] Maksymowych W. P., Jhangri G. S., Fitzgerald A. A., LeClercq S., Chiu P., Yan A., et al. A six-month randomized, controlled, double-blind, dose-response comparison of intravenous pamidronate (60 mg versus 10 mg) in the treatment of nonsteroidal antiinflammatory drug-refractory ankylosing spondylitis. *Arthritis and rheumatism,* 2002;46(3):766-73.

[109] Viapiana O., Gatti D., Idolazzi L., Fracassi E., Adami S., Troplini S., et al. Bisphosphonates vs infliximab in ankylosing spondylitis treatment. *Rheumatology (Oxford, England),* 2014;53(1):90-4.

[110] Clunie G. P., Ginawi A., O'Conner P., Bearcroft P. W., Garber S. J., Bhagat S., et al. An open-label study of zoledronic acid (Aclasta 5 mg iv) in the treatment of ankylosing spondylitis. *Annals of the rheumatic diseases,* 2014;73(6):1273-4.

[111] Reid I. R., Gamble G. D., Mesenbrink P., Lakatos P., Black D. M. Characterization of and risk factors for the acute-phase response after zoledronic acid. *The Journal of clinical endocrinology and metabolism,* 2010;95(9):4380-7.

[112] Setty A. R., Choi H. K. Psoriatic arthritis epidemiology. *Current rheumatology reports,* 2007;9(6):449-54.

[113] Pedreira P. G., Pinheiro M. M., Szejnfeld V. L. Bone mineral density and body composition in postmenopausal women with psoriasis and psoriatic arthritis. *Arthritis research and therapy,* 2011;13(1):R16.

[114] McQueen F., Lloyd R., Doyle A., Robinson E., Lobo M., Exeter M., et al. Zoledronic acid does not reduce MRI erosive progression in PsA but may suppress bone oedema: the Zoledronic Acid in Psoriatic Arthritis (ZAPA) Study. *Annals of the rheumatic diseases,* 2011;70(6):1091-4.

[115] Bolzetta F., Veronese N., Manzato E., Sergi G. Chronic gout in the elderly. *Aging clinical and experimental research,* 2013;25(2):129-37.

[116] Richette P., Bardin T. *Gout. Lancet,* 2010;375(9711):318-28.

[117] Roddy E., Mallen C. D., Doherty M. *Gout. BMJ (Clinical research ed),* 2013;347: f5648.

[118] Roddy E., Choi H. K. Epidemiology of gout. *Rheumatic diseases clinics of North America,* 2014;40(2):155-75.

[119] Dalbeth N., Collis J., Gregory K., Clark B., Robinson E., McQueen F. M. Tophaceous joint disease strongly predicts hand function in patients with gout. *Rheumatology (Oxford, England),* 2007;46(12):1804-7.

[120] Dalbeth N., Clark B., Gregory K., Gamble G., Sheehan T., Doyle A., et al. Mechanisms of bone erosion in gout: a quantitative analysis using plain radiography and computed tomography. *Annals of the rheumatic diseases,* 2009;68(8):1290-5.

[121] Dalbeth N., Aati O., Gamble G. D., Horne A., House M. E., Roger M., et al. Zoledronate for prevention of bone erosion in tophaceous gout: a randomised, double-blind, placebo-controlled trial. *Annals of the rheumatic diseases,* 2014;73(6):1044-51.

[122] Hochberg M. C., Yerges-Armstrong L., Yau M., Mitchell B. D. Genetic epidemiology of osteoarthritis: recent developments and future directions. *Current opinion in rheumatology,* 2013;25(2):192-7.

[123] Suri P., Morgenroth D. C., Hunter D. J. Epidemiology of osteoarthritis and associated comorbidities. *PM & R : the journal of injury, function, and rehabilitation,* 2012;4(5 Suppl.):S10-9.

[124] Zhang Y., Niu J., Kelly-Hayes M., Chaisson C. E., Aliabadi P., Felson D. T. Prevalence of symptomatic hand osteoarthritis and its impact on functional status among the elderly: The Framingham Study. *American journal of epidemiology,* 2002;156(11): 1021-7.

[125] Felson D. T., Naimark A., Anderson J., Kazis L., Castelli W., Meenan R. F. The prevalence of knee osteoarthritis in the elderly. The Framingham Osteoarthritis Study. *Arthritis and rheumatism,* 1987;30(8):914-8.

[126] Chaganti R. K., Parimi N., Lang T., Orwoll E., Stefanick M. L., Nevitt M., et al. Bone mineral density and prevalent osteoarthritis of the hip in older men for the Osteoporotic Fractures in Men (MrOS) Study Group. *Osteoporosis international: a journal established as result of cooperation between the European Foundation for Osteoporosis and the National Osteoporosis Foundation of the USA,* 2010;21(8): 1307-16.

[127] Sinigaglia L., Varenna M., Girasole G., Bianchi G. Epidemiology of osteoporosis in rheumatic diseases. *Rheumatic diseases clinics of North America,* 2006;32(4):631-58.

[128] Sowers M., Lachance L., Jamadar D., Hochberg M. C., Hollis B., Crutchfield M., et al. The associations of bone mineral density and bone turnover markers with osteoarthritis of the hand and knee in pre- and perimenopausal women. *Arthritis and rheumatism,* 1999;42(3):483-9.

[129] Zhang Y., Hannan M. T., Chaisson C. E., McAlindon T. E., Evans S. R., Aliabadi P., et al. Bone mineral density and risk of incident and progressive radiographic knee osteoarthritis in women: the Framingham Study. *The Journal of rheumatology,* 2000;27(4):1032-7.

[130] Arden N. K., Crozier S., Smith H., Anderson F., Edwards C., Raphael H., et al. Knee pain, knee osteoarthritis, and the risk of fracture. *Arthritis and rheumatism,* 2006;55(4):610-5.

[131] Bergink A. P., van der Klift M., Hofman A., Verhaar J. A., van Leeuwen J. P., Uitterlinden A. G., et al. Osteoarthritis of the knee is associated with vertebral and nonvertebral fractures in the elderly: the Rotterdam Study. *Arthritis and rheumatism,* 2003;49(5):648-57.

[132] Prieto-Alhambra D., Javaid M. K., Judge A., Maskell J., Kiran A., de Vries F., et al. Fracture risk before and after total hip replacement in patients with osteoarthritis: potential benefits of bisphosphonate use. *Arthritis and rheumatism,* 2011;63(4):992-1001.

[133] Vestergaard P., Rejnmark L., Mosekilde L. Osteoarthritis and risk of fractures. *Calcified tissue international,* 2009;84(4):249-56.

[134] Hunter D. J., McDougall J. J., Keefe F. J. The symptoms of osteoarthritis and the genesis of pain. *The Medical clinics of North America,* 2009;93(1):83-100, xi.

[135] Walsh D. A., McWilliams D. F., Turley M. J., Dixon M. R., Franses R. E., Mapp P. I., et al. Angiogenesis and nerve growth factor at the osteochondral junction in rheumatoid arthritis and osteoarthritis. *Rheumatology (Oxford, England),* 2010;49(10):1852-61.

[136] Nagae M., Hiraga T., Wakabayashi H., Wang L., Iwata K., Yoneda T. Osteoclasts play a part in pain due to the inflammation adjacent to bone. *Bone,* 2006;39(5):1107-15.

[137] Nagae M., Hiraga T., Yoneda T. Acidic microenvironment created by osteoclasts causes bone pain associated with tumor colonization. *Journal of bone and mineral metabolism,* 2007;25(2):99-104.

[138] Davis A. J., Smith T. O., Hing C. B., Sofat N. Are bisphosphonates effective in the treatment of osteoarthritis pain? A meta-analysis and systematic review. *PloS one,* 2013;8(9):e72714.

[139] Laslett L. L., Dore D. A., Quinn S. J., Boon P., Ryan E., Winzenberg T. M., et al. Zoledronic acid reduces knee pain and bone marrow lesions over 1 year: a randomised controlled trial. *Annals of the rheumatic diseases,* 2012;71(8):1322-8.

[140] Pineda C., Martinez-Lavin M. Hypertrophic osteoarthropathy: what a rheumatologist should know about this uncommon condition. *Rheumatic diseases clinics of North America,* 2013;39(2):383-400.

[141] Jayakar B. A., Abelson A. G., Yao Q. Treatment of hypertrophic osteoarthropathy with zoledronic acid: case report and review of the literature. *Seminars in arthritis and rheumatism,* 2011;41(2):291-6.

[142] Hewitt R. E., Lissina A., Green A. E., Slay E. S., Price D. A., Sewell A. K. The bisphosphonate acute phase response: rapid and copious production of proinflammatory cytokines by peripheral blood gd T cells in response to aminobisphosphonates is inhibited by statins. *Clinical and experimental immunology,* 2005;139(1):101-11.

[143] Apalla Z., Tzellos T., Lallas A., Sotiriou E., Lefaki I. Possible zoledronic acid-induced dermatomyositis. *Clinical and experimental dermatology,* 2012;37(3):309-11.

[144] Tong P. L., Yu L. L., Chan J. J. Drug-induced dermatomyositis after zoledronic acid. *The Australasian journal of dermatology,* 2012;53(4):e73-5.

[145] Metyas S., Ibrahim M., Solyman J., Yeter K. C., Arkfeld D. G. Giant cell arteritis with visual loss following zoledronic acid infusion. *International journal of rheumatic diseases,* 2014;17(1):113-5.

[146] Gonzalez-Gay M. A., Blanco R., Rodriguez-Valverde V., Martinez-Taboada V. M., Delgado-Rodriguez M., Figueroa M., et al. Permanent visual loss and cerebrovascular accidents in giant cell arteritis: predictors and response to treatment. *Arthritis and rheumatism,* 1998;41(8):1497-504.

[147] Werner de Castro G. R., Neves F. S., de Magalhaes Souza Fialho S. C., Pereira I. A., Ribeiro G., Zimmermann A. F. Flare-up of hand osteoarthritis caused by zoledronic acid infusion. *Osteoporosis international : a journal established as result of cooperation between the European Foundation for Osteoporosis and the National Osteoporosis Foundation of the USA,* 2010;21(9):1617-9.

[148] Carneiro S., Sampaio-Barros P. D. SAPHO syndrome. *Rheumatic diseases clinics of North America,* 2013;39(2):401-18.

[149] Kopterides P., Pikazis D., Koufos C. Successful treatment of SAPHO syndrome with zoledronic acid. *Arthritis and rheumatism,* 2004;50(9):2970-3.
[150] Devogelaer J. P., Sambrook P., Reid D. M., Goemaere S., Ish-Shalom S., Collette J., et al. Effect on bone turnover markers of once-yearly intravenous infusion of zoledronic acid versus daily oral risedronate in patients treated with glucocorticoids. *Rheumatology (Oxford, England),* 2013;52(6):1058-69.
[151] Sambrook P. N., Roux C., Devogelaer J. P., Saag K., Lau C. S., Reginster J. Y., et al. Bisphosphonates and glucocorticoid osteoporosis in men: results of a randomized controlled trial comparing zoledronic acid with risedronate. *Bone,* 2012;50(1):289-95.
[152] Reid I. R., Black D. M., Eastell R., Bucci-Rechtweg C., Su G., Hue T. F., et al. Reduction in the risk of clinical fractures after a single dose of zoledronic Acid 5 milligrams. *The Journal of clinical endocrinology and metabolism,* 2013;98(2):557-63.
[153] Zhang J., Wang R., Zhao Y. L., Sun X. H., Zhao H. X., Tan L., et al. Efficacy of intravenous zoledronic acid in the prevention and treatment of osteoporosis: a meta-analysis. *Asian Pacific journal of tropical medicine,* 2012;5(9):743-8.
[154] Chen J., Liu W., Lin Q., Chen L., Yin J., Huang H. Vitamin D deficiency and low bone mineral density in native Chinese rheumatoid arthritis patients. *International journal of rheumatic diseases,* 2014;17(1):66-70.
[155] Lee S. G., Park Y. E., Park S. H., Kim T. K., Choi H. J., Lee S. J., et al. Increased frequency of osteoporosis and BMD below the expected range for age among South Korean women with rheumatoid arthritis. *International journal of rheumatic diseases,* 2012;15(3):289-96.
[156] Dao H. H., Do Q. T., Sakamoto J. Bone mineral density and frequency of osteoporosis among Vietnamese women with early rheumatoid arthritis. *Clinical rheumatology,* 2011;30(10):1353-61.
[157] El Maghraoui A., Rezqi A., Mounach A., Achemlal L., Bezza A., Ghozlani I. Prevalence and risk factors of vertebral fractures in women with rheumatoid arthritis using vertebral fracture assessment. *Rheumatology (Oxford, England),* 2010;49(7): 1303-10.
[158] Zhang J., Redden D. T., McGwin G., Jr., Callahan L. F., Smith E. A., Alarcon G. S., et al. Generalized bone loss as a predictor of three-year radiographic damage in African American patients with recent-onset rheumatoid arthritis. *Arthritis and rheumatism,* 2010;62(8):2219-26.
[159] Haugen I. K., Slatkowsky-Christensen B., Orstavik R., Kvien T. K. Bone mineral density in patients with hand osteoarthritis compared to population controls and patients with rheumatoid arthritis. *Annals of the rheumatic diseases,* 2007;66(12):1594-8.
[160] Westhoff G., Rau R., Zink A. Radiographic joint damage in early rheumatoid arthritis is highly dependent on body mass index. *Arthritis and rheumatism,* 2007;56(11):3575-82.
[161] Nolla J. M., Roig-Vilaseca D., Gomez-Vaquero C., Mateo L., Juanola X., Rodriguez-Moreno J., et al. Frequency of osteoporosis in 187 men with rheumatoid arthritis followed in a university hospital. *The Journal of rheumatology,* 2006;33(8):1472-5.
[162] Orstavik R. E., Haugeberg G., Mowinckel P., Hoiseth A., Uhlig T., Falch J. A., et al. Vertebral deformities in rheumatoid arthritis: a comparison with population-based controls. *Archives of internal medicine,* 2004;164(4):420-5.
[163] Lodder M. C., de Jong Z., Kostense P. J., Molenaar E. T., Staal K., Voskuyl A. E., et al. Bone mineral density in patients with rheumatoid arthritis: relation between disease

severity and low bone mineral density. *Annals of the rheumatic diseases,* 2004;63(12): 1576-80.

[164] Lee J. H., Cho S. K., Han M., Lee S., Kim J. Y., Ryu J. A., et al. Validity and role of vertebral fracture assessment in detecting prevalent vertebral fracture in patients with rheumatoid arthritis. *Joint, bone, spine : revue du rhumatisme,* 2014;81(2):149-53.

[165] Nampei A., Hashimoto J., Koyanagi J., Ono T., Hashimoto H., Tsumaki N., et al. Characteristics of fracture and related factors in patients with rheumatoid arthritis. *Modern rheumatology / the Japan Rheumatism Association,* 2008;18(2):170-6.

[166] Baskan B. M., Sivas F., Alemdaroglu E., Duran S., Ozoran K. Association of bone mineral density and vertebral deformity in patients with rheumatoid arthritis. *Rheumatology international,* 2007;27(6):579-84.

[167] Arai K., Hanyu T., Sugitani H., Murai T., Fujisawa J., Nakazono K., et al. Risk factors for vertebral fracture in menopausal or postmenopausal Japanese women with rheumatoid arthritis: a cross-sectional and longitudinal study. *Journal of bone and mineral metabolism,* 2006;24(2):118-24.

[168] Lee J. J., Aghdassi E., Cheung A. M., Morrison S., Cymet A., Peeva V., et al. Ten-year absolute fracture risk and hip bone strength in Canadian women with systemic lupus erythematosus. *The Journal of rheumatology,* 2012;39(7):1378-84.

[169] Almehed K., Hetenyi S., Ohlsson C., Carlsten H., Forsblad-d'Elia H. Prevalence and risk factors of vertebral compression fractures in female SLE patients. *Arthritis research and therapy,* 2010;12(4):R153.

[170] Lee C., Almagor O., Dunlop D. D., Manzi S., Spies S., Chadha A. B., et al. Disease damage and low bone mineral density: an analysis of women with systemic lupus erythematosus ever and never receiving corticosteroids. *Rheumatology (Oxford, England),* 2006;45(1):53-60.

[171] Bultink I. E., Lems W. F., Kostense P. J., Dijkmans B. A., Voskuyl A. E. Prevalence of and risk factors for low bone mineral density and vertebral fractures in patients with systemic lupus erythematosus. *Arthritis and rheumatism,* 2005;52(7):2044-50.

[172] Yee C. S., Crabtree N., Skan J., Amft N., Bowman S., Situnayake D., et al. Prevalence and predictors of fragility fractures in systemic lupus erythematosus. *Annals of the rheumatic diseases,* 2005;64(1):111-3.

[173] Pineau C. A., Urowitz M. B., Fortin P. J., Ibanez D., Gladman D. D. Osteoporosis in systemic lupus erythematosus: factors associated with referral for bone mineral density studies, prevalence of osteoporosis and factors associated with reduced bone density. *Lupus,* 2004;13(6):436-41.

[174] Singh H. J., Nimarpreet K., Ashima, Das S., Kumar A., Prakash S. Study of bone mineral density in patients with ankylosing spondylitis. *Journal of clinical and diagnostic research: JCDR,* 2013;7(12):2832-5.

[175] Klingberg E., Lorentzon M., Gothlin J., Mellstrom D., Geijer M., Ohlsson C., et al. Bone microarchitecture in ankylosing spondylitis and the association with bone mineral density, fractures, and syndesmophytes. *Arthritis research and therapy,* 2013;15 (6):R179.

[176] Vasdev V., Bhakuni D., Garg M. K., Narayanan K., Jain R., Chadha D. Bone mineral density in young males with ankylosing spondylitis. *International journal of rheumatic diseases,* 2011;14(1):68-73.

[177] Muntean L., Rojas-Vargas M., Font P., Simon S. P., Rednic S., Schiotis R., et al. Relative value of the lumbar spine and hip bone mineral density and bone turnover markers in men with ankylosing spondylitis. *Clinical rheumatology*, 2011;30(5):691-5.
[178] Ghozlani I., Ghazi M., Nouijai A., Mounach A., Rezqi A., Achemlal L., et al. Prevalence and risk factors of osteoporosis and vertebral fractures in patients with ankylosing spondylitis. *Bone*, 2009;44(5):772-6.
[179] van der Weijden M. A., van der Horst-Bruinsma I. E., van Denderen J. C., Dijkmans B. A., Heymans M. W., Lems W. F. High frequency of vertebral fractures in early spondylarthropathies. *Osteoporosis international: a journal established as result of cooperation between the European Foundation for Osteoporosis and the National Osteoporosis Foundation of the USA*, 2012;23(6):1683-90.
[180] Grazio S., Cvijetic S., Vlak T., Grubisic F., Matijevic V., Nemcic T., et al. Osteoporosis in psoriatic arthritis: is there any? *Wiener klinische Wochenschrift*, 2011;123(23-24):743-50.
[181] Borman P., Babaoglu S., Gur G., Bingol S., Bodur H. Bone mineral density and bone turnover in patients with psoriatic arthritis. *Clinical rheumatology*, 2008;27(4):443-7.
[182] Hofbauer L. C., Schoppet M., Christ M., Teichmann J., Lange U. Tumour necrosis factor-related apoptosis-inducing ligand and osteoprotegerin serum levels in psoriatic arthritis. *Rheumatology (Oxford, England)*, 2006;45(10):1218-22.

In: Zoledronic Acid
Editor: Ronald Carman

ISBN: 978-1-63321-525-2

Chapter 8

ZOLEDRONIC ACID AND BENIGN BONE DISEASE: CLINICAL USES, THERAPEUTIC EFFECTS AND PHARMACOKINETICS

P. K. Wong[1] and J. D. Wark[2]

[1]Mid-North Coast Arthritis Clinic, Coffs Harbour, and Rural Clinical School, Faculty of Medicine, University of New South Wales, Kensington, New South Wales, Australia

[2]Department of Medicine, University of Melbourne and Bone and Mineral Medicine, Royal Melbourne Hospital, both in Parkville, Victoria, Australia

ABSTRACT

Bisphosphonates such as alendronate, risedronate and zoledronate have revolutionised the treatment of benign bone disease. Zoledronate (ZLD)/zoledronic acid is a nitrogen containing intravenous (IV) bisphosphonate which is a potent inhibitor of osteoclast mediated bone resorption via several possible mechanisms, but especially by inhibition of the enzyme farnesyl pyrophosphate synthase. Annual administration has been shown to increase bone mineral density at all sites measured, with a concomitant reduction in the risk of vertebral and hip fracture in patients with osteoporosis. Interestingly, IV ZLD has also been shown to lower mortality following hip fracture. The mechanism for this remains unclear, but may be related to a reduction in cardiovascular events. One of the main advantages of ZLD is the convenient annual IV dosing which improves patient compliance. This is of particular importance in the field of osteoporosis where poor compliance with bone protective therapy is well described. However, the long *in vivo* half-life and high potency of ZLD may be responsible for the reported association with delayed dental healing (DDH) and the rare, but potentially devastating complication of osteonecrosis of the jaw (ONJ). The possible association with atypical femoral fractures will also be discussed. This chapter will discuss the clinical use and therapeutic effects of ZLD in benign bone disease, focusing on the treatment of osteoporosis and Paget's disease. The advantages and disadvantages of ZLD relative to the other treatments for osteoporosis will be reviewed. A practical approach to the contentious issue of DDH and ONJ will also be discussed.

INTRODUCTION

Osteoporosis (OSP), the commonest benign bone disease, is characterized by low bone mass and structural deterioration which results in reduced bone strength and increased fracture risk (Holroyd 2008). According to the World Health Organization (WHO) definition of OSP (bone mineral density, BMD T-score < -2.5, that is, 2.5 standard deviations below that for young normal controls as measured by dual x-ray absorptiometry, DXA) approximately 11% of men and 27% of women aged 60 years or over are osteoporotic (WHO 2001). The major complication of OSP is low trauma fracture (LTF, trauma equivalent to a fall from a standing height). Fracture incidence in Australian men and women aged 50 years and over was 1248 and 1916 per 100 000 person-years, respectively (Cooley 2001). Lifetime fracture risk in a person aged 50 years was 27% for men and 44% for women, respectively (Cooley 2001). Osteoporotic fractures are a major public health issue in Western countries and are already an increasing problem in Asia and South America due to an ageing population (Eisman 2012). Patients sustaining a hip fracture have a 33% mortality rate in the subsequent 12 months (Jensen 1979, Keene 1999). This excess mortality persists for up to 10 years following the incident fracture (Bliuc 2009, Haentjens 2010) and up to one third of such patients subsequently require admission to residential care (Marottoli 1994).

Paget's disease of bone (PDB) is the second commonest benign bone disease after OSP and affects up to 3% of people aged 55 years and older with a slightly higher prevalence in men (Eekhoff 2004). It is a progressive monostotic or polyostotic disease characterized by focal abnormal bone remodeling, with increased bone resorption and excessive disorganized new bone formation (Figure 1) (Roodman 2005). Despite thicker bone, there is weakened strength due to abnormal bone architecture manifesting as an irregular mosaic pattern (woven bone) instead of the more usual parallel symmetry seen in normal (lamellar) bone. Osteoclasts usually predominate early in the course of a Pagetic bone focus, resulting in osteolysis, but as the lesion matures this usually progresses to a predominance of osteoblasts (Reid 2011). While PDB is often asymptomatic, it can result in bone symptoms or joint pain from premature osteoarthritis (Figure 1a), bone deformity or even fracture in the affected bone. Despite extensive research, the cause of PDB remains unclear. However, a slow virus infection of bone remains the favoured aetiology (Michou 2011).

Bisphosphonates (BPs) have revolutionised the treatment of both OSP (Black 2007, Lyles 2007, Black 2012) and PDB (Reid 2005, Hosking 2007). These drugs are stable analogues of inorganic pyrophosphate contained in bone in which the P-O-P "backbone" has been replaced by P-C-P (Widler 2002). The oral BPs alendronate (ALN) and risedronate (RSD) and the intravenous (IV) BPs pamidronate (APD) and the more potent zoledronic acid/zoledronate (ZLD) contain at least one nitrogen group ("nitrogen-containing" BPs) in contrast to clodronate, etidronate and tiludronate which do not. The presence of this nitrogen side chain confers a more potent anti-resorptive effect mediated mainly via inhibition of mevalonate metabolism (Widler 2002). Due to its potent anti-resorptive effect, IV ZLD is also used for the treatment of malignant bone disease, for example in myeloma and breast cancer with bone metastases (Coleman 2013, Zwolak 2013, Gnant 2014). However, the use of ZLD in the treatment of malignant bone disease is outside the scope of this paper.

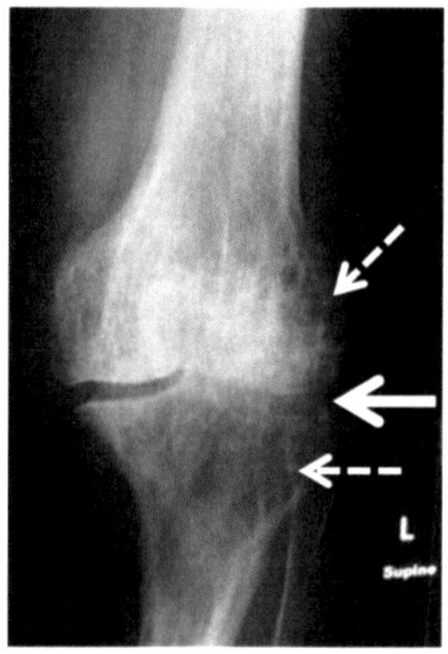

a) AP x-ray of the L knee showing Paget's disease affecting the distal femur and proximal tibia with secondary osteoarthritis of the femoro-tibial articulation (thick arrow).

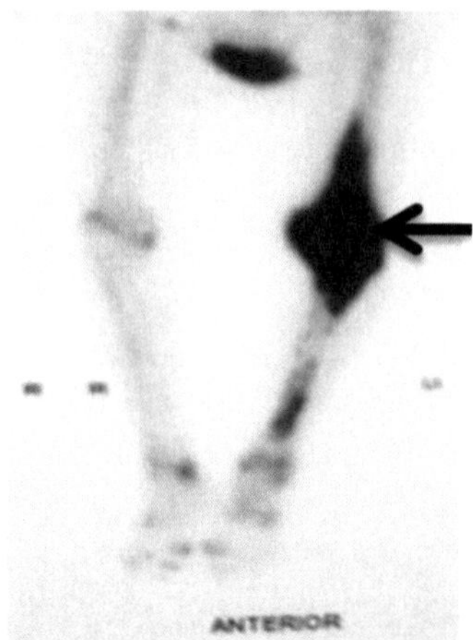

b) Technetium 99m nuclear bone scan showing intense increased uptake in the L distal femur and proximal tibia of the patient in (a) consistent with metabolically active Paget's disease.

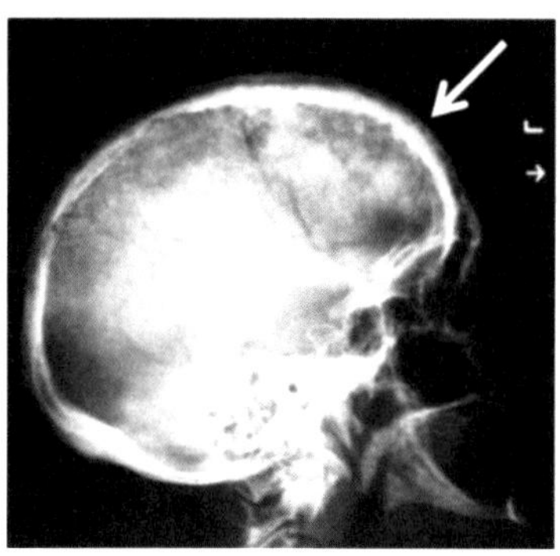

c) Lateral skull x-ray showing Pagetic change in the calvarium especially affecting the fronto-parietal area.

Figure 1. Paget's disease of bone affecting the knee and skull.

Pharmacokinetics

Zoledronic acid was identified as a potent inhibitor of bone resorption following screening of more than 300 novel BPs and reference compounds in the search for a potent bone active drug (Green 1994). The aim was to identify a chemical with an improved therapeutic ratio (potency versus side effects) compared to APD, the first IV BP in widespread clinical use (Green 1994). Zoledronic acid was found to be between 87- and 940-fold more potent than APD in a range of *in vivo* and *in vitro* assays (Green 1994), with a much higher affinity for the hydroxyapatite crystals in bone compared to other BPs (rank order of ZLD > ALN> ibandronate > RSD > etidronate > clodronate) (Nancollas 2006). The observed higher affinity of nitrogen containing BPs such as ZLD, ALN and RSD, for hydroxyapatite means these drugs have a longer *in vivo* bone half-life and continue to exert a biologic effect for some years following their cessation (Watts 2010).

Once deposited in bone, BPs are released during resorption and taken up by osteoclasts, the only cell type capable of bone resorption. This leads to inhibition of protein prenylation and blockade of mevalonate metabolism, which in turn results in impaired osteoclast activation and stimulation of osteoclast apoptosis due to development of cytoskeletal abnormalities (Hughes 1995, Rogers 1999, Russell 1999). Inhibition of the key enzyme in the mevalonate pathway, farnesyl diphosphate synthase (FDS) *in vitro* has been shown to correlate with inhibition of bone resorption *in vivo* (Dunford 2001). Zoledronic acid was found to be a more potent inhibitor of FDS than other BPs, with a rank order of ZLD > RSD > ibandronate > incadronate > ALN > APD (Dunford 2001).

In addition to their potent effect on osteoclasts, BPs possess anti-angiogenic activity (Santini 2002, Wood 2002, Giraudo 2004). They may also inhibit matrix metalloproteinases (the enzymes involved in tumour metastasis and connective tissue remodelling) (Teronen 2000, Ferretti 2005) and inhibit proliferation of oral keratinocytes (Ferretti 2005).

Due to their highly polar nature, oral BPs are poorly absorbed from the gastrointestinal tract and therefore have low bioavailability, often less than 2% (Lin 1996, Licata 2005). This may explain why some patients continue to sustain low trauma fractures despite being adherent with oral BPs. A systematic literature review of multiple databases identified 30 randomized placebo-controlled trials involving 59 209 patients on treatment for post-menopausal OSP and found the highest probability of reducing vertebral, hip or wrist fracture was seen with parenteral agents, specifically ZLD, teriparatide (recombinant human parathyroid hormone analogue 1-34), and denosumab (the novel Receptor Activator of Nuclear Factor kappa-B Ligand, RANKL inhibitor) (Hopkins 2011). The poor oral bioavailability along with the risk of upper gastrointestinal complications and low patient rates of adherence with oral BPs, which will be discussed in more detail later (Caro 2004, Siris 2006, Penning-van Beest 2007, Rabenda 2008, Siris 2009), mean that IV ZLD is often the BP of choice in the treatment of benign bone disease.

Following IV administration, ZLD is mainly eliminated via renal glomerular filtration with up to 40% of the dose being excreted unmetabolized in urine within 24 hours, with approximately 60% of the dose being retained in the skeleton (Chen 2002). This was independent of the duration of infusion, dose or the number of doses administered (Chen 2002). The *in vivo* anti-resorptive effects manifested by suppression of serum and urine bone turnover markers such as C-terminal telopeptide of type-1 collagen (C-telopeptide, CTx) and

N-telopeptide (NTx), hydroxyproline, pyridinoline and deoxypyridinoline were evident within 24 hours following administration (Chen 2002). As there is little inhibition of the human cytochrome P450 family of enzymes, drug interactions are unlikely (De Luca 2011).

ZOLEDRONIC ACID AND POST-MENOPAUSAL OSTEOPOROSIS

Bisphosphonates (BPs) such as ALN, RSD and ZLD are first-line treatments for OSP, especially following LTF (Sambrook 2002). Annual administration of IV ZLD in post-menopausal women was well-tolerated and resulted in increased BMD by up to 5% at 12 months (Reid 2002). A double-blind placebo-controlled trial, the Health Outcomes and Reduced Incidence with Zoledronic Acid Once Yearly-Pivotal Fracture Trial (HORIZON-PFT) recruited patients with a femoral neck BMD T-score of −2.5 or less with or without existing vertebral fracture, or a femoral neck BMD T-score of −1.5 or less, with at least two mild vertebral fractures or one moderate vertebral fracture. The trial randomised 3889 patients to one infusion of ZLD 5 mg and 3876 patients to placebo, each administered at baseline, 12 months and 24 months with follow-up until 36 months (Black 2007). Zoledronic acid lowered the risk of vertebral fracture by 70% at 36 months compared to placebo (3.3% in the ZLD group versus 10.9% in the placebo group; relative risk, RR: 0.30) and reduced hip fracture risk by 41% (1.4% in the ZLD group versus 2.5% in the placebo group; RR: 0.59) (Black 2007). This was associated with a significant improvement in BMD as measured by DXA at the total hip (6.02%; 95% confidence interval, CI, 5.77 to 6.28), lumbar spine (6.71%; 95% CI, 5.69 to 7.74) and femoral neck (5.06%; 95% CI, 4.76 to 5.36) compared to the placebo group ($p<0.001$ for all comparisons). The only significant difference in adverse events was that serious atrial fibrillation occurred more frequently in the ZLD group (50 versus 20 patients, $p<0.001$) (Black 2007).

Extension of the HORIZON-PFT study out to six years allowed longer term examination of the effects of ZLD on BMD and fracture risk. One thousand two hundred and thirty three women who had received ZLD annually for three years were randomised to three more years of ZLD or placebo (Black 2012). In years 3 to 6, femoral neck BMD remained constant after six years of annual IV ZLD but fell slightly in the group who received placebo from year 3-6 (between-treatment difference of 1.04%; 95% CI 0.4-1.7; $p=0.0009$). However, even the latter group maintained their BMD above pre-treatment levels. Unlike in the HORIZON-PFT study, no significant increase in AF was seen in the extension study (Black 2012). The small between-group difference in BMD observed in the extension study suggests treatment with IV ZLD can be stopped after three years in those at low risk of fracture.

The HORIZON Recurrent Fracture Trial (HORIZON-RFT) examined the effect of ZLD following hip fracture and randomized 1065 patients to annual IV ZLD and 1062 patients to placebo, each for three years. At enrolment, over 40% of patients had a T-score of -2.5 or less at the femoral neck. All ZLD infusions were first administered within 90 days following surgical repair of the hip fracture with a median follow-up of 1.9 years. New clinical fracture occurred in 8.6% of the ZLD group and 13.9% of the placebo group, a 35% risk reduction ($p=0.001$) (Lyles 2007). Rates of new clinical vertebral fracture were 1.7% and 3.8% ($p=0.02$), respectively and rates of new non-vertebral fracture were 7.6% and 10.7% ($p = 0.03$), respectively (Lyles 2007). Most importantly, 101 of 1054 (9.6%) patients who received

ZLD and 141 of 1057 (13.3%) patients who received placebo died, a reduction in mortality of 28% following IV ZLD (p = 0.01). There was no difference in adverse effects between the two study arms, in particular, no difference was observed in the rate of AF and no cases of osteonecrosis of the jaw (ONJ) were reported. Interestingly, the reduction in mortality appeared to be due to a beneficial effect on cardiovascular events and pneumonia (Colón-Emeric 2010). Given the well-recognised increase in mortality following hip fracture (Jensen 1979, Keene 1999, Bliuc 2009, Haentjens 2010) this trial provided a strong reason to use IV ZLD for bone protection post-hip fracture.

Post-hoc analysis of patients (n=1367) from these two ZLD intervention trials (HORIZON-PFT and HORIZON-RFT) (Black 2007, Lyles 2007) found that at a mean follow-up of 1.5 years those who had received only one ZLD infusion still had a 32% reduction in clinical fracture compared to those who received placebo (95%CI; 2–53%, p= 0.04). This magnitude of fracture reduction was comparable to that seen in those who had received three or more annual infusions of ZLD. New morphometric vertebral fractures were reduced by 68% in the single-infusion group (p=0.004) (Reid 2013). This result is heartening and means that fracture reduction can be achieved with only one infusion of ZLD. This finding has favourable implications for drug safety, expense and patient compliance.

In a prospective longitudinal study, male and female patients (mean age 60.5 ± 11.0 years) with low BMD (DXA T-score below -2.0 at the lumbar spine or total hip) received one infusion of ZLD 4 mg at baseline (Borba 2007). Median serum levels of the bone turnover markers CTx and bone specific alkaline phosphatase (BSAP) remained suppressed below baseline even at 18 months. This was associated with a significant increase in BMD compared to 12 months (median increase of 6.1% at the lumbar spine and 2.0% for the total hip) (Borba 2007). When administered to 50 post-menopausal women, one infusion of ZLD 5 mg suppressed bone turnover markers (serum osteocalcin, P1NP and CTx and urine NTx) by at least 38% at two years with higher BMD in the ZLD group compared to placebo (Grey 2009). There was also increased BMD by DXA at the lumbar spine (5.7%, 95% CI 4.0–7.4), proximal femur (3.9%, 95% CI 2.2–5.7) and the total body (1.7%, 95% CI 0.8–2.5) ($p < 0.0001$ for each site) (Grey 2009). These findings suggest that although the recommended infusion frequency of ZLD is once every 12 months one infusion of ZLD 4-5 mg appears to inhibit bone turnover for at least 18-24 months. This means that in low risk patients where IV ZLD is stopped, say after three years, the *in vivo* biologic effect may continue for at least two years following cessation.

Zoledronic Acid and Drug Adherence

Patient adherence to medication is a major issue in the treatment of chronic disease (Krueger 2003, Sabatae 2003). This is especially important in the management of OSP which is asymptomatic unless complicated by fracture (Caro 2004, Siris 2006, Penning-van Beest 2007, Rabenda 2008, Siris 2009). A retrospective cohort study using data from health insurance companies collected for the Belgian national social security institute assessed drug persistence (duration of time from initiation to discontinuation of therapy) and compliance (extent to which a patient acts in accordance with the prescribed interval and dose of a dosing regimen) in 29 157 women commenced on a BP (Rabenda 2008). Medication compliance as measured by a medication possession ratio, MPR $\geq$ 80% was 64.7% at 12 months but was higher for patients taking weekly compared to daily ALN (70.5% versus 58.6%, respectively $p<0.001$). At 12 months, only 40% of women continued to take ALN without a gap of more than five weeks. The median duration of medication persistence was only 35.7 weeks (Rabenda 2008). Greater patient medication adherence with a less frequent dosing frequency of BP therapy for the treatment of OSP has also been reported by others (Cramer 2005).

Poor medication adherence results in increased fracture risk. A study using information from the health service database of one of the ten Canadian provinces examined 11,249 women with OSP (mean age at commencement of BP therapy 68.4 years and average follow-up of two years) noted an overall fracture rate of 4.5% per year. Patients with greater drug adherence (drug available to cover > 80% of the time) had a 16% lower fracture rate (Caro 2004).

A retrospective cohort analysis of 35,537 women aged $\geq$ 45 yo who were prescribed a BP and followed up for two years found that forty three percent were compliant (MPR $\geq$ 80) and 20% were persistent with BP therapy at 24 months (Siris 2006). The risk of total, vertebral, non-vertebral and hip fracture was lower by 20-45% in compliant and persistent patients. The probability of fracture risk reduction began to rise at a MPR of 50% and became more marked at a MPR $\geq$ 75%. The converse of this is that women only compliant with BP therapy < 50% of the time gained little from taking a BP. Assuming that BP therapy lowered fracture risk by a conservative figure of 25%, extrapolation of these results to the US population suggested that better adherence to therapy would prevent 300,000 fractures per year leading to a saving of over USD 3 billion per year (Siris 2006, Siris 2009).

Poor adherence with medication is a complex issue and may be due to a range of reasons such as lack of immediate patient-recognized benefits, concern about the risk of adverse effects, drug cost and an inconvenient dosing regime (Siris 2009). In view of these issues, the IV route of administration with ZLD guarantees fracture protection for at least 12 months. This advantage is particularly useful in older patients with poor memory who may forget to regularly take an oral agent. For those patients in residential care an annual IV administration also saves nursing time compared to a regular daily or even weekly oral preparation.

Zoledronic Acid and Male Osteoporosis

Unfortunately, most studies examining the effect of pharmacologic intervention in men with OSP have used surrogate endpoints such as BMD or bone turnover markers to assess efficacy and have therefore been underpowered to detect an effect on fracture reduction – the most important clinical outcome (Orwoll 2003, Boonen 2009. should be, Orwoll 2010). A multi-centre randomized controlled trial in men with OSP of annual IV ZLD 5 mg versus weekly ALN, the most commonly prescribed oral BP, demonstrated non-inferiority of ZLD for change in BMD and suppression of bone turnover markers (Orwoll 2010). Zoledronic acid increased BMD at the lumbar spine, total hip, femoral neck, and trochanter at 24 months with a similar rate of adverse events compared to ALN. Among 275 participants who completed the study questionnaires, 204 (74.2%) preferred annual IV ZLD compared to 42 participants (15.3%) who preferred weekly oral ALN (Orwoll 2010). This was independent of the occurrence of side effects. The main advantage of annual IV ZLD was that it guaranteed 100% drug bioavailability and medication adherence for the subsequent year.

A multi-center double-blind, placebo-controlled trial of 1199 men with OSP reported fewer incident vertebral fractures with ZLD (1.6 versus 4.9%, p= 0.002) over 24 months following two annual infusions of ZLD 5 mg. This equated to a 67% relative risk reduction and was associated with a significant increase in BMD and a decrease in serum levels of bone turnover markers (Boonen 2012). The beneficial effect was seen in both eugonadal and hypogonadal men. This magnitude of relative risk reduction was similar to that observed in postmenopausal women with OSP who received ZLD (relative risk reduction in vertebral fracture of 71% at two years) (Black 2007). This study (Boonen 2012) clearly supported the anti-fracture effectiveness of ZLD in men with OSP and provided strong evidence the protective effect was independent of gender.

ZOLEDRONIC ACID AND GLUCOCORTICOID INDUCED OSTEOPOROSIS

The Health Outcomes and Reduced Incidence with Zoledronic acid Once yearly (HORIZON) study was a one year randomised, double-blind, non-inferiority study to assess the effectiveness of IV ZLD 5 mg versus oral RSD 5 mg/d for prevention (taking corticosteroid for less than three months) and treatment (taking corticosteroid for more than three months) of glucocorticoid-induced osteoporosis (GIOP) (Reid 2009). Approximately two thirds of patients were being treated with corticosteroids for rheumatoid arthritis (RA), polymyalgia rheumatica or systemic lupus erythematosus at a mean dose of prednisone 10 mg/d. Eight hundred and thirty three patients were randomised to receive ZLD (n=416) or RSD (n=417). Zoledronic acid was non-inferior and even more importantly, superior to RSD for increase of lumbar spine BMD in both the treatment (mean 4·06% versus 2·71%, mean difference 1·36% 95% CI 0·67–2·05, p=0·0001) and prevention (mean 2·60% versus 0·64%, mean difference 1·96% 95% CI 1·04–2·88, p<0·0001) groups at 12 months (Reid 2009). Adverse events were more common in the ZLD group, mainly due to flu-like symptoms and fever post-infusion (Reid 2009). The commonest serious adverse event was worsening of RA, which was felt to be severe in six (2%) patients in each group. No cases of AF were deemed by an independent adjudication panel to be related to ZLD. Importantly, almost 80% of patients preferred the IV route of administration for convenience and satisfaction. Zoledronic acid had a faster and greater inhibitory effect on serum bone turnover biomarkers than RSD (Reid 2009). This effect is probably important for prevention of GIOP as reduction in BMD occurs within a few months following commencement of glucocorticoids (van Staa 2006).

Although this short duration (12 months) study was not powered to assess fracture risk reduction and so used surrogate measures of efficacy (bone turnover markers and BMD), it clearly showed that in patients with a range of corticosteroid responsive disorders one infusion of ZLD was more effective than RSD for the treatment and prevention of GIOP. Furthermore, ZLD was preferred by patients for its convenient mode and frequency of administration.

ZOLEDRONIC ACID AND PAGET'S DISEASE OF BONE (PDB)

Bisphosphonates are standard therapy for the treatment of PDB. A randomized, double-blind trial comparing one infusion of ZLD 5 mg to oral RSD 30 mg daily for 60 days in 357 patients with PDB showed normalization of the serum total ALP in 89% of ZLD-treated patients and 58% of RSD-treated patients after six months ($p<0.001$) (Reid 2005). Zoledronic acid was associated with a faster time to therapeutic response (64 versus 89 days, $p<0.001$) with the curves of therapeutic response as measured by serum ALP diverging as early as 10 days (Reid 2005). Response to ZLD was independent of age, sex, baseline serum ALP level and previous treatment for PDB.

The physical-component score of the Medical Outcomes Study 36-item Short-Form General Health Survey, a measure of patient quality of life increased significantly from baseline at both three and six months in the ZLD group with more favourable scores compared to the RSD group at three months. At a median follow-up of 190 days, 21 of 82 patients in the RSD group had lost therapeutic response compared to only one of 113 patients who received ZLD ($p<0.001$) (Reid 2005).

Patients who achieved a therapeutic response defined as a $\geq$ 75% reduction in the excess serum ALP above the mid-point of the reference range at six months were followed to determine the duration of treatment response. After two years, ZLD continued to maintain bone turnover in the reference range (Hosking 2007). In particular, therapeutic response was maintained in 98% of those who received ZLD but only 57% of RSD-treated patients (Hosking 2007). The observed greater efficacy of ZLD versus RSD was thought to be due to greater binding to hydroxyapatite and persistence at bone remodelling sites.

The use of IV ZLD in the treatment of PDB has allowed a more sustained long-term response to be achieved, even after one infusion, compared to a course of an oral BP. Re-treatment is usually indicated when symptoms of PDB recur in parallel with a rising serum ALP.

SAFETY AND TOLERABILITY

The commonest side effects associated with IV ZLD are flu-like symptoms, for example bone pain, nausea, vomiting, fatigue and fever, that are probably related to an acute phase response. These usually occur within 24 hours following the infusion, last less than 48 hours and become less severe with subsequent infusions (Berenson 2005). Analgesics and non-steroidal anti-inflammatories usually provide sufficient relief of these symptoms.

Amino-bisphosphonates such as ZLD, APD and ALN contain a nitrogen group that can activate gamma delta (γ/δ) T cells *in vitro* (Kunzmann 2000) and *in vivo* (Kunzmann 1999). In contrast, non-amino containing BPs such as etidronate and clodronate failed to do so. Activation of γ/δ T cells resulted in release of pro- inflammatory cytokines such as interferon-γ and granulocyte macrophage colony stimulating factor (Kunzmann 2000). While this may be of value in mediating the immune response to malignant cells such as in myeloma or breast cancer, it may also be responsible for the acute phase reaction often seen following ZLD (Kunzmann 1999).

Rarely, this immune response can result in ocular inflammation such as anterior uveitis, episcleritis, and scleritis, or even orbital inflammatory disease (Colucci 2009, Peterson 2012). Orbital inflammatory disease usually occurs within six days of administration when patients presented with ocular pain, diplopia and blurred vision accompanied by lid edema, conjunctival hyperaemia and chemosis. While this may result in permanent visual impairment most patients experienced full recovery following prompt systemic corticosteroid therapy (Peterson 2012).

An uncommon but important adverse event is deterioration in renal function, especially in patients with pre-existing renal function or who were taking co-existent nephrotoxic medication (Berenson 2005). A US Food and Drug Administration (FDA) safety newsletter reported 24 cases of renal impairment and acute renal failure which occurred from April 2007 to February 2009 following the use of IV ZLD 5 mg for the treatment of OSP (US FDA 2009). A subsequent FDA report documenting an additional 11 cases of fatal acute renal failure and nine cases of renal impairment requiring dialysis following ZLD infusion in the period from March 2009 to April 2011 (US FDA 2011) prompted a statement that ZLD was contraindicated in patients with a creatinine clearance (CrCl) <35mL/min as calculated by the Cockcroft-Gault formula (US FDA 2011). Serum electrolytes and renal function should be checked prior to administration and adequate patient hydration should be present with administration over at least 30 minutes rather than the 15 minutes that was initially suggested. In the HORIZON-PFT trial (Black 2012), transient but significant increases in serum creatinine were observed in 12 patients in the ZLD group after the second infusion, mostly in those with an estimated baseline CrCl between 30 and 34 mL/min, compared with one patient in the placebo group (p<0.002). These changes had normalized by 12 months (Boonen 2008, Miller 2013). In the subsequent extension study (Black 2012), more patients had transient rises in serum creatinine 9 to 11 days post IV ZLD in the group who received ZLD for six consecutive years compared to those who received ZLD for three years followed by placebo for three years (n=18 versus n =4; p=0.002) (Miller 2012, Miller 2013). These studies suggested that IV ZLD can be safely used in most patients as long as the eGFR is >35 mL/min) (Miller 2013).

Zoledronic Acid and Osteonecrosis of the Jaw (ONJ)

Multiple case reports since 2003 have raised a possible association between BPs, especially ZLD or APD and ONJ (Figure 2) (Marx 2003, Migliorati 2003, Ruggiero 2004, Bagan 2005, Carter 2005, Purcell 2005, Woo 2006). However, incomplete patient data, lack of long-term follow-up and incomplete reporting of BP dosage parameters made it impossible to accurately estimate the true prevalence of ONJ (Khosla 2007, Pazianas 2007, Migliorati 2011). Unfortunately, in the absence of firm scientific data, intense media scrutiny, often of a sensationalist nature, resulted in at-risk patients frequently refusing therapy with BPs (Sambrook 2010). A major reason for the observed heterogeneity of published data has been loose case definition. This has been rectified by several specialty societies agreeing on a definition of ONJ as "exposed necrotic bone in the maxillofacial region that has persisted for more than 8 weeks" in the absence of a history of radiation therapy to the jaw (Khosla 2007, American Association of Oral and Maxillofacial Surgeons 2007, Ruggiero 2009).

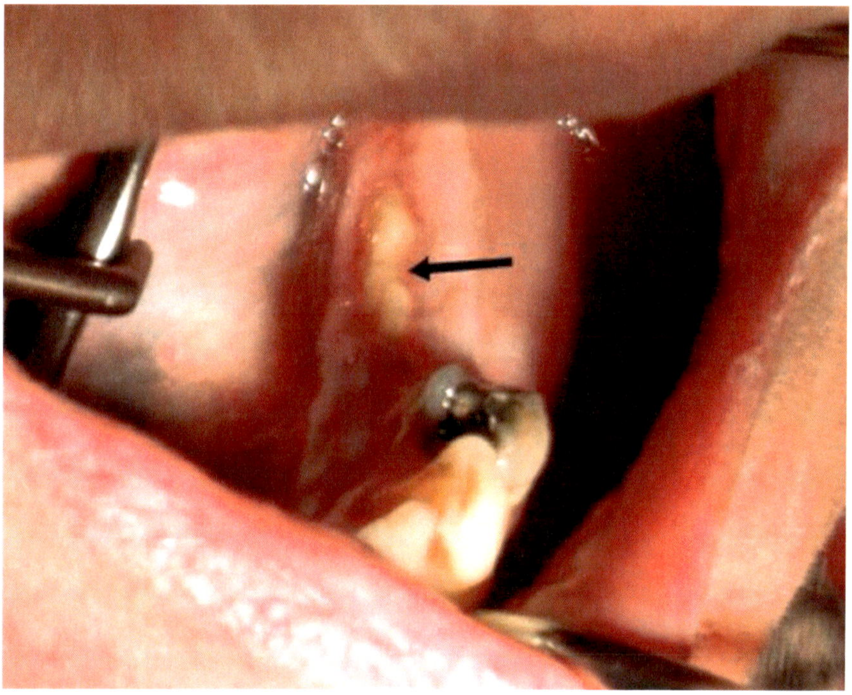

Figure 2. Osteonecrosis of the maxilla in a 51-year-old female patient with Goodpasture's syndrome who had undergone a cadaveric renal transplant 15 years earlier. She had been taking alendronate 70 mg weekly for 4 years for glucocorticoid-induced osteoporosis and presented 4 months following multiple dental extractions with painful areas of non-healing exposed bone (arrow). There was no history of radiotherapy to the area (Wong 2013).

Osteonecrosis of the jaw has been reported mainly in the setting of malignancy, especially multiple myeloma (Lugassy 2004, Durie 2005, Vannuchi 2005) and breast cancer (Wang 2003, Bagan 2005, Carter 2005, Purcell 2005). A major contributory factor is probably the higher cumulative doses of IV BP used (Hoff 2008), for example, ZLD 4 mg IV every four weeks for the treatment of bone metastases from breast cancer (Hillner 2003) compared to ZLD 4 mg IV annually for the treatment of OSP (Reid 2002), respectively. Intravenous ZLD and APD were associated with a 10% and 3% incidence of ONJ at 36 months, respectively in patients with myeloma (Durie 2005). A longitudinal cohort study reported that 1621 patients who received 29 006 doses of IV BP had a crude incidence of ONJ of 8.5%, 3.1%, and 4.9% in patients with myeloma, breast cancer and prostate cancer, respectively (Vahtsevanos 2009). A retrospective study of 2239 cancer patients found a lower prevalence (1.3%) of bisphosphonate related ONJ (BRONJ) (Hoff 2008).

Review of 119 patients with probable BRONJ suggested the mean time to clinical presentation was 14.3 months for APD, 9.4 months for ZLD and three years in patients receiving ALN (Marx 2005). Most of these patients were undergoing treatment with IV BPs for malignant bone disease and ONJ appeared to be preceded by dental trauma, for example tooth extraction or ill-fitting dentures (Marx 2003, Ruggiero 2004, Bagan 2005, Carter 2005). However, potential confounders such as chemotherapy, radiotherapy, corticosteroid use and dental/sinus infections have complicated attribution of causality (Tarassoff 2003).

There appear to be fewer cases of ONJ following treatment for OSP with BPs (Ruggiero 2004, Purcell 2005, Marx 2005, Migliorati 2005, Yarom 2007). The HORIZON-PFT trial involving 3889 patients with postmenopausal OSP who received three infusions of ZLD over a two-year period reported no cases of ONJ (Black 2007). Blinded retrospective adjudication of the clinical trial database yielded one case each of delayed dental healing in the ZLD and control groups. Both cases occurred following dental instrumentation and resolved following antibiotic therapy and gentle debridement (Black 2007). No further cases of ONJ were reported in the three year extension of this study nor following review of data from four other clinical trials involving patients with low BMD treated with ZLD (Grbic 2010, Black 2012).

Osteonecrosis of the jaw is not restricted to patients receiving IV ZLD. Recent case reports have suggested a possible association of ONJ with denosumab, a novel monoclonal antibody which selectively inhibits RANKL, a crucial cytokine promoting osteoclastogenesis (Taylor 2010, Aghaloo 2010). Most of these cases have been described in patients with an underlying malignancy receiving large doses of denosumab (120 mg subcutaneously (s/c) every 4 weeks) rather than the much lower dose of 60 mg s/c every 6 months which is used in the treatment of OSP. However, the association of ONJ with both IV ZLD and s/c denosumab suggest that osteoclast inhibition is important in the pathogenesis of ONJ and this complication is not just related to BP use.

However, the exact risk of ONJ in benign bone disease is uncertain. The ASMBR has suggested a risk estimate of 1:10 000-1:100 000 for patients with OSP taking BPs (Khosla 2007). The higher bioavailability and potency of IV BPs may explain the stronger association with ONJ. However, it is for these very reasons and the convenient mode of administration that IV ZLD is often used.

Management of Osteonecrosis of the Jaw

It is probably wise to arrange a dental review prior to administration of IV ZLD so any invasive dental procedures can be performed (Sambrook 2006, Ruggiero 2009, Borromeo 2011). This applies even to edentulous patients as dentures should to be checked to ensure they are well-fitting and to identify any areas of denture trauma. Patients should be educated regarding the importance of dental hygiene and the need for regular prophylactic dental care as they are often unaware why they have been commenced on BP therapy and the possible impact of BP therapy on dental health (Migliorati 2010). Patients should be strongly advised to promptly report any new dental symptoms to their health care professional, especially dental pain, swelling or exposed bone. Early treatment of dental infection should be undertaken and invasive dental therapy performed only if absolutely necessary, and preferably following consultation with a medical practitioner possessing expertise in the treatment of bone disease. The use of such preventive measures and delaying ZLD administration for 6–8 weeks following any invasive dental procedures to allow wound healing has been shown to reduce the risk of ONJ in oncology patients (Ripamonti 2009, Dimopoulos 2009). While no definite data supports the cessation of BP therapy prior to invasive dental surgery (Woo 2006, Rizzoli 2008), a considered decision should be made in each patient following consultation between members of the treating medical and dental team. The prolonged suppression of bone turnover following cessation of ALN (Bone 2004) means stopping it for even a period of months prior to any invasive dental procedure may not have a meaningful biologic effect. In contrast the shorter *in vivo* half-life of RSD suggests its cessation for some months prior to any invasive dental procedure may be appropriate (Zahrowski 2007). Such a course of action is difficult for ZLD as this is administered on an annual basis with suppression of bone turnover markers occurring up to two years following a single infusion (Bolland 2009).

If ONJ occurs, therapy involving local debridement, irrigation and antibiotics is usually unsuccessful due to difficulty obtaining an acceptable surgical margin that is characterised by viable bleeding bone (Greenberg 2004)(Marx 2005). Unfortunately, surgical debridement is often associated with tissue breakdown which results in fistulae and problematic symptoms such as halitosis and pain (Marx 2004, Greenberg 2004). Conservative therapy is therefore the preferred option with strict control of infection using anti-microbial rinses or systemic antibiotics (Khosla 2007). However, the outcome of ONJ in patients with benign compared to malignant bone disease may be better due to differences in type, dose and route of BP (Favia 2004, Yarom 2007, Wutzl 2012). If required, any necrotic bone and sharp bone edges should be carefully removed under antibiotic cover with as little tissue/bone trauma as possible.

However, it is important to remember that the small absolute risk of ONJ means the benefit-to-risk ratio of BP therapy is high when used to treat OSP in patients who have sustained a LTF (Wong 2013).

Zoledronic Acid and Atypical Femoral Fracture

There has been recent concern regarding the risk of atypical femoral fracture (AFF) following long-term BP use. Unlike ONJ which has been associated with high dose IV BPs, AFFs were first reported following the use of low dose oral BPs for OSP (Goh 2007). Atypical femoral fractures usually occurred just distal to the lesser trochanter but proximal to the supracondylar flare; were associated with minimal/low trauma; and were transverse in orientation and non-comminuted, possibly with a medial spike (Edwards 2013). While the exact pathogenesis remains unclear, the recent ASBMR Taskforce convened to address this issue felt they were most likely stress fractures (Shane 2014).

A nationwide Swedish case control study reviewed radiographs of 1234 of the 1271 women who sustained a subtrochanteric or femoral shaft fracture in 2008 and identified 59 patients with AFFs (Schilcher 2011). National registry data were obtained regarding concomitant medications, especially BP use and coexistent medical conditions. None of the 59 cases appeared to have received IV ZLD. The 59 case patients were compared with 263 control patients who had suffered ordinary subtrochanteric fractures. The increased absolute risk of AFF with BP use was only 5 cases per 10 000 patient-years (95% CI, 4 to 7) (Schilcher 2011). The duration of BP use influenced the risk (odds ratio per 100 daily doses = 1.3; 95% CI, 1.1- 1.6). The excess risk diminished by 70% per year following drug cessation. As BPs concentrate in areas of impending stress fracture, suppression of bone remodelling at the site of an AFF may impair stress fracture healing. Cessation of the BP should therefore lower the risk of an AFF (Shane 2014).

While *post-hoc* analyses should be interpreted with caution, a careful secondary analysis of three large randomised BP intervention trials (the Fracture Intervention Trial (FIT), the FIT

Long-Term Extension (FLEX) trial, and the HORIZON- PFT failed to identify an increased risk of atypical fractures of the femoral shaft for patients on ALN (FIT and FLEX) and ZLD (HORIZON – PFT) (Black 2010). The recent ASBMR Taskforce has estimated the absolute risk of AFFs in patients on BPs at 3.2-50 cases per 100 000 person-years but recognized that long-term use may be associated with higher risk, say 100 cases per 100,000 person-years (Shane 2014). However, as for ONJ the small absolute risk of AFF means the benefit-to-risk ratio of BP therapy for the treatment of OSP is high in those who have previously sustained a LTF.

Other Uses

While ZLD is often the drug of choice in the treatment of OSP and PDB, its potent anti-resorptive effect means it has been successfully used to treat a range of benign metabolic bone disorders including fibrous dysplasia (Mansoori 2010) and osteogenesis imperfecta (Vuorimies 2011, Barros 2012). The close link between the inflammatory cytokine cascade and osteoclast mediated bone destruction seen in RA (McInnes 2011) suggests that osteoclast inhibition may be of value in the treatment of RA independent of its beneficial effect on GIOP. However, while ZLD has been shown to slow the development of bone erosions in early RA (Jarret 2006), a more effective therapeutic intervention in RA has proven to be aggressive use of conventional and biologic disease modifying agents which inhibit inflammation and therefore bone and joint destruction (McInnes 2007).

Other Agents Used to Treat Post-Menopausal Osteoporosis

Careful unravelling of the complex molecular biology of bone turnover has resulted in denosumab, a monoclonal antibody specifically blocking RANKL, a crucial cytokine promoting osteoclastogenesis. Denosumab is administered subcutaneously every six months to treat OSP (Cummings 2009). This is the first "targeted therapy" in the field of bone disease and has been shown to reduce vertebral and hip fractures with few side effects (Cummings 2009). The shorter *in vivo* biologic effect of denosumab compared to IV ZLD may explain the minimal risk of ONJ observed following long-term use of denosumab in patients with post-menopausal OSP (Papapoulos 2012).

Strontium ranelate has been shown to reduce vertebral and non-vertebral fracture risk (Meunier 2004, Reginster 2005). However, recent concern about an increased risk of myocardial infarction has tempered enthusiasm for this drug (European Medicines Agency 2013). Reassuringly, a nested case control study using the United Kingdom Clinical Practice Research Datalink failed to find an increased risk of first definite myocardial infarction, hospitalisation with myocardial infarction or cardiovascular death in those who had used strontium ranelate (Cooper 2014). However, the effective fracture risk reduction and low incidence of side effects seen with both BPs and denosumab make strontium ranelate a second line agent in the treatment of OSP.

Bisphosphonates and denosumab predominantly work on the osteoclast to reduce bone resorption. The other approach to address low bone mass is to stimulate the osteoblast to increase bone formation. The only true bone anabolic agent currently in clinical use is teriparatide (recombinant human parathyroid hormone analogue 1-34) (Neer 2001). This agent results in potent osteoblastic stimulation that leads to a marked increase in BMD and reduced fracture risk (Neer 2001). An early finding from pre-clinical data suggested a dose dependent increased risk of osteosarcoma in rats following administration of teriparatide (Vahle 2002). Reassuringly, the Osteosarcoma Surveillance Study, an ongoing 15-year surveillance study to investigate the implications of this in humans, found that after seven years, there was no association between the use of teriparatide for the treatment of OSP and osteosarcoma (Andrews 2012). However, the need for daily subcutaneous administration and the high cost of this drug limits widespread clinical use. Interestingly, the potent bone anabolic effect may be of clinical utility in promoting bone healing following fracture. One hundred and two post-menopausal women with a dorsally angulated distal radial fracture in need of closed reduction but not surgery, were randomly assigned to eight weeks of once-daily injection of placebo, 20 μg teriparatide (the current dose for treatment of OSP) or 40 μg teriparatide within 10 days of fracture. Both doses of teriparatide reduced the time to first radiographic appearance of complete cortical bridging (Aspenberg 2010).

The arrival of the next generation of bone anabolic agents that specifically block the effect of sclerostin, a key negative regulator of bone formation is eagerly awaited and may revolutionise the treatment of bone disease (Padhi 2011). Drugs such as odanacatib that block cathepsin K, an enzyme released by osteoclasts that degrades type I collagen, the predominant collagen in bone, are currently undergoing clinical trial. A phase II multicenter double-blind randomized placebo-controlled dose-ranging study of odanacatib evaluated the weekly administration of odanacatib in postmenopausal women with low bone mass. A dose-dependent increase in BMD by DXA at the lumbar spine, femoral neck, and total hip was observed after two years, with no significant difference in adverse events compared to placebo (Bone 2010). Phase III trials involving this drug are currently underway and their results will allow us to widen the range of drugs available to treat OSP (Das 2013).

CONCLUSION

Bisphosphonates have revolutionised the treatment of benign bone disease, especially OSP and PDB. The most potent BP is ZLD. Its annual IV administration is convenient, overcomes the poor bioavailability seen with oral BPs and avoids the often questionable patient adherence seen with oral bone protective therapy. The long *in vivo* half-life means there is ongoing fracture protection even following drug cessation. There is good data indicating ZLD reduces fracture risk at all sites and also probably lowers mortality in patients following osteoporotic/low trauma hip fracture. In comparison, the small increased absolute risk of possible complications such as ONJ or AFFs means the benefit:risk ratio of ZLD is high.

FUNDING

The authors declare no relevant conflicts of interest.

REFERENCES

Aghaloo TL, Felsenfeld AL, Tetradis S. Osteonecrosis of the jaw in a patient on Denosumab. *J. Oral Maxillofac. Surg.* 2010;68(5):959-63.

American Association of Oral and Maxillofacial Surgeons Advisory Task Force on Bisphosphonate-Related Ostenonecrosis of the Jaws . American Association of Oral and Maxillofacial Surgeons position paper on bisphosphonate-related osteonecrosis of the jaws. *J. Oral Maxillofac. Surg.* 2007;65(3):369-76.

Andrews EB, Gilsenan AW, Midkiff K, Sherrill B, Wu Y, Mann BH, Masica D. The US postmarketing surveillance study of adult osteosarcoma and teriparatide: study design and findings from the first 7 years. *J. Bone Miner. Res.* 2012;27(12):2429-37.

Aspenberg P, Genant HK, Johansson T, Nino AJ, See K, et al. Teriparatide for acceleration of fracture repair in humans: a prospective, randomized, double-blind study of 102 postmenopausal women with distal radial fractures. *J. Bone Miner. Res.* 2010; 25(2):404–414.

Bagan JV, Murillo J, Jimenez Y, Poveda R, Milian MA, et al. Avascular jaw osteonecrosis in association with cancer chemotherapy. *J. Oral Pathol. Med.* 2005;34(2):120-3.

Barros ER, Saraiva GL, de Oliveira TP, Lazaretti-Castro M. Safety and efficacy of a 1-year treatment with zoledronic acid compared with pamidronate in children with osteogenesis imperfecta. *J. Pediatr. Endocrinol. Metab.* 2012;25(5-6):485-91.

Berenson JR. Recommendations for zoledronic acid treatment of patients with bone metastases. *Oncologist* 2005;10(1):52-62.

Black DM, Delmas PD, Eastell R, Reid IR, Boonen S, et al. Once-yearly zoledronic acid for treatment of postmenopausal osteoporosis. *N. Engl. J. Med.* 2007;356(18):1809-22.

Black DM, Kelly MP, Genant HK, Palermo L, Eastell RN, et al. Bisphosphonates and fractures of the subtrochanteric or diaphyseal femur. *N. Engl. J. Med.* 2010;362:1761-71.

Black DM, Reid IR, Boonen S, Bucci-Rechtweg C, Cauleyet JA, et al. The effect of 3 versus 6 years of zoledronic acid treatment of osteoporosis: a randomized extension to the HORIZON-Pivotal Fracture Trial (PFT). *J. Bone Miner. Res.* 2012;27(2):243-54.

Bliuc D, Nguyen ND, Milch VE, Nguyen TV, Eisman JA, Center JR. Mortality risk associated with low-trauma osteoporotic fracture and subsequent fracture in men and women. *JAMA* 2009;301(5):513-21.

Bone HG, Hosking D, Devogelaer JP, Tucci JR, Emkey RD, et al. Ten years' experience with alendronate for osteoporosis in post-menopausal women. *N. Engl. J. Med.* 2004;350(12): 1189-99.

Bone HG, McClung MR, Roux C, Recker RR, Eisman JA, et al. Odanacatib, a cathepsin-K inhibitor for osteoporosis: a two-year study in postmenopausal women with low bone density. *J. Bone Miner. Res.* 2010;25(5):937–47.

Boonen S, Sellmeyer DE, Lippuner K, Orlov-Morozov A, Abramset K, et al. Renal safety of annual zoledronic acid infusions in osteoporotic postmenopausal women. *Kidney Int.* 2008;74(5):641–8.

Boonen S, Orwoll ES, Wenderoth D, Stoner KJ, Eusebio R, Delmas PD. Once- weekly risedronate in men with osteoporosis: results of a 2-year, placebo-controlled, double-blind, multicenter study. *J. Bone Miner. Res.* 2009;24(4):719-25.

Boonen S, Reginster JY, Kaufman JM, Lippuner K, Zanchetta J, et al. Fracture risk and zoledronic acid therapy in men with osteoporosis. *N. Engl. J. Med.* 2012;367(18):1714-23.

Borba VZ, Paz-Filho G, Kulak CA, Seibel MJ, Bilezikian JP, et al. Bone turnover 18 months after a single intravenous dose of zoledronic acid. *Int. J. Clin. Pract.* 2007; 61:1058–62.

Borromeo GL, Tsao CE, Darby IB, Ebeling PR. A review of the clinical implications of bisphosphonates in dentistry. *Aust. Dent. J.* 2011;56(1):2-9.

Caro JJ, Ishak KJ, Huybrechts KF, Raggio G, Naujoks C. The impact of compliance with osteoporosis therapy on fracture rates in actual practice. *Osteoporos. Int.* 2004;15(12):1003-8.

Carter G, Goss A, Doecke C. Bisphosphonates and avascular necrosis of the jaw: a possible association. *Med. J. Aust.* 2005;182(8):413-5.

Chen T, Berenson J, Vescio R, Swift R, Gilchick A, et al. Pharmacokinetics and pharmacodynamics of zoledronic acid in cancer patients with bone metastases. *J. Clin. Pharmacol.* 2002;42(11):1228-36.

Coleman RE, Rathbone E, Brown JE. Management of cancer treatment-induced bone loss. *Nat. Rev. Rheumatol.* 2013;9(6):365-74.

Colón-Emeric CS, Mesenbrink P, Lyles KW, Pieper CF, Boonen S, et al. Potential mediators of the mortality reduction with zoledronic acid after hip fracture. *J. Bone Miner. Res.* 2010;25(1):91-7.

Colucci A, Modorati G, Miserocchi E, Di Matteo F, Rama P. Anterior uveitis complicating zoledronic acid infusion. *Ocul. Immunol. Inflamm.* 2009;17(4):267-8.

Cooley H, Jones G. A population-based study of fracture incidence in southern Tasmania: lifetime fracture risk and evidence for geographic variations within the same country. *Osteoporos. Int.* 2001;12(2):124–130.

Cooper C, Fox KM, Borer JS. Ischaemic cardiac events and use of strontium ranelate in postmenopausal osteoporosis: a nested case-control study in the CPRD. *Osteoporos. Int.* 2014;25(2):737-45.

Cramer JA, Amonkar MM, Hebborn A, Altman R. Compliance and persistence with bisphosphonate dosing regimens among women with postmenopausal osteoporosis. *Curr. Med. Res. Opin.* 2005;21(9):1453-60.

Cummings SR, San Martin J, McClung MR, Siris ES, Eastell R, et al. FREEDOM Trial. Denosumab for prevention of fractures in postmenopausal women with osteoporosis. *N. Engl. J. Med.* 2009;361:756–765.

Das S, Crockett JC. Osteoporosis - a current view of pharmacological prevention and treatment. *Drug Des. Devel. Ther.* 2013;7:435-48.

De Luca A, Lamura L, Gallo M, Daniele G, D'Alessio A, Giordano P, Maiello MR, Pergameno M, Perrone F, Normanno N. Pharmacokinetic evaluation of zoledronic acid. *Expert Opin. Drug Metab. Toxicol.* 2011;7(7):911-8.

Dimopoulos MA, Kastritis E, Bamia C, Melakopoulos I, Gika D, et al. Reduction of osteonecrosis of the jaw (ONJ) after implementation of preventive measures in patients with multiple myeloma treated with zoledronic acid. *Ann. Oncol.* 2009;20(1):117-20.

Dunford JE, Thompson K, Coxon FP, Luckman SP, Hahn FM, Poulter CD, Ebetino FH, Rogers MJ. Structure-activity relationships for inhibition of farnesyl diphosphate synthase in vitro and inhibition of bone resorption in vivo by nitrogen-containing bisphosphonates. *J. Pharmacol. Exp. Ther.* 2001;296(2):235-42.

Durie B, Katz M, Crowley J. Osteonecrosis of the jaw and bisphosphonates. *N. Engl. J. Med.* 2005;353(1):99-102.

Edwards BJ, Bunta AD, Lane J, Odvina C, Rao DS, et al. Bisphosphonates and nonhealing femoral fractures: analysis of the FDA Adverse Event Reporting System (FAERS) and international safety efforts: a systematic review from the Research on Adverse Drug Events And Reports (RADAR) project. *J. Bone Joint Surg. Am.* 2013; 95(4):297-307.

Eekhoff ME, van der Klift M, Kroon HM, Cooper C, Hofman A, Pols HA, Papapoulos SE. Paget's disease of bone in The Netherlands: A population-based radiological and biochemical survey – the Rotterdam Study. *J. Bone Miner. Res.* 2004;19(4):566–570.

Eisman JA, Bogoch ER, Dell R, Harrington JT, McKinney RE Jr, et al. ASBMR Task Force on Secondary Fracture Prevention. Making the first fracture the last fracture: ASBMR task force report on secondary fracture prevention. *J. Bone Miner. Res.* 2012;27(10): 2039-46.

European Medicines Agency. Recommendation to restrict the use of Protelos/Osseor/strontium ranelate 2013. Available from http://www.ema.europa.eu/ema/index.jsp?curl=pages/news_and_events/news/2013/04/news_detail_001774.jsp&mid=WC0b01ac058004d5c1

Favia G, Pilolli GP, Maiorano E. Osteonecrosis of the jaw correlated to bisphosphonate therapy in non-oncologic patients: clinicopathological features of 24 patients. *J. Rheumatol.* 2009;36(12):2780-7.

Ferretti G, Fabi A, Carlini P, Papaldo P, Cordiali Fei P, et al. Zoledronic-acid-induced circulating level modifications of angiogenic factors, metalloproteinases and proinflammatory cytokines in metastatic breast cancer patients. *Oncology* 2005;69(1):35-43.

Giraudo E, Inoue M, Hanahan D. An amino-bisphosphonate targets MMP-9-expressing macrophages and angiogenesis to impair cervical carcinogenesis. *J. Clin. Invest.* 2004;114(5):623-33.

Gnant M. Role of bisphosphonates in postmenopausal women with breast cancer. *Cancer Treat. Rev.* 2014;40(3):476-84.

Goh SK, Yang KY, Koh JS, Wong MK, Chua SY, Chua DT, Howe TS. Subtrochanteric insufficiency fractures in patients on alendronate therapy: a caution. *J. Bone Joint Surg. Br.* 2007;89(3):349–53.

Grbic JT, Black DM, Lyles KW, Reid DM, Orwoll E, et al. The incidence of osteonecrosis of the jaw in patients receiving 5 milligrams of zoledronic acid: data from the health outcomes and reduced incidence with zoledronic acid once yearly clinical trials program. *J. Am. Dent. Assoc.* 2010;141(11):1365-70.

Green JR, Muller K, Jaeggi KA. Preclinical pharmacology of CGP 42'446, a new, potent, heterocyclic bisphosphonate compound. *J. Bone Miner. Res.* 1994;9(5):745-51.

Greenberg M. Intravenous bisphosphonates and osteonecrosis. *Oral Surg. Oral Med. Oral Pathol. Oral Radiol. Endod.* 2004;98(3): 259-60.

Grey A, Bolland MJ, Wattie D, Horne A, Gamble G, Reid IR. The antiresorptive effects of a single dose of zoledronate persist for two years: a randomized, placebo-controlled trial in osteopenic postmenopausal women. *J. Clin. Endocrinol. Metab.* 2009;94(2):538–44.

Haentjens P, Magaziner J, Colón-Emeric CS, Vanderschueren D, Milisen K, Velkeniers B, Boonen S. Meta-analysis: excess mortality after hip fracture among older women and men. *Ann. Intern. Med.* 2010;152(6):380-90.

Hillner BE, Ingle JN, Chlebowski RT, Gralow J, Yee GC, et al. American Society of Clinical Oncology 2003 update on the role of bisphosphonates and bone health issues in women with breast cancer. *J. Clin. Oncol.* 2003;21(21):4042-57.

Hoff AO, Toth BB, Altundag K, Johnson MM, Warneke CL, et al. Frequency and risk factors associated with osteonecrosis of the jaw in cancer patients treated with intravenous bisphosphonates. *J. Bone Miner. Res.* 2008;23(6):826-36.

Holroyd C, Cooper C, Dennison E. Epidemiology of osteoporosis. *Best Pract. Res. Clin. Endocrinol. Metab.* 2008;22(5):671–85.

Hopkins RB, Goeree R, Pullenayegum E, Adachi JD, Papaioannou A, Xie F, Thabane L. The relative efficacy of nine osteoporosis medications for reducing the rate of fractures in post-menopausal women. *BMC Musculoskelet. Disord.* 2011;Sept 26;12:209.

Hosking D, Lyles K, Brown JP, Fraser WD, Miller P, et al. Long-term control of bone turnover in Paget's disease with zoledronic acid and risedronate. *J. Bone Miner. Res.* 2007;22(1):142–148.

Hughes DE, Wright KR, Uy HL, Sasaki A, Yoneda T, Roodman GD, Mundy GR, Boyce BF. Bisphosphonates promote apoptosis in murine osteoclasts in vitro and in vivo. *J. Bone Miner. Res.* 1995;10(10):1478-87.

Jarrett SJ, Conaghan PG, Sloan VS, Papanastasiou P, Ortmann CE, O'Connor PJ, Grainger AJ, Emery P. Preliminary evidence for a structural benefit of the new bisphosphonate zoledronic acid in early rheumatoid arthritis. *Arthritis Rheum.* 2006;54(5):1410-4.

Jensen JS, Tondevold E. Mortality after hip fractures. *Acta Orthop. Scand.* 1979;50(2):161-7.

Keene GS, Parker MJ, Pryor GA. Mortality and morbidity after hip fractures. *BMJ* 1999;307(6914):1248-50.

Khosla S, Burr D, Cauley J, Dempster DW, Ebeling PR, et al. American Society for Bone and Mineral Research. Bisphosphonate-associated osteonecrosis of the jaw: report of a task force of the American Society for Bone and Mineral Research. *J. Bone Miner. Res.* 2007;22(10):1479-91.

Krueger KP, Felkey BG, Berger BA. Improving adherence and persistence: a review and assessment of interventions and description of steps toward a national adherence initiative. *J. Am. Pharm. Assoc.* 2003;43(6):668-78.

Kunzmann V, Bauer E, Wilhelm M. Gamma/delta T-cell stimulation by pamidronate. *N. Engl. J. Med.* 1999;340(9):737–738.

Kunzmann V, Bauer E, Feurle J, Weissinger F, Tony HP, Wilhelm M. Stimulation of gamma delta T cells by aminobisphosphonates and induction of antiplasma cell activity in multiple myeloma. *Blood* 2000;96(2):384–392.

Licata AA. Discovery, clinical development, and therapeutic uses of bisphosphonates. *Ann. Pharmacother.* 2005;39(4):668-77.

Lin JH. Bisphosphonates: a review of their pharmacokinetic properties. *Bone* 1996;18(2):75-85.

Lugassy G, Shaham R, Nemets A, Ben-Dor D, Nahlieli O. Severe osteomyelitis of the jaw in long-term survivors of multiple myeloma: a new clinical entity. *Am. J. Med.* 2004;117(6):440-1.

Lyles KW, Colón-Emeric CS, Magaziner JS, Adachi JD, Pieper CF, et al. Zoledronic acid in reducing clinical fracture and mortality after hip fracture. *N. Engl. J. Med.* 2007; 357(18):1799-809.

Mansoori LS, Catel CP, Rothman MS. Bisphosphonate treatment in polyostotic fibrous dysplasia of the cranium: case report and literature review. *Endocr. Pract.* 2010;16(5):851-4.

Marottoli RA, Berkman LF, Leo-Summers L, Cooney LM Jr. Predictors of mortality and institutionalisation after hip fracture: The New Haven EPESE cohort. *Am. J. Pub. Health* 1994;84(11):1807-12.

Marx R. Pamidronate (Aredia) and zoledronate (Zometa) induced avascular necrosis of the jaws: a growing epidemic. *J. Oral Maxillofac. Surg.* 2003;61(9):1238-9.

Marx RE, Sawatari Y, Fortin M, Broumand V. Bisphosphonate-induced exposed bone (osteonecrosis/osteopetrosis) of the jaws: risk factors, recognition, prevention, and treatment. *J. Oral Maxillofac. Surg.* 2005;63(11):1567-75.

McInnes IB, Schett G. Cytokines in the pathogenesis of rheumatoid arthritis. *Nat. Rev. Immunol.* 2007;7(6):429-42.

McInnes IB, Schett G. The pathogenesis of rheumatoid arthritis. *N. Engl. J. Med.* 2011;365(23):2205-19.

Meunier PJ, Roux C, Seeman E, Ortolani S, Badurski JE, et al. The effects of strontium ranelate on the risk of vertebral fracture in women with postmenopausal osteoporosis. *N. Engl. J. Med.* 2004;350:459-68.

Michou L, Brown JP. Emerging strategies and therapies for treatment of Paget's disease of bone. *Drug Des. Devel. Ther.* 2011;5:225-39.

Migliorati, CA. Bisphosphonates and oral cavity avascular bone necrosis. *J. Clin. Oncol.* 2003;21(22):4253-4.

Migliorati C. Bisphosphonate-associated oral osteonecrosis. *Oral Surg. Oral Med. Oral Pathol. Oral Radiol. Endod.* 2005;99(2):35.

Migliorati CA, Mattos K, Palazzolo MJ. How patients' lack of knowledge about oral bisphosphonates can interfere with medical and dental care. *J. Am. Dent. Assoc.* 2010;141(5):562-6.

Migliorati CA, Epstein JB, Abt E, Berenson JR. Osteonecrosis of the jaw and bisphosphonates in cancer: a narrative review. *Nat. Rev. Endocrinol.* 2011;7(1):34–42.

Miller PD, Black DM, Hruska J, Boonen S. Renal effects of treatment with zoledronic acid: results from the HORIZON-PFT extension study. *Osteoporos. Int.* 2012;23:S197–8.

Miller PD, Jamal SA, Evenepoel P, Eastell R, Boonen S. Renal safety in patients treated with bisphosphonates for osteoporosis: a review. *J. Bone Miner. Res.* 2013;28(10):2049-59.

Nancollas GH, Tang R, Phipps RJ, Henneman Z, Gulde S, Wu W, et al. Novel insights into actions of bisphosphonates on bone: differences in interactions with hydroxyapatite. *Bone* 2006;38(5):617–27.

Neer RM, Arnaud CD, Zanchetta JR, Prince R, Gaich GA, et al. Effect of parathyroid hormone (1-34) on fractures and bone mineral density in postmenopausal women with osteoporosis. *N. Engl. J. Med.* 2001;344(19):1434-41.

Orwoll ES, Scheele WH, Paul S, Adami S, Syversen U, et al. The effect of teriparatide (human para- thyroid hormone (1-34)) therapy on bone density in men with osteoporosis. *J. Bone Miner. Res.* 2003;18(1):9-17.

Orwoll ES, Miller PD, Adachi JD, Brown J, Adler RA, et al. Efficacy and safety of a once-yearly i.v. infusion of zoledronic acid 5mg versus a once-weekly 70-mg oral alendronate in the treatment of male osteoporosis: a randomized, multicenter, doubleblind, active-controlled study. *J. Bone Miner. Res.* 2010; 25(10):2239–2250.

Padhi D, Jang G, Stouch B, Fang L, Posvar E. Single-dose, placebo controlled, randomized study of AMG 785, a sclerostin monoclonal antibody. *J. Bone Miner. Res.* 2011;26(1):19–26.

Papapoulos S, Chapurlat R, Libanati C, Brandi ML, Brown JP, et al. Five years of denosumab exposure in women with postmenopausal osteoporosis: results from the first two years of the FREEDOM extension. *J. Bone Miner. Res.* 2012;27(3):694–701.

Pazianas M, Miller P, Blumentals WA, Bernal M, Kothawala P. A review of the literature on osteonecrosis of the jaw in patients with osteoporosis treated with oral bisphosphonates: prevalence, risk factors, and clinical characteristics. *Clin. Ther.* 2007;29(8):1548-58.

Penning-van Beest FJ, Erkens JA, Olson M, Herings RM. Loss of treatment benefit due to low compliance with bisphosphonate therapy. *Osteoporos. Int.* 2008;19(4):511-7.

Peterson JD, Bedrossian EH Jr. Bisphosphonate-associated orbital inflammation--a case report and review. *Orbit* 2012;31(2):119-23.

Purcell P, Boyd I. Bisphosphonates and osteonecrosis of the jaw. *Med. J. Aust.* 2005;182(8):417-8

Rabenda V, Mertens R, Fabri V, Vanoverloop J, Sumkay F, et al. Adherence to bisphosphonates therapy and hip fracture risk in osteoporotic women. *Osteoporos. Int.* 2008;19(6):811-8.

Reginster JY, Seeman E, De Vernejoul MC, Adami S, Compston J, et al. Strontium ranelate reduces the risk of nonvertebral fractures in postmenopausal women with osteoporosis: Treatment of Peripheral Osteoporosis (TROPOS) study. *J. Clin. Endocrinol. Metab.* 2005;90(5):2816-22.

Reid IR, Brown JP, Burckhardt P, Horowitz Z, Richardson P, et al. Intravenous zoledronic acid in postmenopausal women with low bone mineral density. *N. Engl. J. Med.* 2002;346(9):653-61.

Reid IR, Miller P, Lyles K, Fraser W, Brown JP, et al. Comparison of a single infusion of zoledronic acid with risedronate for Paget's disease. *N. Engl. J. Med.* 2005;353(9):898-908.

Reid DM, Devogelaer JP, Saag K, Roux C, Lau CS, et al. Zoledronic acid and risedronate in the prevention and treatment of glucocorticoid induced osteoporosis (HORIZON): a multicentre, double- blind, double- dummy, randomised controlled trial. *Lancet* 2009;373(9671):1253–63.

Reid IR, Hosking DJ. Bisphosphonates in Paget's disease. *Bone* 2011;49(1):89-94.

Reid IR, Black DM, Eastell R, Bucci-Rechtweg C, Su G, et al. HORIZON Pivotal Fracture Trial and HORIZON Recurrent Fracture Trial Steering Committees Reduction in the risk of clinical fractures after a single dose of zoledronic Acid 5 milligrams. *J. Clin. Endocrinol. Metab.* 2013;98(2):557-63.

Ripamonti CI, Maniezzo M, Campa T, Fagnoni E, Brunelli C, et al. Decreased occurrence of osteonecrosis of the jaw after implementation of dental preventive measures in solid tumour patients with bone metastases treated with bisphosphonates. The experience of the National Cancer Institute of Milan. *Ann. Oncol.* 2009;20(1):137-45.

Rizzoli R, Burlet N, Cahall D, Delmas PD, Eriksen EF, et al. Osteonecrosis of the jaw and bisphosphonate treatment for osteoporosis. *Bone* 2008;42(5):841-7.

Rogers MJ, Frith JC, Luckman SP, Coxon FP, Benford HL, et al. Molecular mechanisms of action of bisphosphonates. *Bone* 1999;24(5 Suppl):73S-79S.

Roodman GD, Windle JJ. Paget disease of bone. *J. Clin. Invest.* 2005;115(2):200–208.

Ruggiero S, Mehrotra B, Rosenberg TJ, Engroff SL. Ostenecrosis of the jaws associated with the use of bisphosphonates: a review of 63 cases. *J. Oral Maxillofac. Surg.* 2004;62(5): 527-34.

Ruggiero SL, Dodson TB, Assael LA, Landesberg R, Marx RE, et al. American Association of Oral and Maxillofacial Surgeons position paper on bisphosphonate-related osteonecrosis of the jaw - 2009 update. Task Force on Bisphosphonate-Related Osteonecrosis of the Jaws, American Association of Oral and Maxillofacial Surgeons. *Aust. Endod. J.* 2009;35(3):119-30.

Russell RG, Rogers MJ, Frith JC, Luckman SP, Coxon FP et al. The pharmacology of bisphosphonates and new insights into their mechanisms of action. *J. Bone Miner. Res.* 1999;14 Suppl 2:53-65.

Sabatâe E. World Health Organization. Adherence to Long-term Therapies: Evidence for Action. In. Geneva, Switzerland: World Health Organization; 2003:7-10.

Sambrook P, Seeman E, Phillips SR, Ebeling PR, Osteoporosis Australia, et al. Preventing osteoporosis: outcomes of the Australian Fracture Prevention Summit. *Med. J. Aust.* 2002;176:S1-16.

Sambrook P, Olver I, Goss A. Bisphosphonates and osteonecrosis of the jaw. *Aust. Fam. Physician* 2006;35(10):801-3.

Sambrook PN, Chen JS, Simpson JM, March LM. Impact of adverse news media on prescriptions for osteoporosis: effect on fractures and mortality. *Med. J. Aust.* 2010;193(3):154-6.

Santini D, Vincenzi B, Avvisati G, Dicuonzo G, Battistoni F, et al. Pamidronate induces modifications of circulating angiogenetic factors in cancer patients. *Clin. Cancer Res.* 2002;8(5):1080-4.

Schilcher J, Michaëlsson K, Aspenberg P. Bisphosphonate use and atypical fractures of the femoral shaft. *N. Engl. J. Med.* 2011;364(18):1728-37.

Shane E, Burr D, Abrahamsen B, Adler RA, Brown TD, et al. Atypical subtrochanteric and diaphyseal femoral fractures: second report of a task force of the american society for bone and mineral research. *J. Bone Miner. Res.* 2014;29(1):1-23.

Siris ES, Harris ST, Rosen CJ, Barr CE, Arvesen JN, Abbott TA, Silverman S. Adherence to bisphosphonate therapy and fracture rates in osteoporotic women: relationship to vertebral and nonvertebral fractures from 2 US claims databases. *Mayo Clin. Proc.* 2006;81(8):1013-22.

Siris ES, Selby PL, Saag KG, Borgström F, Herings RM, Silverman SL. Impact of osteoporosis treatment adherence on fracture rates in North America and Europe. *Am. J. Med.* 2009;122(2 Suppl):S3-13.

Tarassoff P, Csermak K. Avascular necrosis of the jaws: risk factors in metastatic cancer patients. *J. Oral Maxillofac. Surg.* 2003;61(10):1238-9.

Taylor KH, Middlefell LS, Mizen KD. Osteonecrosis of the jaws induced by anti-RANK ligand therapy. *Br. J. Oral Maxillofac. Surg.* 2010;48 (3):221-3.

Teronen O, Laitinen M, Salo T, Hanemaaijer R, Heikkilä P, et al. Inhibition of matrix metalloproteinases by bisphosphonates may in part explain their effects in the treatment of multiple myeloma. *Blood* 2000;96(12):4006-7.

U.S. Food and Drug Administration (FDA). Drug Safety Newsletter. 2009;Volume 2, Number 2 (Internet). Silver Spring (MD): U.S. Food and Drug Administration; 2009 (cited 2013 Aug 05). Available at: http:// www.fda.gov/downloads/Drugs/DrugSafety/ DrugSafetyNewsletter/ UCM168579.pdf.

U.S. Food and Drug Administration (FDA). FDA Drug Safety Communication: New contraindication and updated warning on kidney impairment for Reclast (zoledronic acid) (Internet). Silver Spring (MD): U.S. Food and Drug Administration; 2011 (cited 2013 Aug 05). Available at: http://www.fda.gov/Drugs/DrugSafety/ucm270199.htm.

Vahle JL, Sato M, Long GG, Young JK, Francis PC, et al. Skeletal changes in rats given daily subcutaneous injections of recombinant human parathyroid hormone (1–34) for 2 years and relevance to human safety. *Toxicol. Pathol.* 2002;30(3):312–21.

Vahtsevanos K, Kyrgidis A, Verrou E, Katodritou E, Triaridis S, et al. Longitudinal cohort study of risk factors in cancer patients with bisphosphonate-related osteonecrosis of the jaw. *J. Clin. Oncol.* 2009;27(32):5356-62.

Vannuchi A, Ficarra G, Antonioli E, Bosi A. Osteonecrosis of the jaw associated with zoledronate therapy in a patient with multiple myeloma. *Br. J. Haem.* 2005;128(6):738.

van Staa TP. The pathogenesis, epidemiology and management of glucocorticoid-induced osteoporosis. *Calcif. Tissue Int.* 2006; 79(3): 129–37.

Vuorimies I, Toiviainen-Salo S, Hero M, Mäkitie O. Zoledronic acid treatment in children with osteogenesis imperfecta. *Horm. Res. Paediatr.* 2011;75(5):346-53.

Wang J, Goodger NM, Pogrel MA. Osteonecrosis of the jaws associated with cancer chemotherapy. *J. Oral Maxillofac. Surg.* 2003;61(9):1104-7.

Watts NB, Diab DL. Long-term use of bisphosphonates in osteoporosis. *J. Clin. Endocrinol. Metab.* 2010;95(4):1555-65.

Widler L, Jaeggi KA, Glatt M, Müller K, Bachmann R, et al. Highly potent germinal bisphosphonates. From pamidronate disodium (Aredia) to zoledronic acid (Zometa). *J. Med. Chem.* 2002;45(17):3721–38.

Wong PK, Borromeo GL, Wark JD. Bisphosphonate-related osteonecrosis of the jaw in non-malignant bone disease. *Rheumatol. Int.* 2013;33(9):2189-98.

Woo SB, Hellstein JW, Kalmar JR. Systematic review: bisphosphonates and osteonecrosis of the jaws. *Ann. Intern. Med.* 2006;144(10):753-61.

Wood J, Bonjean K, Ruetz S, Bellahcène A, Devy L, Foidart JM, Castronovo V, Green JR. Novel antiangiogenic effects of the bisphosphonate compound zoledronic acid. *J. Pharmacol. Exp. Ther.* 2002;302(3):1055-61.

World Health Organization Assessment of fracture risk and its application to screening for postmenopausal osteoporosis: Report of a WHO Study Group. Geneva: WHO, 1994 (Technical Report Series 843). *JAMA* 2001; 285:785–95.

Wutzl A, Pohl S, Sulzbacher I, Seemann R, Lauer G, Ewers R, Drach J, Klug C. Factors influencing surgical treatment of bisphosphonate-related osteonecrosis of the jaws. *Head Neck* 2012;34(2):194-200.

Yarom N, Yahalom R, Shoshani Y, Hamed W, Regev E, Elad S. Osteonecrosis of the jaw induced by orally administered bisphosphonates: incidence, clinical features, predisposing factors and treatment outcome. *Osteoporos. Int.* 2007;18(10):1363-70.

Zahrowski JJ. Comment on the American Association of Oral and Maxillofacial Surgeons statement on bisphosphonates. *J. Oral Maxillofac. Surg.* 2007;65(7):1440-1.

Zwolak P, Dudek AZ. Antineoplastic activity of zoledronic acid and denosumab. *Anticancer Res.* 2013;33(8):2981-8.

In: Zoledronic Acid
Editor: Ronald Carman
ISBN: 978-1-63321-525-2

Chapter 9

ZOLEDRONIC ACID AND BISPHOSPHONATE RELATED OSTEONECROSIS OF THE JAW

Dileep Sharma*[*], *Stephen Hamlet*,
Eugen Bogdan Petcu and Saso Ivanovski
Griffith Health Institute, MBOD group,
School of Dentistry and Oral Health, Australia

ABSTRACT

Zoledronic acid is the most potent bisphosphonate (BP) currently available for use in various clinical conditions. This increasing use of the high potency drug has led to an elevated incidence of a unique but well-documented oral adverse effect termed "bisphosphonate-related osteonecrosis of the jaws (BRONJ)".

BRONJ, as a clinical entity, is classically described as a non-healing ulcer on the jaw bone (maxillae or mandible) in a patient with a history of BP use in the absence of radiotherapy. Initially, the aetiology of BRONJ was considered to be related to direct suppression of osteoclastic activity in the jaw bone. However, recent literature suggests that a host of factors are involved in the pathogenesis of this complex condition and a wide variation exists in its occurrence, mainly based on the potency of the BP used. BRONJ is specifically reported in jaw bones and zoledronic acid, due to its high potency is the most commonly implicated drug. A thorough knowledge of BRONJ is important for a dental surgeon as it is essential for initial identification, prompt diagnosis and successful management of this unique condition.

This chapter comprises an overview of BRONJ as a clinical entity, classification and staging, various etio-pathological theories, and general guidelines in management of zoledronic acid induced BRONJ.

---

[*] Corresponding author: Dileep Sharma. Griffith Health Institute, MBOD group, School of Dentistry and Oral Health, Griffith University Gold Coast campus QLD 4222.

INTRODUCTION

The use of BPs, similar to any drugs predominately used in cancer patients, has been associated with a host of adverse effects. Orally administered BPs are known to induce a host of adverse effects ranging from recurrent ulcers, burning sensation and blisters in the oral cavity to oesophagitis, oesophageal stenosis, gastric ulcerations and abdominal pain [1-4].

However, the more severe debilitating adverse effect seen in jaw bones termed "Bisphosphonate-related osteonecrosis of the jaw bone" (BRONJ) is seen most commonly, although not exclusively, after using the higher potency intravenous BPs, Pamidronate and Zoledronate [5, 6]. Ever since the first reported case of BRONJ more than a decade ago, there has been an increasing focus by researchers and dental professionals to identify the precise etio-pathogenesis, and develop possible preventive modalities [7].

Clinical Definition

BRONJ is defined as an area of exposed bone in the maxillofacial region that does not heal within 8 weeks after identification by a healthcare provider, in a patient who has been receiving or has been exposed to a BP and has no previous history of radiation therapy to the craniofacial region. [8] BRONJ symptoms range from painless exposed bone to severe jaw pain, and concomitant tissue infection. [9] However, clinical staging of BRONJ has evolved over the past decade (Table 1) and recent classifications include forms of BRONJ which do not necessarily present with bone exposure [10-13].

A thorough medical history recording is of paramount importance in the differential diagnosis of BRONJ and more common conditions like gingivitis, periodontitis, mucositis, pulpo-periapical lesions, osteomyelitis, primary and metastatic osseous malignancies (Table 2) [14].

Putative Risk Factors for BRONJ (Figure 1)

I. Pharmacological Factors

a Potency, dosage and multiple BPs use: Nitrogen containing BPs (the intravenously used Zoledronate and pamidronate and the orally administered alendronate) are the most common drugs associated with BRONJ. [15-17]. Drug combination and higher dosage of BPs also seem to influence the incidence of BRONJ [18-20]

b Purpose and duration of use: The duration of BP use depends on the clinical indication. In general, the BPs used in malignant bone diseases, primary or metastatic, have shown highest BRONJ incidence as compared to their use in non-malignant conditions [16, 21, 22]. This may be due to the fact that usually, intravenous NBPs are used in malignant conditions in contrast to the use of oral BPs in non-malignant bone diseases. In a recent comprehensive review by Palaska et al., the mean duration of incidence of BRONJ after use of zoledronate was reported to be 22 months, with minimum time of 10 months. In the case on pamidronate, the mean duration was 34 months with a minimum of 18 months, while for oral BPs, including alendronate and risedronate, the mean duration of onset was reported to be 55 months, with a minimum of 36 months for BRONJ to occur [23]

c Co-medications: Often, patients on BPs are also on other medications, most commonly steroids for pain and other chronic diseases. This can significantly shorten the time required for occurrence of BRONJ in such cases [17, 24, 25]. Furthermore, prospective studies have shown that a previous history of chemotherapy and steroid administration increases the risk of BRONJ if BPs are administered subsequently [26, 27].

Table 1. Clinical staging of BRONJ

Stage	Description	References
Stage 1 Stage 2 Stage 3	Exposed necrotic bone that is asymptomatic Exposed necrotic bone associated with pain and infection Exposed necrotic bone in patients with pain infection and pathologic fracture extraoral fistula or osteolysis extending to the inferior border	Ruggiero et al. 2006 [11]
At risk category Stage 0 Stage 1 Stage 2 Stage 3	No apparent necrotic bone in patients who have been treated with either oral or IV bisphosphonates No clinical evidence of necrotic bone, but non-specific clinical findings and symptoms Exposed and necrotic bone in patients who are asymptomatic and have no evidence of infection Exposed and necrotic bone associated with infection as evidenced by pain and erythema in the region of the exposed bone with or without purulent drainage Exposed and necrotic bone in patients with pain, infection and one or more of the following: exposed and necrotic bone extending beyond the region of alveolar bone (i.e. inferior border and ramus in the mandible, maxillary sinus and zygoma in the maxilla) resulting in pathologic fracture, extra-oral fistula, oral antral/oral nasal communication, or osteolysis extending to the inferior border of the mandible of sinus floor	Ruggiero et al. 2009 [12]
Stage 1 Focal BRONJ Stage 2 Diffuse BRONJ discharge) Stage 3 Complicated BRONJ	Clinical signs and symptoms: bone exposure; sudden dental mobility; nonhealing postextraction socket; mucosal fistula; swelling; abscess formation; trismus; gross mandibular deformity and/or hypoesthesia/paraesthesia of the lips Stage 1 can be Asymptomatic or Symptomatic (pain and purulent discharge) Clinical signs and symptoms: same as Stage 1 diffuse osteosclerosis, with or without the prominence of the inferior alveolar nerve canal; periosteal reaction; sinusitis; sequestra formation; and/or oro-antral fistula on CT Stage 1 can be Asymptomatic or Symptomatic (pain and purulent discharge) Same as Stage 2, with clinical signs and symptoms: extra-oral fistula; displaced mandibular stumps; nasal leakage of fluids CT findings can be osteosclerosis of adjacent bones (zygoma, hard palate); pathologic mandibular fracture; and/or osteolysis extending to the sinus floor.	Bedogni et al. 2012 [13]

Table 2. Possible clinical signs and symptoms associated but not limited to BRONJ

Exposed necrotic jaw bone*
Pain in tooth or bone
Suppuration
Swelling
Sinus and fistula related to jaw bone
Mobility of teeth
Trismus
Non-healing extraction sockets
Soft tissue ulcerations
Gross mandibular deformity
Sequestration of bone

*Classical sign of BRONJ.

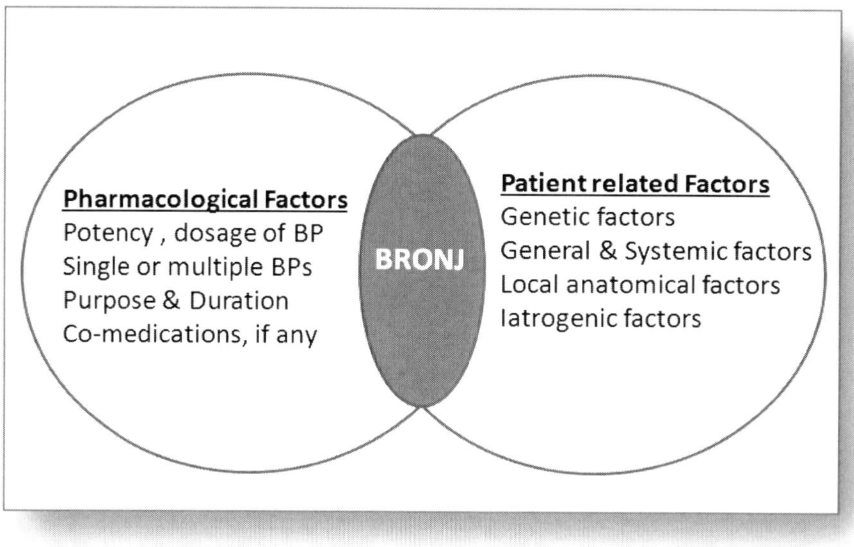

Figure 1. Putative risk factors for BRONJ.

II. Patient Related Factors

a Genetic factors: Single nucleotide polymorphism (SNP) studies have isolated various genetic factors that can increase the incidence of BRONJ. Specifically, polymorphisms of the cytochrome P450 CYP2C8 and a combined presence of COL1A1, RANK, MMP2, OPG and OPN SNPs have been identified as risk factors for BRONJ [28-30]. Vairaktaris et al. (2009) described BRONJ in a case with mutation in the prothrombin gene G21020A [31]. In a recent study by Arduino et al. that comparing female patients with BRONJ and those without, a haplotype effect of VEGF polymorphisms was noted only in BRONJ patients [32]. Another study conducted on Caucasian patients treated with zoledronic acid targeting the gene encoding for the farnesyl pyrophosphate synthase (A/C rs2297480 polymorphism) showed that AA genotype was positively correlated with occurrence of BRONJ [33] This essentially meant that the presence of an AA pair on the rs2297480 loci of the FPS enzyme encoding gene resulted in higher occurrence of BRONJ. However, more studies with a higher sample size and in various populations are essential to confirm the role of SNPs in BRONJ.

b General and systemic factors: Age has been found to be a significant risk factor for BRONJ in many studies, both prospective and retrospective [34, 35]. Some reports found a female predilection whereas others found no gender association of BRONJ [16, 21, 24, 26]. Apart from the disease for which the BPs are indicated, tobacco smoking and obesity were also identified as strong risk factors for BRONJ if zoledronate was administered which could have a role in BRONJ etiopathogenesis [37]. Other less reported conditions include anemia, hypoxemia, diabetes, infection, hypothyroidism, ethylism, renal dialysis and immune deficiency [16, 38-40] although the exact mechanism for this association are unclear.

c Local anatomical factors: In general, studies have reported higher BRONJ incidence in the mandible than in the maxilla [15, 16, 21, 26]. The precise reason is not clear but can be attributed to the fact that the maxilla is more vascular in comparison to the mandible, reducing the risk of BONJ. Further, areas where the mucosal covering is thin and less vascularized, for example on tori or exostosis in either of the jaws, and mylohyoid ridge in mandible, are more prone to BRONJ [34, 41, 42].

d Iatrogenic factors: These include any dental procedures done immediately before or during the intake of BPs. Invariably, most cases which develop BRONJ had a history of dental surgical treatment including extractions, dental implants, apical surgery, dental caries and root canal therapy, periodontitis and periodontal surgery involving bone [16, 42-44]. It is estimated that dental treatment increases the risk of BRONJ more than seven times as against those without any procedure, on treatment with intravenous NBPs [18, 34]. However "spontaneous BRONJ" without a history of any surgical treatments have also been reported [45, 46].

The Ever Puzzling Etiopathogenic Theories of BRONJ

Although many cases of BRONJ have been reported, there has been no causal relationship established between the use of BPs and the occurrence of BRONJ. The multitude of actions of BPs could represent various potential etiopathogenic mechanisms of BRONJ (Figure 2). However, at present there is no clear understanding of this condition, which in fact represents a side effect of BPs therapy.

Impaired Bone Remodelling

a. Effects on Osteoclasts

Due to their high affinity to mineralized tissues, BPs are adsorbed onto the crystals of hydroxyapatite of bone and are released in the acidic pH of osteoclastic bone resorption into the resorption lacunae [47]. This is taken up by the osteoclast by fluid-phase endocytosis resulting in apoptosis of osteoclasts [48], Figure 3.

In case of NNBPs like etidronate, apoptosis is mediated by intracellular accumulation of analogues of adenosine triphosphate (ATP) a metabolite which is non-hydrolyzable and cytotoxic, resulting in inhibition of essential metabolic pathways [49].

On the contrary, NBPs like pamidronate, alendronate and zoledronate inhibit the function of osteoclasts by interfering in the mevalonate pathway at the level of farnesyl pyrophosphate synthase action that is essential in prenylation of small GTP binding proteins. These binding proteins are involved in intracellular trafficking and cytoskeletal organization of osteoclasts, and NBPs essentially impair this and subsequently result in impaired osteoclastic action [50].

Furthermore, specific BPs have been shown to have additional mechanisms to affect osteoclasic bone resorption. Murakami et al. studied the effect of Tiludronate, a NNBP, in mouse culture systems and reported that it did not exert any inhibitory effect on osteoclast recruitment, but preferentially inhibited pit formation by polarized osteoclasts having ruffled borders [51]. Further, histological studies showed that osteoclasts increased in numbers in patients receiving NBPs as the cumulative dose of the drug increased. However, about 25-40% of these detached osteoclasts displayed pyknotic nuclei suggesting apoptosis [52]. Risedronate and alendronate use has been shown to result in a significant reduction in the number and degree of differentiation of osteoclast precursors, formation, vitality and activity of osteoclast in a recent longitudinal study on osteoporosis cases [53, 54].

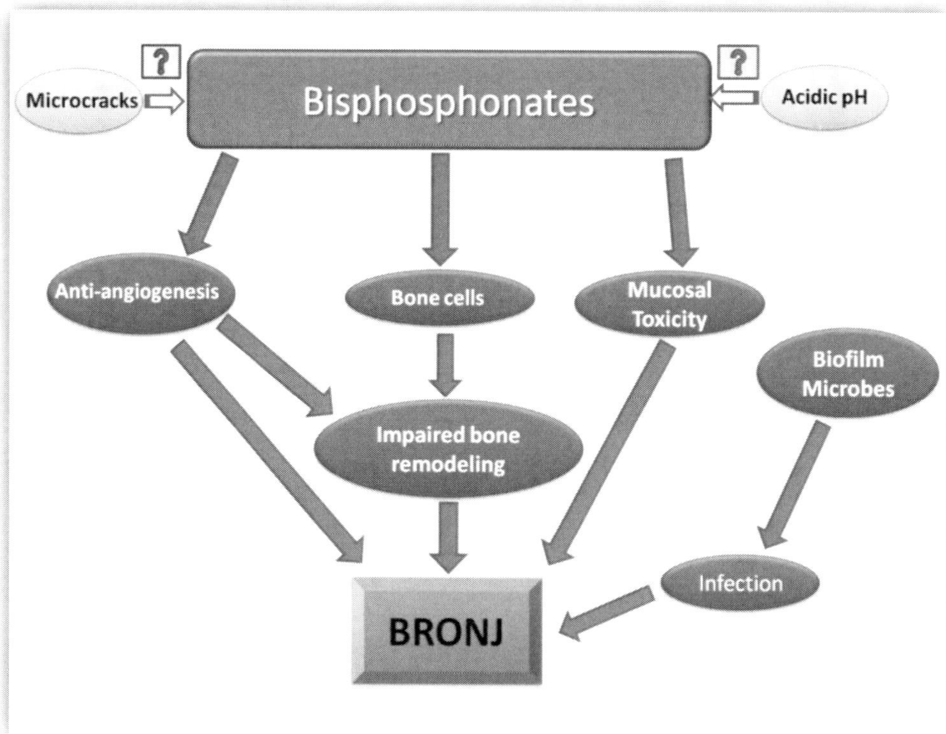

Figure 2. Theories of BRONJ etio-pathogenesis.

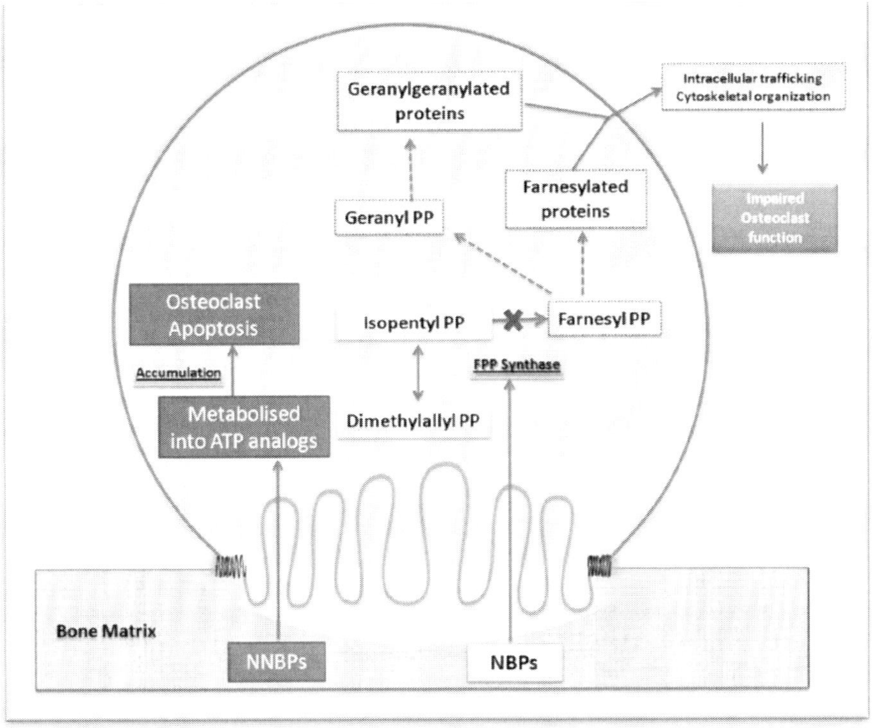

Figure 3. Effect of BPs on osteoclats.

However, there is some evidence that bone remodelling is not affected in BRONJ. Cathepsin K is an enzyme that plays a significant role in mediated proteolytic degradation of type I collagen in bone matrix during resorption [55]. Hansen et al. reported that osteoclasts expressing Cathepsin K are increased in patients on risedronate resulting in BRONJ as compared to those with osteoradionecrosis and controls [55].

b. Effects on Osteoblasts

Recent studies have suggests that BPs affect bone not only by their toxic action on osteoclasts, but also by affecting osteoblasts. NBPs such as risedronate, pamidronate and zoledronate have been shown to influence osteoblast function right from the stage of its differentiation from mesenchymal stem cells and its expression of receptor activator of Nuclear Factor-κB ligand (RANKL) in an in vitro human mesencymal stem cell study [56-58].

Risedronate also affected dose dependant variation in its effect on gene expression by osteoblasts [58]. Birc1b gene, an apoptosis inhibitor was reduced at both high and low levels of risedronate.When human osteoblast cell lines were exposed to pamidronate at ≥ 60 μMol/L, it was observed to significantly decreased cell viability, proliferation, osteogenesis, and wound healing along with apoptosis in $1/5^{th}$ of cells [59]. Similar results were seen when alendronate was used at concentrations $\geq$ 10 mMol/L [60].

Recently, Walter et al. compared NNBP and NBP effect on migration of osteoblasts in vitro and noticed that NBP, particularly pamidronate and zoledronate, affect cell viability, cell migration and induce apoptosis of osteoblasts [61].

However, anabolic and anti-apoptotic effects of NBPs on osteoblasts along with enhancement of osteoblast proliferation and differentiation from bone marrow stem cells have also been reported [62, 63].

It has been reported that specific novel analogs of BPs lack pro-apoptotic effects on osteoclast but have an anti-apoptotic effect on osteoblasts through opening of connexin 43 hemichannels and activation of the extracellular signal regulated kinases ERKs [64-66].

c. Effects on Osteocytes

Osteocytes are resting osteoblasts surrounded by bone matrix and communicating with each other through their canaliculi [67]. Absence of osteocytes either due to natural death or otherwise leads to a vacant osteocyte "lacunae" and results in non-viable bone, a pattern also seen in the case of BPs-induced osteocyte apoptosis [68].

In a beagle dog model, clinical doses of oral alendronate administered for one or three years, was compared with zoledronate for six months. Although there was no clinical bone exposure, mandibular histological examination revealed areas without osteocytes and patent canaliculi, suggestive of bone necrosis [69, 70]. However, zoledronate has been shown to suppress the formation of bone without causing death of osteocytes in a mouse model [71].

Based on above data, it can be concluded that although it seems to be the most obvious and plausible, the action of BPs on bone cells alone cannot completely account for the etiopathogenesis of BRONJ and other factors might have a significant role.

Anti-Angiogenic Effects of Zoledronate

Vascularity is essential for tissue homeostasis, local immunity and adequate regeneration or repair of all vital tissues of the body, more so in the case of bone due to its high turnover rate. Angiogenesis or formation of new blood capillaries is considered an essential factor in wound healing, as well as invasion of normal tissues by malignant cells [72]. It has been suggested that BPs could have an anti-angiogenic action, thus warranting their use in malignant conditions such as multiple myeloma, breast cancer and other invasive lesions of the bone [73]. This mode of action has also been implicated in the pathogeneisis of BRONJ. In fact, BRONJ represents an avasular necrosis of the jaw bone, as evidenced by the lack of blood vessels in the necrotic areas [74].

Circulating vascular endothelial growth factor (VEGF) levels, as well as local mRNA expression, are considered classic measures of angiogenesis. Zoledronate was recently tested for its in vitro effects on a non-small-cell lung cancer cell line, and it was shown that mRNA and protein expression of VEGF was substantially reduced [75]. Serum VEGF levels and other cytokines involved in angiogenesis, such as Interleukin-17, have also been found to be affected by the use of BPs like zoledronate and pamidronate [76-78].

In animal models, the anti-angiogenic effect has been studied on rats with experimental periodontitis and found that a short duration of risedronate treatment can inhibit bone resorption, but at higher dose for longer duration, risedronate can cause impaired angiogenesis [79]. This anti-angiogenic effect of NBPs has also been reported to be independent of FPPS pathways in an in vitro study using the potent BPs zoledronate and risedronate [80].

NBPs have a significant anti-angiogenic effect, as demonstrated in various cell culture models. Hasmim et al. showed that zoledronate inhibits human umbilical vein endothelial cells (HUVEC) adhesion, survival, migration and actin stress fiber formation by interfering with protein prenylation [81]. Similar findings were reported on proliferation and adhesion of human endothelial cells by Wood et al. [82].

In a recent study by Wehrhan et al., mucoperiosteal tissue samples from BRONJ cases and controls were assessed for vascularization (CD31 staining) and neo-angiogenesis (CD105 staining). It was reported that although there was no difference in vascularization between sample groups, there were significantly fewer CD105-positive vessels in BRONJ samples suggesting that neo-angiogenesis was suppressed in BRONJ cases [83].

Toxic Effects on Soft Tissue Cells

The toxic effects of oral BPs on GI tract soft tissue is well established, necessitating specific precautions while and after ingesting them. Indeed, regulatory requirements have made it a requirement for these precautions to be made available on the products' label [2-4]. In oral keratinocyte cell studies, BPs were shown to induce senescence and apoptosis, as wll as inhibit cell growth, by blocking the FPPS enzyme of the cholesterol biosynthetic pathway [84-89]. This is the same mechanism through which NBPs inhibit osteoclast function, as well as induce apoptosis and prevent invasion of tumor cells. Specifically, the NBPs, like potent pamidronate and zoledronate, had a strong negative effect on cell viability, migration ability, and apoptosis compared with the NNBP clodronate, which actually increased cell viability [86].

Similar effects were seen when cancer cell lines were studied following exposure to varying doses of pamidronate and zoledronate, although this occurred via inhibition of anti-apoptotic bcl-2 gene expression [90, 91]. Further, a tissue examination of BRONJ cases showed reduced numbers of basal epithelial progenitor cells compared to controls. The proposed mechanism for this finding ia a reduction in p53 gene expression through the mevalonate pathway [92].

These toxic effects can delay the healing capacity of oral mucosa either after trauma or surgical manipulation such aslike dental extraction [92]. An immunohistochemical tissue study on dogs also showed that MMP-9 was significantly decreased following zoledronate treatment, along with increased expression of caspase 3 increase, thus suggesting that higher levels of BPs can increase epithelial cell apoptosis along with decreasing soft tissue remodeling, thus resulting in BRONJ [93]. The effects of BPs on fibroblasts have also been reported to be similar [61]. When the effects of zoledronate were studied on fibroblast cell lines, it was found that cell mobility was reduced, in addition to inhibition of both type 1 collagen COL1A1 and COL1A2 chain expression, resulting in collagen loss as determined by immunofluorescence [94]. The resultant reduction in extracellular matrix production by human gingival fibroblasts cell under BPs exposure warrents further observation [95].

The in vitro exposure of periodontal fibroblasts to higher concentrations of zoledronate also resulted in cell apoptosis and necrosis [96].

Further, the chemical mediators of inflammation that are produced by gingival fibroblasts and are essential for creating the local milieu conducive for bone homeostasis. Increased production of IL-6 and OPG ($p \leq 0.04$) and decreased production of RANKL ($p \leq 0.02$), suggestive of reduced bone resorption signalling, were noted when alendronate and pamidronate treated gingival fibroblasts were studied [97].

The fact that anti-BPs agents and the addition of growth factors can limit the effect of BPs on soft tissues further confirms the role of toxicity in BRONJ pathogenesis. In vitro, gingival fibroblast mobility was found to be more sensitive to zoledronate compared withpamidronate, and the effect was reported to be reversible on exposure to 10 ng/ mL recombinant human platelet-derived growth factor BB and 50-μmol/L geranylgeraniol [98].

Oral Pathogens and BRONJ

Although hundreds of different bacteria species and viruses are known to be present in the oral cavity, few have been found to be pathogenic. In the case of BRONJ, a prominent group of oral microbes associated with its presence and its local effects are a group of filamentous Gram-positive anaerobic bacteria, Actinomyces. In one of the earliest papers, Lugassy et al. reported the presence of Actinomyces in the histological examination of severe osteomyelitis of the jaw in long-term survivors of multiple myeloma [99]. This was further confirmed by Hensen et al. who reported that out of 45 cases with Actinomycosis they studied, 93.5% suffered from BRONJ in comparison with infected osteoradionecrosis [100]. To examine the presence of the biofilm associated with BRONJ sites, sequestred bone tissue was evaluated using conventional histopathologic techniques and scanning electron microscopy and found various bacterial morphotypes embedded in a polymeric matrix, including Fusobacterium, bacillus, actinomyces, Staphylococcus, Streptococcus, Selenomonas, Treponemes in co-aggregation along with Candidal yeasts [101].

Further evidence of the presence of Actinomyces group in many case series and reports strengthened the hypothesis that their presence in BRONJ sites may be more than just a coincidence [102, 103].

Other Theories

Apart from the above extensively studied etiopathogenic theories, there are a few recent theories that need to be explored further. Otto et al. suggested that although the current theories explain the pathogenesis to an extent, none of them do so completely [104].

Further, they opined that the jaws may be more susceptible to BRONJ as a result of the acidic milieu that is created either due to an infection or surgical treatment, that can subsequently lead to the release the BPs bound to bone and locally affect osteoclasts. This was shown in the case of NBPs as the acidification could activate the nitrogen containing group to a much more potent toxic derivative of NBP, thus increasing the chances of BRONJ. This was one of the mechanisms that could explain the fact that NBPs are more commonly associated with BRONJ compared with NNBPs [104]. However, this theory needs to be explored further.

Another recently proposed and much debated model of BRONJ pathogenesis is the role of "microdamage" or "fatigue" that could be accumulated in bone due to suppressed bone remodelling in patients on BPs [105-107]. However, the precise methodology to detect the existence of such physical defect is questionable and needs more refinement [108, 109].

MANAGEMENT OF PATIENTS ON BPS IN DENTAL PRACTICE

In terms of preventative measures to minimise the chances of BRONJ, the role of the dental professional begins before a patient is put on BPs (Table 3).

Before BP is Started

The general protocol is that the physician prescribing the BPs should first refer the patient to a dentist for evaluation of the oral health status. If there are any infected teeth or periodontal disease, they need to be addressed before the commencement of BPs. If endodontic, periapical and subsequent restorative therapy is needed, it should be completed at least 4-6 weeks before initiation of BPs to ensure adequate osseous healing. Also, the prevention and/or early treatment of mucosal trauma lesions is essential as exposure of bone, in any form, can lead to BRONJ. Dental implant therapy is not contraindicated in these patients but the patient needs to be informed that BPs can affect the long term survival of the prosthesis.

At Risk Category

Frequently, patients with a recent history of dental manipulation exhibit increased risk of BRONJ occurrence. This risk rises significantly if the patient is on an intravenous BP like Zoledronate as against oral BPs, as the latter needs more prolonged exposure to cause BRONJ. Frequent visits to a dentist and stringent oral hygiene practice can ensure that the chances of BRONJ are minimal. Elective surgical treatments should be mostly avoided until they are absolutely essential. Serum C-terminal telopeptide (CTX) analysis may be used in monitoring patients on BPs. It is an indirect measure of bone turnover suppression and a value of 150 pg/mL or greater suggests minimal suppression of bone turnover. If the CTX value is less than 100 pg/mL it is recommended to avoid any surgical treatment and to seek the physician's opinion on a possible "drug holiday". However, close consultion between the dentist and the physician is required to determine if the risk of BRONJ outweighs the ill-effects of BP withdrawal.

Table 3. Suggested Treatment regimens for BRONJ

Stage 0 and Stage 1	Daily oral antimicrobial rinses (0.12% chlorhexidine) and regular clinical follow-up
Stage 2	Antimicrobial therapies based on culture and sensitivity data; analgesia and daily oral antimicrobial rinses (0.12% chlorhexidine) Low level laser therapy Ozone therapy Hyperbaric Oxygen Therapy
Stage 3	Serum CTX evaluation and Surgical debridement of necrotic bone, antimicrobial therapy (oral or intravenous), and pain killers and daily oral rinses (0.12% chlorhexidine)

Established BRONJ

Radiographic evaluation of the suspected lesion should, to some extent, help in the diagnosis of BRONJ. Biopsy of the site must be avoided until BRONJ is completely ruled out, and it needs to be determined whether the benefit of biopsy outweighs the risk of initiating a BRONJ lesion. The only possible indication would be when a malignant tumour is suspected and needs to be confirmed histologically.

Stage 1 can be managed with mouthwashes (chlorhexidine 0.12%) and any concomitant infection with antibiotics based on the culture from the suspected site (stage 2 BRONJ).

Stage 3 or complicated BRONJ is a condition where the management of the patient would essentially involve surgical debridement to remove bony sequestra and promote healing of the "unaffected" bone. However the fact remains that the "unaffected" bone is still exposed to systemically administered BPs and thus has the potential to become necrotic due to surgical exposure. Meticulous surgical planning is essential to prevent this and conservative approaches need to be followed in such cases.

References

[1] De Groen, P. C., Lubbe, D. F., Hirsch, L. J., et al. Esophagitis associated with the use of alendronate. *N. Engl. J. Med.* 1996;335:1016–1021.

[2] Kaye, P. S. Gastric hemorrhage and ulceration in hiatal hernia sac associated with alendronate (letter) *Dig. Dis. Sci.* 1999;44:903–904.

[3] Lanza, F. L., Hunt, R. H., Thomson, A. B., et al. Endoscopic comparison of esophageal and gastroduodenal effects of risedronate and alendronate in postmenopausal women. *Gastroenterology* 2000;119:631-638.

[4] Abraham, S. C., Cruz-Correa, M., Lee, L. A., Yardley, J. H., Wu, T. T. Alendronate-associated esophageal injury: pathologic and endoscopic features. *Mod. Pathol.* 1999; 12:1152-1157.

[5] Watters, A. L. 1, Hansen, H. J., Williams, T., Chou, J. F., Riedel, E., Halpern, J., Tunick, S., Bohle, G., Huryn, J. M., Estilo, C. L. Intravenous bisphosphonate-related osteonecrosis of the jaw: long-term follow-up of 109 patients. *Oral Surg. Oral Med. Oral Pathol. Oral Radiol.* 2013 Feb.;115(2):192-200. doi: 10.1016/j.oooo.2012.05.017. Epub. 2012 Oct. 1.

[6] Fortuna, G., Ruoppo, E., Pollio, A., et al. Multiple myeloma vs. breast cancer patients with bisphosphonates-related osteonecrosis of the jaws: a comparative analysis of response to treatment and predictors of outcome. *J. Oral Pathol. Med.* 2012;41(3):222-228.

[7] Marx, R. E. Pamidronate (Aredia) and zoledronate (Zometa) induced avascular necrosis of the jaws: a growing epidemic. *J. Oral Maxillofac. Surg.* 2003;61:1115-1117.

[8] Khosla, S., Burr, D., Cauley, J., et al. Bisphosphonate-associated osteonecrosis of the jaw: report of a task force of the american society for bone and mineral research. *J. Bone Miner. Res.* 2007;22:1479-1491.

[9] Sambrook, P., Olver, I., Goss, A. Bisphosphonates and osteonecrosis of the jaw. *Aust. Fam. Physician* 2006;35:801-803.

[10] Junquera, L., Gallego, L. Nonexposed bisphosphonate-related osteonecrosis of the jaws: another clinical variant? *J. Oral Maxillofac. Surg.* 2008 Jul.;66(7):1516-7.

[11] Ruggiero, S. L., Fantasia, J., Carlson, E. Bisphosphonate-related osteonecrosis of the jaw: background and guidelines for diagnosis, staging and management. *Oral Surg. Oral Med. Oral Pathol. Oral Radiol. Endod.* 2006 Oct.;102(4):433-41.

[12] Ruggiero, S. L., Dodson, T. B., Assael, L. A., Landesberg, R., Marx, R. E., Mehrotra, B.; American Association of Oral and Maxillofacial Surgeons. American Association of Oral and Maxillofacial Surgeons position paper on bisphosphonate-related osteonecrosis of the jaws-2009 update. *J. Oral Maxillofac. Surg.* 2009;67(5 Suppl.):2-12.

[13] Bedogni, A., Fusco, V., Agrillo, A., Campisi, G. Learning from experience. Proposal of a refined definition and staging system for bisphosphonate-related osteonecrosis of the jaw (BRONJ). *Oral Dis.* 2012 Sep.;18(6):621-3.

[14] Sharma, D., Ivanovski, S., Slevin, M., Hamlet, S., Pop, T. S., Brinzaniuc, K., Petcu, E. B., Miroiu, R. I. Bisphosphonate-related osteonecrosis of jaw (BRONJ): diagnostic criteria and possible pathogenic mechanisms of an unexpected anti-angiogenic side effect. *Vasc. Cell* 2013 Jan. 14;5(1):1. doi: 10.1186/2045-824X-5-1.

[15] Mavrokokki, T., Cheng, A., Stein, B., Goss, A. Nature and frequency of bisphosphonate-associated osteonecrosis of the jaws in Australia. *J. Oral Maxillofac. Surg.* 2007;65:415-423.

[16] Filleul, O., Crompot, E., Saussez, S. Bisphosphonate-induced osteonecrosis of the jaw: a review of 2,400 patient cases. *J. Cancer Res. Clin. Oncol.* 2010;136:1117-1124.

[17] Park, W., Kim, N. K., Kim, M. Y., Rhee, Y. M., Kim, H. J. Osteonecrosis of the jaw induced by oral administration of bisphosphonates in Asian population: five cases. *Osteoporos. Int.* 2010;21:527-533.

[18] Badros, A., Weikel, A., Salama, A., et al. ONJ in multiple myeloma patients: clinical features and risk factors. *J. Clin. Oncol.* 2006;24:945-952.

[19] Oizumi, T., Funayama, H., Yamaguchi, K., et al. Inhibition of necrotic actions of nitrogen-containing bisphosphonates (NBPs) and their elimination from bone by etidronate (a non-NBP): a proposal for possible utilization of etidronate as a substitution drug for NBPs. *J. Oral Maxillofac. Surg.* 2010;68:1043-1054.

[20] Barasch, A., Cunha-Cruz, J., Curro, F. A., et al. Risk factors for osteonecrosis of the jaws: a case-control study from the CONDOR dental PBRN. *J. Dent. Res.* 2011;90:439-444.

[21] Otto, S., Schreyer, C., Hafner, S., et al. Bisphosphonate-related osteonecrosis of the jaws - Characteristics, risk factors, clinical features, localization and impact on oncological treatment. *J. Craniomaxillofac. Surg.* 2012;40:303-309.

[22] Boonyapakron, T., Schirmer, I., Reichart, P. A., Sturm, I., Massenkeil, G. Bisphosphonate-induced osteonecrosis of the jaws: prospective study of 80-patients with multiple myeloma and other malignancies. *Oral Oncol.* 2008;44:857-869.

[23] Palaska, P. K., Cartsos, V., Zavras, A. I. Bisphosphonates and time to osteonecrosis development. *Oncologist* 2009;14:1154-1166.

[24] Chiu, C. T., Chiang, W. F., Chuang, C. Y., Chang, S. W. Resolution of oral bisphosphonate and steroid-related osteonecrosis of the jaw--a serial case analysis. *J. Oral Maxillofac. Surg.* 2010;68:1055-1063.

[25] Ruggiero, S. L. Bisphosphonate-related osteonecrosis of the jaw: an overview. *Ann. NY Acad. Sci.* 2011;1218:38-46.

[26] Abu-Id, M. H., Warnke, P. H., Gottschalk, J., Springer, I., Wiltfang, J., Acil, Y., et al. "Bis-phossy jaws" – high and low risk factors for bisphosphonate-induced osteonecrosis of the jaw. *J. Craniomaxillofac. Surg.* 2008;36:95-103.

[27] Grant, B. T., Amenedo, C., Freeman, K., Kraut, R. A. Outcomes of placing dental implants in patients taking oral bisphosphonates: a review of 115 cases. *J. Oral Maxillofac. Surg.* 2008; 66:223-230.

[28] Sarasquete, M. E., García-Sanz, R., Marín, L., et al. Bisphosphonate-related osteonecrosis of the jaw is associated with polymorphisms of the cytochrome P450 CYP2C8 in multiple myeloma: a genome-wide single nucleotide polymorphism analysis. *Blood* 2008;112:2709-2712.

[29] Katz, J., Gong, Y., Salmasinia, D., et al. Genetic polymorphisms and other risk factors associated with bisphosphonate induced osteonecrosis of the jaw. *Int. J. Oral Maxillofac. Surg.* 2011;40:605-611.

[30] Lehrer, S., Montazem, A., Ramanathan, L., et al. Bisphosphonate-induced osteonecrosis of the jaws, bone markers, and a hypothesized candidate gene. *J. Oral Maxillofac. Surg.* 2009;67:159-161.

[31] Vairaktaris, E., Vassiliou, S., Avgoustidis, D., Stathopoulos, P., Toyoshima, T., Yapijakis, C. Bisphosphonate-induced avascular osteonecrosis of the mandible associated with a common thrombophilic mutation in the prothrombin gene. *J. Oral Maxillofac. Surg.* 2009;67:2009-2012.

[32] Arduino, P. G., Menegatti, E., Scoletta, M., et al. Vascular endothelial growth factor genetic polymorphisms and haplotypes in female patients with bisphosphonate-related osteonecrosis of the jaws. *J. Oral Pathol. Med.* 2011;40:510-515.

[33] Marini, F., Tonelli, P., Cavalli, L., et al. Pharmacogenetics of bisphosphonate-associated osteonecrosis of the jaw. *Front. Biosci.* (Elite Ed.) 2011;3:364-370.

[34] Ruggiero, S. L., Dodson, T. B., Assael, L. A., Landesberg, R., Marx, R. E., Mehrotra, B.; American Association of Oral and Maxillofacial Surgeons. American Association of Oral and Maxillofacial Surgeons position paper on bisphosphonate-related osteonecrosis of the jaws-2009 update. *J. Oral Maxillofac. Surg.* 2009;67(5 Suppl.):2-12.

[35] Pozzi, S., Marcheselli, R., Sacchi, S., et al.; Gruppo Italiano Studio Linfomi. Bisphosphonate-associated osteonecrosis of the jaw: a review of 35 cases and an evaluation of its frequency in multiple myeloma patients. *Leuk. Lymphoma* 2007;48:56-64.

[36] Urade, M., Tanaka, N., Furusawa, K., et al. Nationwide survey for bisphosphonate-related osteonecrosis of the jaws in Japan. *J. Oral Maxillofac. Surg.* 2011;69:e364-71.

[37] Wessel, J. H., Dodson, T. B., Zavras, A. I. Zoledronate, smoking, and obesity are strong risk factors for osteonecrosis of the jaw: a case-control study. *J. Oral Maxillofac. Surg.* 2008;66:625-631.

[38] Assael, L. A. Oral bisphosphonates as a cause of bisphosphonate-related osteonecrosis of the jaws: clinical findings, assessment of risks, and preventive strategies. *J. Oral Maxillofac. Surg.* 2009;67(5 Suppl.):35-43.

[39] Thumbigere-Math, V., Tu, L., Huckabay, S., et al. A Retrospective study evaluating frequency and risk factors of osteonecrosis of the jaw in 576 cancer patients receiving intravenous bisphosphonates. *Am. J. Clin. Oncol.* 2011 Mar. 25. [Epub. ahead of print].
[40] Jadu, F., Lee, L., Pharoah, M., Reece, D., Wang, L. A retrospective study assessing the incidence, risk factors and comorbidities of pamidronate-related necrosis of the jaws in multiple myeloma patients. *Ann. Oncol.* 2007;18:2015-2019.
[41] Goldman, M. L., Denduluri, N., Berman, A. W., et al. A novel case of bisphosphonate-related osteonecrosis of the torus palatinus in a patient with metastatic breast cancer. *Oncology* 2006;71:306-308.
[42] Marx, R. E., Sawatari, Y., Fortin, M., Broumand, V. Bisphosphonate-induced exposed bone (osteonecrosis/osteopetrosis) of the jaws: risk factors, recognition, prevention, and treatment. *J. Oral Maxillofac. Surg.* 2005;63:1567-1575.
[43] Saia, G., Blandamura, S., Bettini, G., et al. Occurrence of bisphosphonate-related osteonecrosis of the jaw after surgical tooth extraction. *J. Oral Maxillofac. Surg.* 2010; 68:797-804.
[44] Bedogni, A., Bettini, G., Totola, A., Saia, G., Nocini, P. F. Oral bisphosphonate-associated osteonecrosis of the jaw after implant surgery: a case report and literature review. *J. Oral Maxillofac. Surg.* 2010;68:1662-1666.
[45] Vescovi, P., Campisi, G., Fusco, V., et al. Surgery-triggered and non surgery-triggered Bisphosphonate-related Osteonecrosis of the Jaws (BRONJ): A retrospective analysis of 567 cases in an Italian multicenter study. *Oral Oncol.* 2011;47:191-194.
[46] Badros, A., Terpos, E., Katodritou, E., et al. Natural history of osteonecrosis of the jaw in patients with multiple myeloma. *J. Clin. Oncol.* 2008; 26: 5904–5909.
[47] Sato, M., Grasser, W., Endo, N., et al. Bisphosphonate action. Alendronate localization in rat bone and effects on osteoclast ultrastructure. *J. Clin. Invest.* 1991;88:2095-2105.
[48] Thompson, K., Rogers, M. J., Coxon, F. P., et al. Cytosolic entry of bisphosphonate drugs requires acidification of vesicles after fluid-phase endocytosis. *Mol. Pharmacol.* 2006;69:1624–1632.
[49] Rogers, M. J., Ji, X., Russell, R. G. G., et al. Incorporation of bisphosphonates into adenine nucleotides by amoebae of the cellular slime mould dictyostelium discoideum. *Biochem. J.* 1994;303:303-311.
[50] Van Beek, E. R., Cohen, L. H., Leroy, I. M., et al. Differentiating the mechanisms of antiresorptive action of nitrogen containing bisphosphonates. *Bone* 2003; 33: 805-811.
[51] Murakami, H., Takahashi, N., Sasaki, T., et al. A possible mechanism of the specific action of bisphosphonates on osteoclasts: tiludronate preferentially affects polarized osteoclasts having ruffled borders. *Bone* 1995;17:137-144.
[52] Weinstein, R. S., Roberson, P. K., Manolagas, S. C. Giant osteoclast formation and long-term oral bisphosphonate therapy. *N. Engl. J. Med.* 2009;360:53-62.
[53] D'Amelio, P., Grimaldi, A., Cristofaro, M. A., et al. Alendronate reduces osteoclast precursors in osteoporosis. *Osteoporos. Int.* 2010;21:1741-1750.
[54] D'Amelio, P., Grimaldi, A., Di Bella, S., et al. Risedronate reduces osteoclast precursors and cytokine production in postmenopausal osteoporotic women. *J. Bone Miner. Res.* 2008;23:373-379.
[55] Hansen, T., Kirkpatrick, C. J., Walter, C., Kunkel, M. Increased numbers of osteoclasts expressing cysteine proteinase cathepsin K in patients with infected osteoradionecrosis

and bisphosphonate-associated osteonecrosis--a paradoxical observation? *Virchows Arch.* 2006;449:448-454.

[56] Fujita, H., Kurokawa, K., Ogino, T., et al. Effect of risedronate on osteoblast differentiation, expression of receptor activator of NF-κB ligand and apoptosis in mesenchymal stem cells. *Basic Clin. Pharmacol. Toxicol.* 2011;109:78-84.

[57] Reinholz, G. G., Getz, B., Pederson, L., Sanders, E. S., Subramaniam, M., Ingle, J. N., Spelsberg, T. C. Bisphosphonates directly regulate cell proliferation, differentiation, and gene expression in human osteoblasts. *Cancer Res.* 2000;60:6001-6007.

[58] Wang, J., Stern, P. H. Dose-dependent differential effects of risedronate on gene expression in osteoblasts. *Biochem. Pharmacol.* 2011;81:1036-1042.

[59] Marolt, D., Cozin, M., Vunjak-Novakovic, G., Cremers, S., Landesberg, R. Effects of pamidronate on human alveolar osteoblasts in vitro. *J. Oral Maxillofac. Surg.* 2012;70: 1081-1092.

[60] García-Moreno, C., Serrano, S., Nacher, M., et al. Effect of alendronate on cultured normal human osteoblasts. *Bone* 1998;22:233-239.

[61] Walter, C., Pabst, A., Ziebart, T., Klein, M., Al-Nawas, B. Bisphosphonates affect migration ability and cell viability of HUVEC, fibroblasts and osteoblasts *in vitro. Oral Dis.* 2011;17:194-199.

[62] Von Knoch, F., Jaquiery, C., Kowalsky, M., et al. Effects of bisphosphonates on proliferation and osteoblast differentiation of human bone marrow stromal cells. *Biomaterials* 2005;26:6941-6949.

[63] Plotkin, L. I., Weinstein, R. S., Parfitt, A. M., Roberson, P. K., Manolagas, S. C., Bellido, T. Prevention of osteocyte and osteoblast apoptosis by bisphosphonates and calcitonin. *J. Clin. Invest.* 1999;104:1363-1374.

[64] Plotkin, L. I., Manolagas, S. C., Bellido, T. Dissociation of the pro-apoptotic effects of bisphosphonates on osteoclasts from their anti-apoptotic effects on osteoblasts/ osteocytes with novel analogs. *Bone* 2006;39:443-452.

[65] Plotkin, L. I., Bivi, N., Bellido, T. A bisphosphonate that does not affect osteoclasts prevents osteoblast and osteocyte apoptosis and the loss of bone strength induced by glucocorticoids in mice. *Bone* 2011;49:122-127.

[66] Lezcano, V., Bellido, T., Plotkin, L. I., Boland, R., Morelli, S. Role of connexin 43 in the mechanism of action of alendronate: dissociation of anti-apoptotic and proliferative signaling pathways. *Arch. Biochem. Biophys.* 2012;518:95-102.

[67] Noble, B. S., Reeve, J. Osteocyte function, osteocyte death and bone fracture resistance. *Mol. Cell. Endocrinol.* 2000; 159:7-13.

[68] Qiu, S., Phipps, R. J., Ebetino, F. H., Palnitkar, S., Sudhaker Rao, D. Effect of risedronate on osteocyte viability and bone turnover in paired iliac bone biopsies from early postmenopausal women. *Calcif. Tissue Int.* 2010;87:392-397.

[69] Burr, D. B., Allen, M. R. Mandibular necrosis in beagle dogs treated with bisphosphonates. *Orthod. Craniofac. Res.* 2009;12:221-228.

[70] Lesclous, P., Abi Najm, S., Carrel, J. P., Baroukh, B., Lombardi, T., Willi, J. P., Rizzoli, R., Saffar, J. L., Samson, J. Bisphosphonate-associated osteonecrosis of the jaw: a key role of inflammation? *Bone* 2009;45:843-852.

[71] Huja, S. S., Fernandez, S. A., Phillips, C., Li, Y. Zoledronic acid decreases bone formation without causing osteocyte death in mice. *Arch. Oral Biol.* 2009;54:851-856.

[72] Liekens, S., De Clercq, E., Neyts, J. Angiogenesis: regulators and clinical applications. *Biochem. Pharmacol.* 2001;61(3):253-270.

[73] Green, J. R. Anti-tumor potential of bisphosphonates. *Med. Klin.* 2000;95:23-28.

[74] Bertè, R., Arcari, A., Bernuzzi, P., et al. Jaw avascular bone necrosis associated with long-term use of bisphosphonates. *Tumori* 2006;92:361.

[75] Di Salvatore, M., Orlandi, A., Bagalà, C., et al. Anti-tumour and anti-angiogenetic effects of zoledronic acid on human non-small-cell lung cancer cell line. *Cell Prolif.* 2011;44:139-146.

[76] Ferretti, G., Fabi, A., Carlini, P., et al. Zoledronic-acid-induced circulating level modifications of angiogenic factors, metalloproteinases and proinflammatory cytokines in metastatic breast cancer patients. *Oncology* 2005;69:35-43.

[77] Santini, D., Vincenzi, B., Avvisati, G., et al. Pamidronate induces modifications of circulating angiogenetic factors in cancer patients. *Clin. Cancer Res.* 2002;8:1080-1084.

[78] Oteri, G., Allegra, A., Bellomo, G., et al. Reduced serum levels of Interleukin 17 in patients with osteonecrosis of the jaw and in multiple myeloma subjects after bisphosphonates administration. *Cytokine* 2008;43:103-104.

[79] Cetinkaya, B. O., Keles, G. C., Ayas, B., Gurgor, P. Effects of risedronate on alveolar bone loss and angiogenesis: a stereologic study in rats. *J. Periodontol.* 2008;79:1950-1961.

[80] Stresing, V., Fournier, P. G., Bellahcène, A., et al. Nitrogen-containing bisphosphonates can inhibit angiogenesis in vivo without the involvement of farnesyl pyrophosphate synthase. *Bone* 2011;48:259-266.

[81] Hasmim, M., Bieler, G., Rüegg, C. Zoledronate inhibits endothelial cell adhesion, migration and survival through the suppression of multiple, prenylation-dependent signaling pathways. *J. Thromb. Haemost.* 2007;5:166-173.

[82] Wood, J., Bonjean, K., Ruetz, S., et al. Novel antiangiogenic effects of the bisphosphonate compound zoledronic acid. *J. Pharmacol. Exp. Ther.* 2002;302:1055-1061.

[83] Wehrhan, F., Stockmann, P., Nkenke, E., et al. Differential impairment of vascularization and angiogenesis in bisphosphonate-associated osteonecrosis of the jaw-related mucoperiosteal tissue. *Oral Surg. Oral Med. Oral Pathol. Oral Radiol. Endod.* 2011;112:216-221.

[84] Kim, R. H., Lee, R. S., Williams, D., et al. Bisphosphonates induce senescence in normal human oral keratinocytes. *J. Dent. Res.* 2011;90:810-816.

[85] Reszka, A. A., Halasy-Nagy, J., Rodan, G. A. Nitrogen-bisphosphonates block retinoblastoma phosphorylation and cell growth by inhibiting the cholesterol biosynthetic pathway in a keratinocyte model for esophageal irritation. *Mol. Pharmacol.* 2001;59:193-202.

[86] Pabst, A. M., Ziebart, T., Koch, F. P., Taylor, K. Y., Al-Nawas, B., Walter, C. The influence of bisphosphonates on viability, migration, and apoptosis of human oral keratinocytes--in vitro study. *Clin. Oral Investig.* 2012;16:87-93.

[87] Virtanen, S. S., Väänänen, H. K., Härkönen, P. L., Lakkakorpi, P. T. Alendronate inhibits invasion of PC-3 prostate cancer cells by affecting the mevalonate pathway. *Cancer Res.* 2002;62:2708-2714.

[88] Oades, G. M., Senaratne, S. G., Clarke, I. A., Kirby, R. S., Colston, K. W. Nitrogen containing bisphosphonates induce apoptosis and inhibit the mevalonate pathway, impairing Ras membrane localization in prostate cancer cells. *J. Urol.* 2003;170:246-252.

[89] Suri, S., Mönkkönen, J., Taskinen, M., et al. Nitrogen-containing bisphosphonates induce apoptosis of Caco-2 cells in vitro by inhibiting the mevalonate pathway: a model of bisphosphonate-induced gastrointestinal toxicity. *Bone* 2001;29:336-343.

[90] Iguchi, K., Tatsuda, Y., Usui, S., Hirano, K. Pamidronate inhibits antiapoptotic bcl-2 expression through inhibition of the mevalonate pathway in prostate cancer PC-3 cells. *Eur. J. Pharmacol.* 2010;641:35-40.

[91] Tamura, T., Shomori, K., Nakabayashi, M., Fujii, N., Ryoke, K., Ito, H. Zoledronic acid, a third-generation bisphosphonate, inhibits cellular growth and induces apoptosis in oral carcinoma cell lines. *Oncol. Rep.* 2011;25:1139-1143.

[92] Scheller, E. L., Baldwin, C. M., Kuo, S., et al. Bisphosphonates inhibit expression of p63 by oral keratinocytes. *J. Dent. Res.* 2011;90:894-899.

[93] Allam, E., Allen, M., Chu, T. M., Ghoneima, A., Jack Windsor, L. In vivo effects of zoledronic acid on oral mucosal epithelial cells. *Oral. Dis.* 2011 Apr.;17(3):291-7.

[94] Ravosa, M. J., Ning, J., Liu, Y., Stack, M. S. Bisphosphonate effects on the behavior of oral epithelial cells and oral fibroblasts. *Arch. Oral Bio.* 2011;56:491-498.

[95] Simon, M. J., Niehoff, P., Kimmig, B., Wiltfang, J., Açil, Y. Expression profile and synthesis of different collagen types I, II, III, and V of human gingival fibroblasts, osteoblasts, and SaOS-2 cells after bisphosphonate treatment. *Clin. Oral Investig.* 2010; 14(1):51-58.

[96] Agis, H., Blei, J., Watzek, G., Gruber, R. Is zoledronate toxic to human periodontal fibroblasts? *J. Dent. Res.* 2010;89:40-45.

[97] Tipton, D. A., Seshul, B. A., Dabbous, M. Kh. Effect of bisphosphonates on human gingival fibroblast production of mediators of osteoclastogenesis: RANKL, osteoprotegerin and interleukin-6. *J. Periodontal. Res.* 2011 Feb.;46(1):39-47.

[98] Cozin, M., Pinker, B. M., Solemani, K., et al. Novel therapy to reverse the cellular effects of bisphosphonates on primary human oral fibroblasts. *J. Oral Maxillofac. Surg.* 2011;69:2564-2578.

[99] Lugassy, G., Shaham, R., Nemets, A., Ben-Dor, D., Nahlieli, O. Severe osteomyelitis of the jaw in long-term survivors of multiple myeloma: a new clinical entity. *Am. J. Med.* 2004;117:440-441.

[100] Hansen, T., Kunkel, M., Springer, E., et al. Actinomycosis of the jaws histopathological study of 45 patients shows significant involvement in bisphosphonate-associated osteonecrosis and infected osteoradionecrosis. *Virchows Arch.* 2007;451:1009-1017.

[101] Sedghizadeh, P. P., Kumar, S. K., Gorur, A., Schaudinn, C., Shuler, C. F., Costerton, J. W. Identification of microbial biofilms in osteonecrosis of the jaws secondary to bisphosphonate therapy. *J. Oral Maxillofac. Surg.* 2008; 66:767-775.

[102] Bisdas, S., Chambron Pinho, N., Smolarz, A., et al. Biphosphonate-induced osteonecrosis of the jaws: CT and MRI spectrum of findings in 32 patients. *Clin. Radiol.* 2008;63:71-77.

[103] Naik, N. H., Russo, T. A. Bisphosphonate-related osteonecrosis of the jaw: the role of actinomyces. *Clin. Infect. Dis.* 2009;49:1729-1732.

[104] Otto, S., Hafner, S., Mast, G., et al. Bisphosphonate-related osteonecrosis of the jaw: is pH the missing part in the pathogenesis puzzle? *J. Oral Maxillofac. Surg.* 2010; 68: 1158-1161.

[105] Hoefert, S., Schmitz, I., Tannapfel, A., Eufinger, H. Importance of microcracks in etiology of bisphosphonate-related osteonecrosis of the jaw: a possible pathogenetic model of symptomatic and non-symptomatic osteonecrosis of the jaw based on scanning electron microscopy findings. *Clin. Oral Investig.* 2010;14:271-284.

[106] yrgidis, A., Vahtsevanos, K. "Fatigue" having a role in the pathogenesis of osteonecrosis of the jaws. *Clin. Oral Investig.* 2009;13:479-480.

[107] Kyrgidis, A., Verrou, E. Fatigue in bone: a novel phenomenon attributable to bisphosphonate use. *Bone* 2010;46:556.

[108] Burr, D. B., Allen, M. R. Reply to: fatigue in bone: a novel phenomenon attributable to bisphosphonate use. *Bone* 2010;47:455.

[109] Allen, M. R. Studying the role of microcracks in the pathophysiology of BRONJ. *Clin. Oral Investig.* 2009;13:481-482.

In: Zoledronic Acid
Editor: Ronald Carman

ISBN: 978-1-63321-525-2

Chapter 10

CLINICAL USES OF ZOLEDRONIC ACID

Colin Phipps[1], Ooi Wei Seong[2], Vin Cci Ng[3] and Daryl Tan[1,2,*]
[1]Department of Haematology, Singapore General Hospital, Singapore
[2]Raffles Cancer Centre, Raffles Hospital, Singapore
[3]Department of Pharmacy, Singapore General Hospital, Singapore

ABSTRACT

Zoledronic acid (ZA) is a potent nitrogen-containing bisphosphonate that was the first in its class to demonstrate efficacy in patients with bone metastases from solid tumors other than breast cancer. It is also used in multiple myeloma as well as non-malignant diseases associated with high bone turnover. This chapter focuses on the biology, pharmacokinetics, and toxicities of ZA and reviews efficacy data that lead to registration for its current clinical use.

INTRODUCTION

Zoledronic acid is a nitrogen-containing bisphosphonate that is widely used in the treatment of hypercalcemia of malignancy (HCM), cancer bone metastases, multiple myeloma (MM), and osteoporosis. It was developed to increase compliance by overcoming the frequent and burdensome dosing requirements of oral bisphosphonates. The core structure of bisphosphonates is formed by two phosphonate groups attached to a single carbon atom (P-C-P structure), similar to endogenous pyrophosphates but are non-hydrolyzable and much more stable. The P-C-P structure allows binding to divalent metal ions like Ca^{2+}. After administration, bisphosphonates concentrate in the skeleton, particularly at sites of active remodeling due to their high affinity for hydroxyapatite crystals in the bone matrix. The main pharmacological action of active bisphosphonates is the inhibition of bone resorption. This has been demonstrated by altered ^{45}Ca and hydroxyproline excretion, and inhibition of metaphyseal modeling-remodeling in growing mice. [1,2] These early studies used non-

* Corresponding Author.: Daryl Tan. Raffles Cancer Centre, 585 North Bridge Road, #13-00 Raffles Hospital, Singapore 188770, Republic of Singapore. Email: tan_daryl@rafflesmedical.com ; Fax : 65-63111181.

nitrogen containing bisphosphonates which act through generation of non-hydrolyzable ATP analogues that accumulate to high concentrations in the cytosol of osteoclasts and induce apoptosis. [3] In contrast, ZA has a nitrogen-containing heterocyclic ring placed at a critical distance from the central carbon which confers a different mode of osteoclast inhibition and increased potency.

Zoledronic acid (CGP42'446) was developed by Novartis Pharmaceuticals after preclinical studies showed potent *in vitro* inhibitory activity on bone resorption in mouse calvarial cultures and *in vivo* in 1,25-hydroxyvitamin D3-induced hypercalcemia in thyroparathyroidectomized (TPTX) rats. These studies revealed that ZA was 850-fold more potent than pamidronate at reducing calcium levels by 50% in TPTX rats. [4] Zoledronic acid entered clinical testing in the mid 1990's with the first therapeutic trial performed in patients with tumor-induced hypercalcemia. This phase I, multicenter study reported normalization of calcium levels in all 5 treated patients after a single-dose of 0.02 or 0.04 mg/kg. [5]

Nitrogen-containing bisphosphonates like ZA mainly act by inhibiting farnesyl diphosphate (FPP) synthase, a key regulatory enzyme in the mevalonate pathway. This inhibition occurs through binding to the geranyl diphosphate (GPP) binding site on FPP synthase, with the nitrogen moiety forming stable bonds with threonine and lysine residues on the enzyme. [6] FPP synthase inhibition prevents downstream generation of FPP resulting in decreases in the production of its derivate, geranylgeranyl diphosphate (GGPP). GGPP is needed for post-translational transfer of farnesyl or geranylgeranyl lipid groups onto a cysteine residue in carboxy-terminal motifs, a process called prenylation that results in farnesylated and geranylgeranyl proteins. Small GTPases, which are mostly geranylgeranyl proteins, play an important role in regulating signaling of a number of crucial processes within precursor and mature osteoclasts, including endosome trafficking, membrane ruffling and apoptosis. Inhibition of protein prenylation by nitrogen-containing bisphosphonates has been demonstrated through *in vitro* studies by failure of incorporation of [^{14}C]mevalonate into small GTPases in purified osteoclasts and accumulation of unprenylated form of small GTPase Rap1A. [7,8]

Apart from its effects on bone resorption, numerous *in vitro* studies have shown direct and indirect anti-tumor activity of bisphosphonates. The direct cytotoxic effect has been demonstrated in several tumor cell lines, including leukemia, and myeloma cell lines. The induction of apoptosis in myeloma cells seems to be due to inhibition of protein prenylation as evidenced by the accumulation of the unprenylated form of small GTPase Rap1A in tumor homogenates. [9] When ZA was given to mice injected with murine myeloma cells, a decrease in paraprotein concentrations and tumor burden was seen resulting in increased survival compared with controls. [10] Beyond the cytotoxic effect on tumor cells, bisphosphonates also have anti-angiogenic effects, demonstrated by reduced endothelial cell proliferation and induction of apoptosis *in vitro* as well as inhibition of revascularization of the prostate in mice under testosterone stimulation. [11] More specifically, ZA sensitizes endothelial cells to tumor necrosis factor-induced, caspase-independent programmed cell death, alluding to FAK-PKB/Akt pathway as a target of ZA. [12] Another indirect anti-tumor effect that has been observed is through sensitization, activation and potentiation of lysis by Vγ9/Vδ2 T-cells. [13] This immunomodulatory effect occurs at significantly lower doses of ZA than that needed for anti-angiogenic and proapoptotic activity. Sensitization of tumor cells to Vγ9/Vδ2 T-cell killing is thought to be through the effects of ZA on the mevalonate pathway resulting in the accumulation of metabolites that are similar to the phosphorylated non-peptide ligands recognized by Vγ9/Vδ2 T-cells.

This chapter will discuss the pharmacokinetics and toxicities of ZA as well as its clinical use in multiple myeloma, solid organ malignancies, and non-malignant bone disease.

PHARMACOKINETICS OF ZOLEDRONIC ACID

Pharmacokinetics of ZA has been evaluated in patients with cancer and bone metastases. Zoledronic acid exhibits a triphasic pharmacokinetic profile best described as a three-compartmental model. [14,15] The drug is given intravenously and achieves its maximum serum concentration (C_{max}) at the end of the infusion. This is followed by a rapid decline to <10% of C_{max} at 4 hours and <1% at 24 hours after the infusion. Zoledronic acid has an early biphasic distribution phase with half-lives of 14 minutes ($t_{1/2\alpha}$), followed by 1.87 hours ($t_{1/2\beta}$). A prolonged terminal phase then ensues with $t_{1/2\gamma}$ of at least 146 hours and persistently low serum concentration of ≤0.1% of C_{max} until day 28. This may indicate that zoledronic acid is primarily bound to bone tissues and is very slowly released into the systemic circulation.

The area under the plasma concentration versus time curve (AUC_{24h}) of ZA was dose proportional from 2 mg to 6 mg. [14,15] After intravenous infusion of ZA 4 mg over 15 minutes, it achieved a C_{max} of 264 ng/mL and AUC_{24h} of 420 ng.h/mL. Additionally, ZA exhibits little accumulation after multiple infusions. After 3 cycles of ZA given every 28 days, the mean AUC_{24h} ratios for the 2nd and 3rd dose compared to the 1st dose were 1.13 and 1.16, respectively. The plasma protein binding of ZA is low. *In-vitro* studies indicated that 28% (at 200 ng/mL) to 53% (at 50 ng/mL) of the drug is protein bound and its mean blood to plasma concentration ratio is 0.59.

Zoledronic acid showed negligible metabolism or biotransformation in the liver. [14,15] The effect of hepatic impairment on its pharmacokinetics was not studied. In addition, no dose adjustment recommendation is provided by the manufacturer for patients with hepatic impairment. The elimination of ZA occurs exclusively by the kidney through glomerular filtration. [14,15] Approximately 40% of the administered dose was excreted unchanged in the urine within 24 hours and only traces of the dose were detected after 48 hours. Most of the drugs were distributed into the bone (~60%) and <3% were eliminated via faeces. Renal clearance within 24 hours post-infusion is 3.7 L/h. Although the total clearance of ZA is independent of its dose, population kinetics in patient with bone metastases described a correlation with creatinine clearance (CrCl); estimated by the Cockcroft-Gault formula. On the basis of a comparison of AUC_{24h}, patients with mild to moderate renal impairment had 15% to 43% higher exposure (AUC_{24h}) to ZA than patients with normal renal function. However, no plasma accumulations were documented in patient with renal impairment following multiple doses of zoledronic acid. Currently, there are limited safety and efficacy data on ZA use in patients with severe renal impairment. Hence, its use is not recommended in patients with CrCl <30 mL/min.

Pharmacokinetics of ZA in the paediatric population was studied in 10 patients aged 3 to 17 years old with severe osteogenesis imperfecta. [15] All patients received ZA 0.05 mg/kg intravenous infusion over 30 minutes. Mean C_{max} and AUC_{24h} was 167 ng/mL and 220 ng.h/mL, respectively. Thus, paediatric pharmacokinetics profiles are similar to adult patients at equivalent mg/kg dose of ZA. Beside age, patient's gender, ethnicity, and body weight also had no effect on the pharmacokinetics of ZA as documented in subsequent pharmacokinetics studies in these specialized populations. [15,16]

Drug Interactions

In-vitro studies showed no cytochrome P450 enzymes inhibition or induction by ZA. However, no *in-vivo* drug-drug interaction studies were available. Caution is advised on co-administration of ZA with aminoglycosides, loop diuretics, or nephrotoxic agents (e.g. NSAIDS) due to documented risk of nephrotoxicity and prolonged hypocalcemia in case reports. [16]

Use in Pregnancy

Zoledronic acid most likely crosses the placenta as it has a low molecular weight (290 g/mol in hydrated form), lacks metabolism, has low plasma protein binding, and is associated with a prolonged terminal elimination half-life. There is limited evidence available on the use of ZA in pregnant woman (FDA pregnancy category D). One case report documented its use in a 33 year-old woman with metastatic breast cancer, who was given 2 doses of ZA intravenous infusion as well as concurrent palliative chemotherapy. She had a healthy and normal developing infant at 12 months of age. [17] However, animal data suggested teratogenic risk with ZA use during pregnancy; decrease in viable fetuses, fetal skeletal, visceral, and external malformations. [15,16] The reproductive toxicity findings with ZA are likely to be related to its therapeutic mechanism through sequestration of calcium and inhibition of bone resorption. Therefore, until more data is available on ZA use during pregnancy, it should be discontinued in women of reproductive potential as early as possible prior to a planned pregnancy due to the possible extended low-level exposure to the fetus. Some data suggest withholding bisphosphonate for 6 months to at least 1 year prior to pregnancy. Although ZA use in pregnant woman is not recommended, inadvertent exposure during early pregnancy does not appear to present a major risk to the embryo-fetus development. [18,19] Nevertheless, monitoring of serum calcium levels during pregnancy and lactation is imperative for the successful outcome of pregnancy.

Side Effects and Toxicities

1. Acute-Phase Reactions

Intravenous infusion of ZA may illicit an acute systemic immune reaction via cytokines (IL-1, IL-6, tumor necrosis factor-a, C-reactive protein) released from activated macrophages and gamma/delta T cells ($\gamma\delta$T cells). [20] The resulting reaction is called an acute-phase reaction. It is typically characterized by flu-like symptoms (e.g. arthralgia, myalgia, low-grade fever, fatigue, and malaise) and has been reported in approximately 40% of patients receiving ZA infusion. [21] Acute-phase reactions generally occur only after the first dose of ZA and is often self-limiting with most of the symptoms resolving within 3 to 4 days. However, some acute-phase reactions have been reported to persist for a longer duration (7 to 14 days). Mild analgesic (e.g. acetaminophen) given prior to first infusion and for 72 hours post-infusion may reduce these symptoms. This reaction usually diminishes with subsequent drug administrations.

2. Acute and Chronic Nephrotoxicity

Nephrotoxicity has been reported with ZA administration. Most incidences were observed with higher doses and shorter durations of infusion, i.e. ZA 8 mg given over 5 minutes versus the FDA-approved dosing schedule of 4 mg over 15 minutes. [22] Transient rise in serum creatinine after ZA administration is commonly observed. However, clinically significant increase in serum creatinine and development of acute nephrotoxicity leading to renal failure and the need for dialysis are rare. [23,24] The exact mechanism of ZA-induced nephrotoxicity is unknown. Nevertheless, it is postulated to be a result of ZA accumulation in proximal tubular epithelial cells and leading to toxic acute tubular necrosis, which is characterized by tubular cell degeneration, loss of brush border, and apoptosis. [25] This is in contrast to pamidronate-induced nephrotoxicity, which is associated with renal cellular injury and collapsing focal segmented glomerulosclerosis evident on renal biopsies. [26] The incidence of nephrotoxicity varies from 9% to 24%. [15,16] Post-marketing reports to the FDA in 2001 to 2003 had documented 72 cases of renal failure associated with ZA administration; 42 patients with myeloma, 39 patients had serum creatinine > 1.4 mg/dl at baseline, and 45 patients had previously received pamidronate therapy. [24] The onset of renal dysfunction occurs at a median of 2 months after the first infusion. In December 2004, Novartis Pharmaceutical petitioned to FDA for labelling changes based on pharmacokinetics profile of ZA, specifically in patients with estimated creatinine clearance between 30 to 60 ml/min. In general, treatment with ZA is not recommended in patients with serum creatinine greater than 3 mg/dl or CrCl less than 30 ml/min. [27] Risk factors for ZA-induced nephrotoxicity include multiple administrations of ZA, prior bisphosphonates therapy, and preexisting renal impairment. Therefore, avoidance of concurrent nephrotoxic agents (e.g. NSAIDs, diuretics), ensuring adequate pre-hydration, dose reduction in accordance with the degree of renal dysfunction, and withholding therapy in the presence renal deterioration have largely reduced the risks of nephrotoxicity. Prolonging the infusion duration of ZA from 5 minutes in previous pivotal trials to 15 minutes now, has profoundly reduced the incidence of renal toxicity specifically in patients requiring repeated or chronic bisphosphonate administration. After the change, the incidence of ZA-induced nephrotoxicity appeared to be similar to the incidence of nephrotoxicity among patients on placebo in a trial exploring the use of ZA in patients with metastatic bone disease. [28] However, there is no evidence to support a lower incidence of nephrotoxicity with the increase of ZA infusion duration to 30 minutes. [29] Therefore, ZA should be infused over at least 15 minutes. The recommended dose adjustments according to creatinine clearance (CrCl) calculated using the Cockcroft-Gault formula are listed in Table 1.

Table 1. Recommended dose adjustments for zolendronic acid according to creatinine clearance

Indication	Baseline creatinine clearance (CrCl)	Zoledronic acid dose
Multiple myeloma, Metastatic bone lesions from solid tumors	> 60 ml/min	4 mg
	50 - 60 ml/min	3.5 mg
	40 - 49 ml/min	3.3 mg
	30 - 39 ml/min	3 mg
	< 30 ml/min	Use is not recommended
Hypercalcemia of malignancy	Mild to moderate	No dose adjustment
	Severe impairment (Scr > 4.5 mg/dL or 400 μmol/L)	Evaluate risk versus benefit

Serum creatinine level should be monitored prior to each dose of ZA. In patients with bone metastases and multiple myeloma, significant deterioration of renal function after ZA infusion was defined as serum creatinine increase by at least 0.5 mg/dL (44 μmol/L) from normal baseline renal function or serum creatinine increase by at least 1 mg/dL (88 μmol/L) from abnormal baseline serum creatinine. Zoledronic acid treatment should be withheld until serum creatinine has improved to within 10% of baseline. Nevertheless, for patients presenting with concurrent hypercalcemia of malignancy (HCM) and renal impairment (Scr <4.5 mg/dl or 400 μmol/L), ZA 4 mg infusion over 15 minutes had been safely administered in clinical trials. [32] It is crucial to initiate aggressive intravenous saline hydration to correct intravascular volume depletion and to improve glomerular filtration rate prior to starting bisphosphonate therapy as initial management strategy of HCM. The American Society of Clinical Oncology (ASCO) recommends the monitoring of albuminuria every 3 to 6 months during ZA therapy for all patients. [33] For multiple myeloma patients with unexplained albuminuria (> 500 mg albumin over 24 hours), interruption of ZA therapy until resolution of albuminuria is recommended. Then after, more frequent monitoring prior to each ZA dose is suggested.

3. Osteonecrosis of the Jaw (ONJ)

According to the American Association of Oral and Maxillofacial Surgeons (AAOMS), ONJ is defined as an area of exposed bone in the oral cavity that does not heal within 8 weeks of adequate treatment in patients without prior radiation therapy to the region and had no evidence of malignancy. [34] ONJ typically presents with localized pain or numbness, soft tissues swelling, inflammation, loose teeth, and bone infections. It often affects the mandible and maxillofacial region, and rarely the soft palate. The risk of ONJ with intravenous bisphosphonate therapy (ZA and pamidronate) was first reported in 2003. [35] Subsequently, multiple case reports documenting the association of bisphosphonate therapy with ONJ were published. The incidence of ONJ in cancer patients varies from 0.8% to 12%, with higher occurrences among patients with multiple myeloma (8.5%) compared to patients with breast (3.1%) or prostate (4.9%) cancers. The pathogenesis of ONJ-related to bisphosphonate administration is not fully elucidated. Two main hypotheses were proposed: bisphosphonate has profound anti-resorptive effect that directly reduces bone turnover via osteoclast inhibition and its anti-angiogenic effect leads to bone vascular insufficiency. [36] Higher jaw bone vascularization and bone turnover rate due to the presence of teeth compared to other bones resulted in greater bisphosphonate exposure and increased susceptibility to osteonecrosis of the jaw bones. Consequently, minor insult is more likely to progress into non-healing wound and widespread necrosis due to compromised vascular supply to the area. This potentially serious but rare complication of bisphosphonate therapy is influenced by the multiple factors. Prolonged bisphosphonate administration especially with use beyond 2 years appears to be associated with higher risk of ONJ. A number of studies have also suggested that ZA is correlated with a greater risk of ONJ compared to pamidronate, possibly due to its greater potency and prolonged inhibition of bone resorption. [37-39] However, this should not be a basis for recommendation of pamidronate over ZA as the higher risks of ONJ with ZA is based on observational studies and pamidronate has also been reported to cause ONJ. [35] Patients undergoing invasive dental procedures who were also receiving intravenous bisphosphonate therapy were at least 7 times more likely to develop ONJ. [37] Thus, when possible, major dental procedures should be completed before the initiation of therapy. For patients who are already on ZA treatment, the manufacturer and various clinical practice guidelines provided no guidance on the most appropriate management. Some practitioners may withhold bisphosphonate therapy during and after major dental procedures. The most recent American Dental Association recommendations in 2011 do not suggest withholding bisphosphonates in these cases because of their long half-lives and the lack of evidence to support this practice. [40] However, the International Myeloma Working Group (IMWG) 2013 consensus guideline recommends disrupting bisphosphonates for 90 days before and after invasive dental procedures, which include tooth extraction, dental implants, or jaw surgery (grade D recommendation). [41] Other risk factors such as older age, Caucasian race, diagnosis of multiple myeloma or breast cancer, corticosteroids therapy, smoking, alcohol use, and poor oral hygiene were also found to correlate with ONJ development. Prevention of ONJ should be the priority. However, if ONJ has occurred it should be managed conservatively. Topical and systemic antibiotics or surgical debridement may be required based on symptoms and severity of ONJ. [42] The AAOMS's updated recommendations in 2009 categorized patients with ONJ according to different levels of severity and provided guidance on the appropriate management options as summarized in Table 2. [43] The proposed treatment strategies were based on expert opinions and were not evidence-based. There are currently no prospective studies with long-term follow-up to guide the management of ONJ. However, bisphosphonates therapy discontinuation might be beneficial in stabilizing the progression of ONJ in these patients and the decision to rechallenge later with bisphosphonate is often based on physicians' discretions.

4. Electrolytes Abnormalities

Inhibition of osteoclastic function by ZA may disrupt normal regulatory mechanisms of calcium, leading to the development of hypocalcemia, hypophosphatemia, and hypomagnesemia. Zoledronic acid-induced hypocalcemia has been reported in 5 to 10% of patients. [15,16] Most cases were mild to moderate in severity with grade 3 or 4 occuring in ≤1% of patients. They were typically transient and did not result in clinical symptoms or necessitated any dose modification or interruption. Patients were often times asymptomatic and electrolytes disturbances typically occured within the first 6 months of therapy. Parathyroid hormone is usually able to compensate for low serum calcium by increasing renal absorption of vitamin D and calcium. However, patients with pre-existing vitamin D deficiency, hypothyroidism, previous parathyroid resection, and renal impairment are at higher risk for developing ZA-induced hypocalcemia. Hypomagnesemia and hypophosphatemia are less frequently reported with ZA. Hence, regular monitoring of serum electrolytes, especially serum calcium level prior to ZA acid infusion is recommended to prevent ZA-induced electrolytes abnormalities. [15,16] Serum calcium levels should also be corrected prior to the initiation of ZA infusion. Supplementation with calcium ≥ 500 mg daily and vitamin D ≥ 400 IU daily in patients with metastatic disease or multiple myeloma are highly recommended to prevent hypocalcemia.

Table 2. Staging and recommended management of bisphosphonate-related ONJ*

Stage	Findings	Recommendations
At-risk category	No apparent exposed/necrotic bone in patients who have been treated with either oral or IV bisphosphonates	• No treatment indicated • Patient education
Stage 0	Nonspecific clinical findings and symptoms such as jaw pain or osteosclerosis but no clinical evidence of exposed bone	• Systemic management, including use of pain medication and antibiotics
Stage 1	Exposed/necrotic bone in patients who are asymptomatic and have no evidence of infection	• Antibacterial mouth rinse • Clinical follow-up on quarterly basis • Patient education and review of indications for continued bisphosphonate therapy
Stage 2	Exposed/necrotic bone associated with infection as evidenced by pain and erythema in the region of the exposed bone with or without purulent drainage	• Symptomatic treatment with oral antibiotics • Oral antibacterial mouth rinse • Pain control • Superficial debridement to relieve soft tissue irritation
Stage 3	Exposed/necrotic bone in patients with pain, infection, and one or more of the following: pathologic fracture, extra oral fistula, or osteolysis extending to the inferior border or sinus floor	• Antibacterial mouth rinse • Antibiotic therapy and pain control • Surgical debridement/resection for longer term palliation of infection and pain

* Data from Advisory Task Force on Bisphosphonate-Related Osteonecrosis of the Jaws. American Association of Oral and Maxillofacial Surgeons position paper on bisphosphonate-related osteonecrosis of the jaws. [34].

5. Others

On rare occasions, ZA has been associated with musculoskeletal pain, atrial fibrillation, stroke, anterior uveitis, and atypical fracture of the femur. [15,16] These side effects have been reported in post-marketing studies of ZA.

Multiple Myeloma

Registration Studies

Zoledronic acid gained United States Food and Drug Administration (US FDA) approval for treatment of patients with multiple myeloma in February 2002. The approval was based on the demonstration of non-inferiority of ZA (4 mg) in preventing a skeletal-related event compared with the pamidronate effect that was seen in previously conducted placebo-controlled trials. [44] In the latter studies, skeletal-related events were defined as pathological fractures, radiotherapy for local bone pain, surgery to stabilize near-fractures, or spinal cord compression. [45-47] Using a composite of clinical benefit end-points, 'skeletal-related events' and a reduction thereof, to define sufficient clinical benefit for US FDA approval represented a regulatory precedent for the bisphosphonate class. [48] The registration study for ZA was an international, multicenter, double-blinded study in 1648 patients with stage IV breast cancer or Durie-Salmon stage III multiple myeloma (N = 513) randomized 1:1:1 to receive either ZA 4 mg, ZA 8 mg, or pamidronate 90mg every 3 to 4 weeks for 12 months. [22] The non-inferiority design required an active control (pamidronate) and the assumption that had this been substituted with a placebo, ZA would demonstrate superiority. In the final analysis considering the treatment effect seen from the three previous pamidronate trials and a comparison between ZA and pamidronate in the randomized trial, ZA retained at least 49.3% of the pamidronate-versus-placebo effect with a similar safety profile, providing adequate evidence for the US FDA to approve ZA 4 mg for the treatment of patients with multiple myeloma. Based on the above trials, the European regulatory authorities also granted marketing approval for ZA use for prevention of skeletal complications in patients with advanced bone malignancies in July 2002.

Demonstration of Safety and Efficacy through Randomized Trials and an Anti-myeloma Effect

Myeloma bone disease is due to interactions between myeloma cells and the bone marrow microenvironment resulting in osteoclast proliferation and increased bone resorption through numerous cytokines, including interleukin-6, interleukin-1 beta, and tumor necrosis factor alpha, which have prominent osteoclast activating functions. Bony lesions affect most patients with advanced stage multiple myeloma causing significant morbidity of debilitating pain, fractures, impaired mobility, spinal cord compression and hypercalcemia. The survival of multiple myeloma patients has increased over the last decade, with median survival of 6 to 7 years reported. Up to one third of newly diagnosed patients would have already suffered their first pathologic fracture. Therefore, long term control of skeletal-related complications is necessary. Zoledronic acid activity against myeloma bone disease has been demonstrated in several randomized clinical trials.

Berenson et al. reported findings from their multicenter, randomized, double-blinded trial comparing three doses of zoledronic acid (0.4 mg, 2 mg, 4 mg) in 280 patients with osteolytic lesions due to either breast cancer or multiple myeloma and used pamidronate 90 mg as an internal control for efficacy and tolerability.[49] The primary efficacy endpoint was the proportion of patients who received radiation to bone in the 10-month study observation period while secondary endpoints were the proportion of patients who developed pathologic fractures and hypercalcemia. Their intent-to-treat analysis showed ZA at doses of 2 mg and 4 mg and pamidronate 90 mg significantly reduced the need for radiation therapy to bone, pathologic fractures and hypercalcemia compared with 0.4 mg of ZA. They also found a dose-response effect of ZA on the mean antero-posterior lumbar spine bone mineral density with an increase of 6.2% in the 0.4 mg ZA group to 9.6% in the 4 mg ZA group ($P < .05$). The increase of 9.6% in bone mineral density was not significantly different from the increase seen with pamidronate in their study (increase of 9.2%). To date, there have been two large randomized trials comparing ZA with another bisphosphonate. The first was the US FDA registration study as described previously but with extended follow up after 25 months reported. [22] Apart from the ZA (4 mg and 8 mg) and pamidronate that were given in a 1:1:1 randomization, patients received standard antineoplastic therapy. The extension phase of this trial confirmed the safety and efficacy of ZA and demonstrated durability of the initial clinical benefit that was observed. The proportion of patients who experienced at least one skeletal-related event (primary endpoint) was similar between the ZA and pamidronate groups but a significantly lower proportion of patients treated with ZA required radiotherapy to bony lesions ($P = .037$). The time to a first skeletal-related event was comparable between the treatment groups in the subset of myeloma patients. In the ZA group, the mean annual incidence of skeletal complications was significantly lower at 0.47 events per year versus 0.71 events in the pamidronate group ($P = .015$). The long-term safety profile of 4 mg ZA given over 15 minutes was comparable to pamidronate 90 mg given over 2 hours, with no increase in incidence of renal impairment. The second study was the United Kingdom Medical Research Council (MRC-IX Myeloma) trial that was conducted on 1960 patients with multiple myeloma. This study compared ZA 4 mg every 3 to 4 weeks with oral clodronate 1600 mg daily combined with anti-myeloma therapy. [50] This study involved 2 broad treatment groups of intensive therapy culminating in autologous transplantation as post-induction therapy and another group that did not undergo transplantation. Within these groups there were 2 randomization steps. The first was to conventional chemotherapy or thalidomide-combination therapy with each of these groups receiving either ZA or clodronate, and the second randomization step was thalidomide maintenance versus no maintenance. Each maintenance group also received either ZA or clodronate. The primary endpoints set were overall survival, progression-free survival, and overall response rate while secondary endpoints included skeletal-related events and toxic effects. After a median follow up of 3.7 years, overall survival was found to be significantly improved in patients who received ZA compared with clodronate, with a reduction in mortality of 16%. This difference was seen starting as early as the first 4 months of therapy. Overall, ZA extended the median overall survival by 5.5 months to 50 months compared to the 44.5 months survival seen with clodronate. Zoledronic acid was also shown to improve progression-free survival by 12%

and extended the median progression-free survival by 2 months to 19.5 months. In terms of skeletal-related events, ZA reduced this risk by 26% compared with clodronate regardless of the anti-myeloma therapy that patients received. The occurrence of most adverse events was similar between patients receiving either bisphosphonate although confirmed ONJ was higher in the ZA group (4% versus less than 1%). This trial demonstrated an overall survival advantage of ZA independent of the reduction in skeletal-related events, suggesting an anti-myeloma effect. The overall survival benefit that emerged within the first few month of therapy alludes to a possible synergistic action of ZA with the anti-myeloma treatment that was given. In this trial, patients received bisphosphonates for a median of 350 days (range 137 to 632 days). At variance with the latter study, a recent Cochrane meta-analysis found that no bisphosphonate showed superior survival over another but ZA was the only bisphosphonate that had an overall survival advantage over placebo. [51]

Usage of ZA in Multiple Myeloma

Initiation of Therapy

Zoledronic acid should be used to prevent skeletal-related events in patients with symptomatic multiple myeloma regardless of the presence of bone lesions as defined by conventional radiography. Lesions usually become evident on x-rays only when over 20% of trabecular bone has been lost and it is not known whether ZA will benefit symptomatic myeloma patients where bone disease has been excluded by more sensitive imaging modalities like magnetic resonance imaging or positron emission tomography. [52] The suggested dose of ZA is 4 mg over a 15 minute infusion every 3 to 4 weeks, provided there is adequate renal function. Its use in myeloma patients without bone lesions on skeletal survey is supported by the MRC-IX Myeloma trial that found a reduction in skeletal-related events in the ZA group patients regardless of the presence of bone disease at diagnosis. [50] The use of ZA in patients with asymptomatic multiple myeloma has been shown to increase bone mineral density at the lumbar spine and in one study showed a reduction in skeletal-related events at the time of disease progression but without influencing the risk of progression. [53,54] Therefore, most guidelines do not recommend the use of ZA in asymptomatic myeloma except where there is age-related osteoporosis, a dose of 5mg yearly can be given.

Duration of Therapy and ONJ

In all of the randomized, placebo-controlled trials, bisphosphonate therapy was limited to 2 years. Accordingly, guidelines from the International Myeloma Working Group, European Myeloma Network and the American Society of Clinical Oncology recommend ZA treatment for a period not exceeding 2 years due to the unknown clinical benefit of continued therapy and the risk of ONJ which is seen in 1.3 to 4% of patients continuing on ZA beyond 2 years. [55,56] This risk of ONJ of the jaw is higher with ZA compared to other bisphosphonates among myeloma patients. In a single institution study, Zervas et al reported that ZA produced a 9.5-fold higher risk of developing osteonecrosis of the jaw than pamidronate (P =.042). [57] Preventive dental measures to maintain strict oral hygiene, minimize invasive dental procedures and assessments carried out by an experienced dental team has shown to decrease the incidence of ONJ among myeloma patients by almost three-fold. [58] It is noteworthy that there were no reports of ONJ in any trial of bisphosphonates before US FDA approval. The above notwithstanding, subset analysis from the MRC-IX Myeloma trial showed continued benefit in terms of a reduction in skeletal-related events and improvement in overall survival in ZA patients continuing therapy beyond 2 years compared with patients receiving clodronate.

Renal Impairment

Myeloma patients commonly present with renal impairment. Zoledronic acid is not metabolized and is excreted unchanged via the kidney and therefore randomized trials with ZA have specifically excluded patients with an elevated serum creatinine of more than 3 mg/dL due to the risk of renal deterioration. In the MRC-IX Myeloma trial, 5 to 7% of patients developed acute renal failure and trials of treatment for bone metastases reported rates of renal deterioration of 9 to 15%. Therefore, ZA is not recommended for myeloma patients with a creatinine clearance of less than 30 milliliters per minute and doses should be attenuated where levels are between 30 to 60 milliliters per minute. When using zoledronic acid, all patients should be kept well hydrated, their serum creatinine checked and the drug stopped should there be deterioration in renal function until the creatinine clearance has returned to within 10% of the baseline level.

Role of ZA in Solid Tumors

The main role for any bisphosphonates in solid tumor is to prevent and delay the onset of skeletal-related events. [59] These include pathological bone fractures, bone pain needing radiation or surgery, and spinal cord compression. Bone is one of the commonest sites of metastases for solid tumors especially breast, lung, prostate and thyroid cancers. They may be predominantly osteolytic, osteoblastic, or mixed. Skeletal-related events are often debilitating, affecting patients' mobility and rendering them dependent on others for activities of daily living. The associated pain may result in decreased quality of life and depression. Zolendroni acid is also used in the management of hypercalcemia of malignancies, to reduce the levels of serum calcium. The first approval for ZA's use for patients with solid tumors and bone metastases was granted by the FDA in 2002. [60] The recommended dose is similar to that used in multiple myeloma.

Breast Cancer

Bone metastases occur in 65-75% of patients with stage 4 breast carcinoma and they are mostly osteolytic in nature. [61] The complication rates are high if they are left untreated. For instance, in the placebo arm of an earlier pamidronate study, 52% of patients with predominantly osteolytic bone lesions secondary to breast carcinoma developed pathologic fractures, 37% required palliative radiation therapy, 13% developed hypercalcemia of malignancy, and 11% required orthopaedic surgery over a period of 2 years. [62] Patients with bone metastases from breast cancer often experience substantial debilitating bone pain which often lead to a poorer quality of life. Zoledronic acid is a potent inhibitor of osteoclastic bone resoption for breast cancer patients with bone metastasis.

Multiple trials had shown superior benefits with ZA when compared with placebo, and at least equilvalence or superiority when compared to other bisphosphonates such as pamidronate or ibandronate. In an early randomized trial, 280 patients with either breast cancer or myeloma were allocated treatment with ZA at 0.4, 2, 4 mg or 90 mg of pamidronate. [49] It was found that for all arms of the trial, when compared with 0.4 mg ZA, there were significant reduction in the subsequent need for bone radiation, the primary endpoint of that trial. Serum N-telopeptide (NTX), a bone resorption marker, was also decreased in all treatment groups. In a subsequent study, 4mg of ZA was compared with 90mg of pamidronate in 767 breast cancer patients with bone metastases. [63] The primary endpoint was the proportion of patients who developed a skeletal-related event. Patients were stratified according to whether they were being treated with hormonal therapy or chemotherapy for their cancer. Zoledonic acid was found to be as effective as pamidronate, and the proportion of ZA-treated patients with a skeletal-related event (42% in the hormonal therapy strata and 44% in the chemotherapy strata) was comparable to the original studies comparing pamidronate to placebo. A separate trial conducted in Japan randomized patients to monthly ZA versus placebo. [64] Treatment duration was 1 year for the study. Zoledronic acid was found to reduce SRE by 39% at 1 year when compared to placebo. The absolute reduction in percentage of SRE was from 49.6% to 29.8%. There was also delayed time-to-first skeletal-related event (364 days in placebo arm and not reached for ZA arm). Among the breast cancer patients (n=412) enrolled in the large randomized, double-blind, phase III study conducted by Rosen et al alluded to earlier, skeletal-related events occurred in 46% and 49% of patients on ZA and pamidronate respectively. [22] At 2 years, the reduction in skeletal-related event risk favored ZA. [65] In particular, ZA (4 mg) was found to significantly decreased the need for radiation therapy to the bone. In addition, breast cancer patients who were only on hormonal therapy had significantly extended time to first skeletal-related event with the use of ZA (415 days vs 370 days for pamidronate, P=0.047).

A study involving 101 breast cancer patients with one or more bone metastasis on hormonal therapy only was done to compare the efficacy and safety of ZA administration in the community setting versus the hospital setting. [66] To measure pain scores, physical, emotional and social functioning, the Brief Pain Inventory (BPI) and the European Organization for Research and Treatment of Cancer Quality of Life Core Questionnaire 30 (EORTC QLQ-C30) were used to assess the potential benefits of ZA therapy in the 2 settings. Interestingly, there were consistently greater improvements in pain scores after treatment in the community setting compared to the hospital crossover setting for worst pain (P=0.021), average pain (P=0.003), and interference with general activity (P=0.001). As efficacy and the incidence of adverse events including renal toxicity between the two settings were comparable, the study informs that ZA may be safely administered in the community setting.

In the ZA versus Ibandronate Comparative Evaluation (ZICE) trial, over 1400 patients with at least one radiologically confirmed bone metastasis were randomly assigned to either monthly ZA or daily oral ibandronate for 2 years. [67] The primary non-inferiority endpoint was the frequency and timing of skeletal-related events over 96 weeks. The annual rates of skeletal-related events were 0.499 and 0.435 with ibandronate and ZA respectively (rate ratio: 1.15, 95% CI 0.97-1.36). As the upper CI was greater than the margin of non-inferiority of 1.08, ibandronate hence appeared to be inferior to ZA. However, more patients in the ZA group had renal toxic adverse reactions compared to the ibandronate group (32% vs 24%). The rates of ONJ were comparably uncommon in both groups (<1 and 1 percent, respectively). These results support the use of ZA over oral ibandronate for women with metastatic breast cancer involving the bones. However, for patients who are at increased risk of renal toxicity and those who prefer the convenience of an oral regimen, oral ibandronate is a reasonable alternative.

A meta-analysis of 34 randomized trials comparing both oral and intravenous bisphosphonates with placebo in breast cancer patients showed that overall, bisphosphonates were able to reduce skeletal-related events by 15% compared to placebo. The benefits were more apparent with the intravenous preparations. In addition, bisphosphonates also delayed the time to development of an skeletal-related event. [68] To date, there is still insufficient evidence recommending the use of ZA or any bisphosphonates in advanced breast cancer patients without clinically evident bone metastases. There is insufficient evidence to support the use of bisphosphonates as adjuvant treatment in reducing bone or visceral metastases, preventing recurrence or improving survival.

Another indication for ZA in cancer patients is the management of treatment-related bone loss. Breast cancer patients on adjuvant aromatase inhibitor therapy, prostate cancer patients undergoing androgen deprivation and females with premature chemotherapy induced menopause or on prolonged steroid therapy are at higher risk. The use of ZA in early breast cancer lies in the premise that it should prevent treatment related bone loss. In the Cancer and Leukemia Group B (CALGB) Trial 79809 study, 166 females were randomly assigned to upfront ZA (4 mg every three months), delayed ZA (same dose starting one year after randomization) or no treatment. [69] These patients had stage I to III breast cancer and chemotherapy-induced ovarian failure. All women were prescribed calcium (1000 mg) and vitamin D (400 iu). The primary end-point was the percentage change in bone mineral density (BMD) in the lumbar spine (LS) in 12 months. After a median follow-up of one year, ZA resulted in a significant increase in lumbosacral BMD (1.2% gain versus 6.7% loss). The authors concluded that ZA every 3 months prevents rapid bone loss related to cancer treatment and should be started together with adjuvant chemotherapy. The Austrian Breast and Colorectal Cancer Study Group (ABCSG)-12 trial sought to examine whether ZA could prevent bone loss associated with adjuvant endocrine therapy in premenopausal patients. [70] Four hundred and one premenopausal women who were receiving adjuvant GnRH therapy with goserelin plus either tamoxifen or anastrozole in the bone mineral density (BMD) sub-protocol of the study were also treated with either ZA (4 mg every six months) or placebo. Serial BMD measurements were taken at 0, 6, 12, 24, and 36 months. Statistically significant bone loss (mean loss of 14.4% in BMD) was evident in the placebo group while women receiving ZA had stable BMD throughout the study period. [70] This suggests that ZA at 4 mg every 6 months effectively inhibited bone loss and hence, it is recommended that regular BMD measurements should be done for patients undergoing adjuvant endocrine therapy and initiation of bisphosphonate therapy should be considered if there is evidence of bone loss. The dosing intervals of ZA is shorter for treatment of metastases due to the need to rapidly inhibit osteoclastic destruction of the bones while the dosing interval for prevention of bone loss is usually longer at about 3 to 6 months. [69,70] The optimal dose interval was further explored in an Italian phase III study where over 400 breast cancer patients who had one or more bone metastases and had completed 12-15 months of monthly treatment with ZA, were randomly assigned to ZA 4 mg every 12 weeks or ZA 4 mg every 4 weeks. [71] The skeletal morbidity rate (skeletal-related events per patient per year) were not significantly different at 0.26 (95% CI 0.15-0.37) and 0.22 (0.14-0.29) for the 12-weekly and the 4-weekly groups respectively. This suggests that the administration of ZA may be stretched to a 3 monthly interval during the second year without affecting the efficacy of treatment. Further studies are ongoing to validate this observation.

For patients in whom osteoclast inhibitor therapy is indicated, the American Society of Clinical Oncology (ASCO) guidelines recommended to continue treatment indefinitely, in the absence of excessive toxicity and as long as treatment is consistent with both the patient's and the clinician's joint treatment goals. [72] As the treatment of the cancer with anti-neoplastic agents frequently takes precedence over supportive bone care, the administration of bisphosphonates could frequently be overlooked for breast cancer patients with metastatic bone disease. [73]

There are also currently no evidence-based guidelines on the approach after the development of skeletal-related event while on bisphophonates. For patients treated with an oral bisphosphonate, a switch to intravenous ZA can be considered. In one prospective trial, 31 women who developed new skeletal-related events while on clodronate or pamidronate were switched to ZA. [74] This resulted in significant improvement in pain scores which were independent of any change in their anticancer treatment. Changes in urinary NTX also correlated well with improvement in pain control. [74] For patients with progressive skeletal-related events while on ZA, a switch to subcutaneous denosumab would be reasonable.

Lung Cancer

The majority of the earlier trials involved mostly breast cancer and myeloma patients. There are however, a few trials that examined the role of ZA in other tumor types. It should be borne in mind that at this point, the FDA's approval extends to bone metastases of all tumor types. In a double-blind, placebo-controlled phase III trial, Rosen et al randomized 773 patients with skeletal metastases from cancers other than breast and prostate (including non-small cell and small cell lung, renal cell, thyroid, and head and neck cancers) to ZA every 3 weeks for 9 months or placebo. The treatment group had a significant reduction in the number of skeletal-related events (38 versus 47 percent) and a significantly longer time to first event (230 versus 163 days, p=0.03). [75] These benefits persisted with continuing treatment and follow-up, indicating that the efficacy of ZA is apparent in these other tumor types. [76] Additional data lending support to use of bisphosphonates in lung cancer came from a retrospective medical claims analysis where 365 patients with bone metastases treated with ZA were compared to 2174 who did not receive ZA. [77] The monthly rate of skeletal complications in ZA-treated patients versus untreated patients was 0.29 +/- 0.3 per month versus 0.43 +/- 0.4 per month, respectively ($P < .001$). Persistent ZA use was associated with longer follow-up duration ($P < .05$) and a greater probability of continuing follow-up. The authors concluded that this study provided real-world evidence indicating that ZA reduced the skeletal morbidity rate and delayed the time to skeletal complications.

Prostate Cancer

Unlike breast cancer and multiple myeloma, the bone metastases from prostate cancer are mostly sclerotic in nature. To demonstrate that ZA is as efficacious in this setting, a randomized phase III study compared ZA 4mg to placebo in 422 men with hormone-refractory prostate cancer with bone metastases. [78,79] Among 22 patients who had completed 24 months of treatment, 38% in the ZA group developed a skeletal-related event compared to 49% in the placebo group. The median time to the first skeletal-related events was 488 days for the ZA group versus 321 days for the placebo group ($P = 0.009$). In addition, the effects of ZA were apparent at 3 months, where only 12% of ZA-treated patients had a skeletal-related event versus 23% for the placebo group ($P = 0.003$). At 6 months, the proportions were 21 vs. 31% for placebo ($P = 0.025$). Interestingly, the same benefit could not be demonstrated in similar groups of patient treated with pamidronate. [80]

The adjuvant use of bisphosphonates in patients with castrate-resistant prostate cancer to decrease the incidence of bone metastases was explored in the phase III Zometa European Study (ZEUS) trial. A thousand four hundred and thirty-three patients with high-risk prostate cancer (defined as PSA ≥20 ng/mL, Gleason 8-10, or node positive disease) were randomly assigned to 3-monthly ZA or placebo for four years. [81] After a median follow-up of 4.8 years, there was no significant difference in the incidence of bone metastases (14.7% versus 13.2%. $p=0.65$). Hence, there is no evidence to recommend ZA in the adjuvant setting. The role of ZA in prevention of bone loss among prostate cancer patients with no metastases and beginning androgen deprivation therapy was also explored. [82] Mean lumbar BMD increased by 5.6% among patients randomized to receive ZA group and decreased by 2.2% in the placebo group (mean difference 7.8%, 95% confidence interval 5.6%-10.0%, $p <0.001$). A similar trend was also observed with the BMD changes in the trochanter.

Role of ZA in Benign Conditions

Zolendronic acid is approved globally for 6 indications: treatment of postmenopausal osteoporosis in women to reduce the incidence of hip, vertebral, and nonvertebral fractures and to increase BMD, prevention of clinical fractures after hip fracture in men and women, treatment of osteoporosis in men, treatment and prevention of glucocorticoid-induced osteoporosis, prevention of postmenopausal osteoporosis (in the US) and the treatment of Paget's disease of bone. For benign indications several clinical studies have documented that a single infusion of intravenous ZA resulted in decreased bone turnover and improved bone density for at least 12 months post infusion. The key efficacy data for ZA in the treatment of benign bone conditions are summarised in table 3. [83-91]

Table 3. Key efficacy data for ZA in the treatment of benign bone conditions

Author/reference	Study	Result	Conclusions
Black et al (83)	(HORIZON-PFT) Double-blind, placebo-controlled trial where patients with postmenopausal osteoporosis were randomized between a ZA (5 mg) or placebo at baseline, at 12 months, and at 24 months Primary end points were new vertebral fracture (in patients not taking concomitant osteoporosis medications) and hip fracture (in all patients). Secondary end points included bone mineral density, bone turnover markers, and safety outcomes.	70% reduction in morphometric vertebral fractures, 41% reduction in hip fractures and 25% reduction in nonvertebral fractures over 3 years	Annual infusion of zoledronic acid during a 3-year period significantly reduced the risk of vertebral, hip, and other fractures
Lyles et al (84)	(HORIZON-RFT) Randomized, double-blind, placebo-controlled trial where patients who had already sustained hip fracture were assigned to receive yearly intravenous ZA (5 mg) or placebo. The primary end point was a new clinical fracture. Median follow-up was 1.9 years	28% reduction in mortality after hip fracture, 35% risk reduction of all new clinical fractures, 46% risk reduction of all new clinical vertebral fractures and 27% risk reduction in new nonvertebral fractures. ZA improved BMD at total hip and femoral neck	Annual infusion of ZA within 90 days after repair of a low-trauma hip fracture was associated with a reduction in the rate of new clinical fractures and improved survival
McClung et al (85)	Double-blind, double-dummy trial where postmenopausal osteoporosis patients women with low BMD previously been treated alendronate were randomized between a single dose of IV ZA (5 mg) or oral alendronate (70 mg weekly)	Lumbar spine BMD remained stable with both treatments at 12 months but 78.7% of patients preferred the once a-year infusion to weekly oral therapy	Patients can be switched from oral alendronate to ZA infusion with maintenance of therapeutic effect for at least 12 months and that patients prefer a once yearly infusion to weekly oral therapy.
Saag et al (86)	Double-blind, double-dummy, trial where postmenopausal osteoporosis patients with low BMD were randomized between a single infusion of ZA (5 mg) or weekly oral alendronate. The effects of these therapies on other markers of bone turnover, patient preference and adverse events were also assessed	Significantly greater relative change in urine NTx values at week 1 with ZA vs alendronate. Significantly lower mean urine NTx values throughout the 24-week study and greater and more rapid reduction in BTMs with ZA compared with weekly alendronate	A single infusion of ZA 5 mg reduced urine NTX levels more rapidly than weekly oral alendronate. The majority of study patients preferred an intravenous treatment regimen of ZA 5 mg over weekly osteoporosis therapy with alendronate 70 mg.

Table 3. (Continued)

Author/reference	Study	Result	Conclusions
Reid et al (87)	1-year randomised, double-blind, double-dummy, non-inferiority study testing the effectiveness of 5 mg intravenous infusion of ZA acid versus 30 mg of oral risedronate for prevention and treatment of glucocorticoid-induced osteoporosis.	ZA demonstrated superior BMD increase at 12 months compared with oral daily risedronate. ZA significantly decreased levels of β-CTx and P1NP compared with oral daily risedronate in both the prevention and the treatment subpopulations. 84% of all patients preferred annual IV over daily oral pills	A single 5 mg intravenous infusion of zoledronic acid is non-inferior, possibly more effective, and more acceptable to patients than is 5 mg of oral risedronate daily for prevention and treatment of bone loss that is associated with glucocorticoid use.
Reid et al (Paget's disease core study) (88)	Two identical, randomized, double-blind, actively controlled trials comparing one 15-minute infusion of 5 mg of ZA with 60 days of oral risedronate (30 mg per day). The primary efficacy end point was the rate of therapeutic response at six months, defined as a normalization of alkaline phosphatase levels or a reduction of at least 75 percent in the total alkaline phosphatase excess. The results of the studies were pooled.	96% of patients achieved therapeutic response with ZA vs 74% with risedronate at 6 months. 88.6% of patients achieved normal alkaline phosphatase with ZA vs 57.9% with risedronate. ZA produced significantly greater reductions in alkaline phosphatase than risedronate	A single infusion of ZA produces more rapid, more complete, and more sustained responses in Paget's disease than does daily treatment with risedronate.
Hosking et al (Paget's disease extension study) (89)	Eligible patients from both core studies reexamined 24 months after treatment to compare the ability of ZA vs risedronate to maintain long-term control of bone turnover.	98% of those given ZA maintained therapeutic response vs 57% of those given risedronate at 24 months	ZOL maintains bone turnover within the reference range over 24 months from the initiation of treatment. A reduction in the incidence and severity of long-term complications may require persistent normalization of bone turnover over many years, and ZA is effective in this regard.
Boonen et al (geriatric osteoporosis) (90)	Post hoc subgroup analysis of pooled data from the Health Outcome and Reduced Incidence with ZA (HORIZON) Pivotal Fracture Trial and the HORIZON Recurrent Fracture Trial.	At 3 years, incidence of any clinical, vertebral and non-vertebral fracture was significantly lower in ZA group compared with placebo group (10.8% vs 16.6%, 1.1% vs 3.7%, and 9.9% vs 13.7%, respectively).	Once-yearly intravenous ZA(5mg) was associated with a significant reduction in the risk of new clinical fractures (vertebral and nonvertebral) in elderly postmenopausal women with osteroporosis.
Orwoll et al (male osteoporosis) (91)	Double-blind, active-controlled, parallel-group study where hypogonadal men were randomized to receive either once-yearly ZA 5 mg or weekly oral alendronate 70 mg for 24 months.	ZA increased BMD at lumbar spine, total hip, femoral neck, and trochanter and was noninferior to alendronate at 24 months. At month 12, the median changes from the baseline of markers for bone resorption β-CTx, urine NTx and P1NP formation, serum BSAP were comparable between ZA and alendronate groups	A once-yearly infusion of ZA 5 mg increased bone density and decreased bone turnover markers similarly to once-weekly oral alendronate 70 mg in men with low bone density.

CONCLUSION

Zoledronic acid is highly effective for the prevention of skeletal morbidity in advanced cancers with bone metastases and treatment of hypercalcemia. It prevents bone loss in both the benign and malignant settings, and may influence the metastatic process when administered in the adjuvant setting for some cancer patients. Side effects are usually mild and ZA is very well tolerated. Safety precautions remain of importance and monitoring of renal function especially in the elderly and attention to dental hygiene will reduce the side effect profile further. The dosing regimen used in malignancy is considerably more intensive than that used for osteoporosis or Paget's disease. Its use in both oncology and non-oncology patients has had a major positive impact on the quality of life.

REFERENCES

[1] Reynolds JJ, Minkin C, Morgan DB, Spycher D, Fleisch H. The effect of two diphosphonates on the resorption of mouse calvaria in vitro. *Calcif Tissue Res.* 1972;10(4):302-313.
[2] Schenk R, Merz WA, Muhlbauer R, Russell RG, Fleisch H. Effect of ethane-1-hydroxy-1,1-diphosphonate (EHDP) and dichloromethylene diphosphonate (Cl 2 MDP) on the calcification and resorption of cartilage and bone in the tibial epiphysis and metaphysis of rats. *Calcif Tissue Res.* 1973;11(3):196-214.
[3] Roelofs AJ, Thompson K, Gordon S, Rogers MJ. Molecular mechanisms of action of bisphosphonates: current status. *Clin Cancer Res.* 2006;12(20 Pt 2):6222s-6230s.
[4] Green JR, Muller K, Jaeggi KA. Preclinical pharmacology of CGP 42'446, a new, potent, heterocyclic bisphosphonate compound. *J Bone Miner Res.* 1994;9(5):745-751.
[5] Body JJ FJ, Vigneron AM. A dose finding study of zoledronate intravenous infusion in patients with tumour induced hypercalcemia. *Journal of Bone and Mineral Research;* 1996:S485.
[6] Kavanagh KL, Guo K, Dunford JE, et al. The molecular mechanism of nitrogen-containing bisphosphonates as antiosteoporosis drugs. *Proc Natl Acad Sci U S A.* 2006;103(20):7829-7834.
[7] Coxon FP, Helfrich MH, Van't Hof R, et al. Protein geranylgeranylation is required for osteoclast formation, function, and survival: inhibition by bisphosphonates and GGTI-298. *J Bone Miner Res.* 2000;15(8):1467-1476.
[8] Thompson K, Rogers MJ, Coxon FP, Crockett JC. Cytosolic entry of bisphosphonate drugs requires acidification of vesicles after fluid-phase endocytosis. *Mol Pharmacol.* 2006;69(5):1624-1632.
[9] Guenther A, Gordon S, Tiemann M, et al. The bisphosphonate zoledronic acid has antimyeloma activity in vivo by inhibition of protein prenylation. *Int J Cancer.* 2010;126(1):239-246.
[10] Croucher PI, De Hendrik R, Perry MJ, et al. Zoledronic acid treatment of 5T2MM-bearing mice inhibits the development of myeloma bone disease: evidence for decreased osteolysis, tumor burden and angiogenesis, and increased survival. *J Bone Miner Res.* 2003;18(3):482-492.

[11] Fournier P, Boissier S, Filleur S, et al. Bisphosphonates inhibit angiogenesis in vitro and testosterone-stimulated vascular regrowth in the ventral prostate in castrated rats. *Cancer Res*. 2002;62(22):6538-6544.
[12] Bezzi M, Hasmim M, Bieler G, Dormond O, Ruegg C. Zoledronate sensitizes endothelial cells to tumor necrosis factor-induced programmed cell death: evidence for the suppression of sustained activation of focal adhesion kinase and protein kinase B/Akt. *J Biol Chem*. 2003;278(44):43603-43614.
[13] Mariani S, Muraro M, Pantaleoni F, et al. Effector gammadelta T cells and tumor cells as immune targets of zoledronic acid in multiple myeloma. *Leukemia*. 2005;19(4):664-670.
[14] Chen T, Berenson J, Vescio R, et al. Pharmacokinetics and pharmacodynamics of zoledronic acid in cancer patients with bone metastases. *J Clin Pharmacol*. 2002;42(11):1228-1236.
[15] Zometa [package insert]. East Hanover, NJ: Novartis Pharmaceuticals Corp; 2014.
[16] Micromedex Healthcare Series [database online]. Greenwood Village, CO: Thomson Reuters (Healthcare), Inc; 2012. http://www.thomsonhc.com/hcs/librarian. Accessed April 21, 2014.
[17] Andreadis C, Charalampidou M, Diamantopoulos N, Chouchos N, Mouratidou D. Combined chemotherapy and radiotherapy during conception and first two trimesters of gestation in a woman with metastatic breast cancer. *Gynecol Oncol*. 2004;95(1):252-255.
[18] Djokanovic N, Klieger-Grossmann C, Koren G. Does treatment with bisphosphonates endanger the human pregnancy? *J Obstet Gynaecol Can*. 2008;30(12):1146-1148.
[19] Stathopoulos IP, Liakou CG, Katsalira A, et al. The use of bisphosphonates in women prior to or during pregnancy and lactation. *Hormones (Athens)*. 2011;10(4):280-291.
[20] Kunzmann V, Bauer E, Feurle J, Weissinger F, Tony HP, Wilhelm M. Stimulation of gammadelta T cells by aminobisphosphonates and induction of antiplasma cell activity in multiple myeloma. *Blood*. 2000;96(2):384-392.
[21] Olson K, Van Poznak C. Significance and impact of bisphosphonate-induced acute phase responses. *J Oncol Pharm Pract*. 2007;13(4):223-229.
[22] Rosen LS, Gordon D, Kaminski M, et al. Zoledronic acid versus pamidronate in the treatment of skeletal metastases in patients with breast cancer or osteolytic lesions of multiple myeloma: a phase III, double-blind, comparative trial. *Cancer J*. 2001;7(5):377-387.
[23] Chang JT, Green L, Beitz J. Renal failure with the use of zoledronic acid. *N Engl J Med*. 2003;349(17):1676-1679.
[24] Munier A, Gras V, Andrejak M, et al. Zoledronic Acid and renal toxicity: data from French adverse effect reporting database. *Ann Pharmacother*. 2005;39(7-8):1194-1197.
[25] Markowitz GS, Fine PL, Stack JI, et al. Toxic acute tubular necrosis following treatment with zoledronate (Zometa). *Kidney Int*. 2003;64(1):281-289.
[26] Kunin M, Kopolovic J, Avigdor A, Holtzman EJ. Collapsing glomerulopathy induced by long-term treatment with standard-dose pamidronate in a myeloma patient. *Nephrol Dial Transplant*. 2004;19(3):723-726.
[27] Medwatch. Food and Drug Administration Web site .www.fda.gov/downloads/safety /medwatch/safetyinformation/safetyalertsforhumanmedicalproducts/ucm164908.pdf. Accessed April 18, 2014.

[28] Saad F, Gleason DM, Murray R, et al. A randomized, placebo-controlled trial of zoledronic acid in patients with hormone-refractory metastatic prostate carcinoma. *J Natl Cancer Inst*. 2002;94(19):1458-1468.
[29] Berenson JR, Boccia R, Lopez T, et al. Results of a multicenter open-label randomized trial evaluating infusion duration of zoledronic acid in multiple myeloma patients (the ZMAX trial). *J Support Oncol*. 2011;9(1):32-40.
[30] Berenson JR. Recommendations for zoledronic acid treatment of patients with bone metastases. *Oncologist*. 2005;10(1):52-62.
[31] Shah SR, Jean GW, Keisner SV, Ussery SM, Dowell JE. Risk of renal failure in cancer patients with bone metastasis treated with renally adjusted zoledronic acid. *Support Care Cancer*. 2012;20(1):87-93
[32] Major P, Lortholary A, Hon J, et al. Zoledronic acid is superior to pamidronate in the treatment of hypercalcemia of malignancy: a pooled analysis of two randomized, controlled clinical trials. *J Clin Oncol*. 2001;19(2):558-567.
[33] Berenson JR, Hillner BE, Kyle RA, et al. American Society of Clinical Oncology clinical practice guidelines: the role of bisphosphonates in multiple myeloma. *J Clin Oncol*. 2002;20(17):3719-3736.
[34] Advisory Task Force. American Association of Oral and Maxillofacial Surgeons position paper on bisphosphonate-related osteonecrosis of the jaws. *J Oral Maxillofac Surg*. 2007;65(3):369-376.
[35] Marx. Pamidronate (Aredia) and zoledronate (Zometa) induced avascular necrosis of the jaws: a growing epidemic. *J Oral Maxillofac Surg*. 2003;61(9):1115-1117.
[36] Palant CE, Stern N, Meyer A, Tuck ML, Lee DB, Yanagawa N. Modulation of aortic smooth muscle cell membrane potential by extracellular calcium. *Hypertension*. 1989;14(5):549-55.
[37] Saussez S, Javadian R, Hupin C, et al. Bisphosphonate-related osteonecrosis of the jaw and its associated risk factors: a Belgian case series. *Laryngoscope*. 2009;119(2):323-329.
[38] Bamias A, Kastritis E, Bamia C, et al. Osteonecrosis of the jaw in cancer after treatment with bisphosphonates: incidence and risk factors. *J Clin Oncol*. 2005;23(34):8580-8587.
[39] Filleul O, Crompot E, Saussez S. Bisphosphonate-induced osteonecrosis of the jaw: a review of 2,400 patient cases. *J Cancer Res Clin Oncol*. 2010;136(8):1117-1124.
[40] Hellstein JW, Adler RA, Edwards B, et al. Managing the care of patients receiving antiresorptive therapy for prevention and treatment of osteoporosis: executive summary of recommendations from the American Dental Association Council on Scientific Affairs. *J Am Dent Assoc*. 2011;142(11):1243-1251.
[41] Terpos E, Morgan, Dimopoulos MA, et al. International Myeloma Working Group recommendations for the treatment of multiple myeloma-related bone disease. *J Clin Oncol*. 2013;31(18):2347-2357.
[42] Ruggiero SL. Emerging concepts in the management and treatment of osteonecrosis of the jaw. *Oral Maxillofac Surg Clin North Am*. 2013;25(1):11-20.
[43] Ruggiero SL, Dodson TB, Assael LA, et al. American Association of Oral and Maxillofacial Surgeons position paper on bisphosphonate-related osteonecrosis of the jaws--2009 update. *J Oral Maxillofac Surg*. 2009;67(5 Suppl):2-12.

[44] Ibrahim A, Scher N, Williams G, et al. Approval summary for zoledronic acid for treatment of multiple myeloma and cancer bone metastases. *Clin Cancer Res.* 2003;9(7):2394-2399.

[45] Theriault RL, Lipton A, Hortobagyi GN, et al. Pamidronate reduces skeletal morbidity in women with advanced breast cancer and lytic bone lesions: a randomized, placebo-controlled trial. Protocol 18 Aredia Breast Cancer Study Group. *J Clin Oncol.* 1999;17(3):846-854.

[46] Hortobagyi GN, Theriault RL, Lipton A, et al. Long-term prevention of skeletal complications of metastatic breast cancer with pamidronate. Protocol 19 Aredia Breast Cancer Study Group. *J Clin Oncol.* 1998;16(6):2038-2044.

[47] Berenson JR, Lichtenstein A, Porter L, et al. Long-term pamidronate treatment of advanced multiple myeloma patients reduces skeletal events. Myeloma Aredia Study Group. *J Clin Oncol.* 1998;16(2):593-602.

[48] Johnson JR, Williams G, Pazdur R. End points and United States Food and Drug Administration approval of oncology drugs. *J Clin Oncol.* 2003;21(7):1404-1411.

[49] Berenson JR, Rosen LS, Howell A, et al. Zoledronic acid reduces skeletal-related events in patients with osteolytic metastases. *Cancer.* 2001;91(7):1191-1200.

[50] Morgan GJ, Davies FE, Gregory WM, et al. First-line treatment with zoledronic acid as compared with clodronic acid in multiple myeloma (MRC Myeloma IX): a randomised controlled trial. *Lancet.* 2010;376(9757):1989-1999.

[51] Mhaskar R, Redzepovic J, Wheatley K, et al. Bisphosphonates in multiple myeloma: a network meta-analysis. *Cochrane Database Syst Rev.* 2012;5:CD003188.

[52] Durie BG, Salmon SE. A clinical staging system for multiple myeloma. Correlation of measured myeloma cell mass with presenting clinical features, response to treatment, and survival. *Cancer.* 1975;36(3):842-854.

[53] Berenson JR, Yellin O, Boccia RV, et al. Zoledronic acid markedly improves bone mineral density for patients with monoclonal gammopathy of undetermined significance and bone loss. *Clin Cancer Res.* 2008;14(19):6289-6295.

[54] Musto P, Petrucci MT, Bringhen S, et al. A multicenter, randomized clinical trial comparing zoledronic acid versus observation in patients with asymptomatic myeloma. *Cancer.* 2008;113(7):1588-1595.

[55] Morgan GJ, Davies FE, Gregory WM, et al. Effects of induction and maintenance plus long-term bisphosphonates on bone disease in patients with multiple myeloma: the Medical Research Council Myeloma IX Trial. *Blood.* 2012;119(23):5374-5383.

[56] Henry DH, Costa L, Goldwasser F, et al. Randomized, double-blind study of denosumab versus zoledronic acid in the treatment of bone metastases in patients with advanced cancer (excluding breast and prostate cancer) or multiple myeloma. *J Clin Oncol.* 2011;29(9):1125-1132.

[57] Zervas K, Verrou E, Teleioudis Z, et al. Incidence, risk factors and management of osteonecrosis of the jaw in patients with multiple myeloma: a single-centre experience in 303 patients. *Br J Haematol.* 2006;134(6):620-623.

[58] Dimopoulos MA, Kastritis E, Bamia C, et al. Reduction of osteonecrosis of the jaw (ONJ) after implementation of preventive measures in patients with multiple myeloma treated with zoledronic acid. *Ann Oncol.* 2009;20(1):117-120.

[59] Hortobagyi GN, Theriault RL, Porter L, et al. Efficacy of pamidronate in reducing skeletal complications in patients with breast cancer and lytic bone metastases. Protocol

19 Aredia Breast Cancer Study Group. The New England journal of medicine 1996;335:1785-91.
[60] Cohen MH, Dagher R, Griebel DJ, et al. U.S. Food and Drug Administration drug approval summaries: imatinib mesylate, mesna tablets, and zoledronic acid. The oncologist 2002;7:393-400.
[61] Coleman RE. Skeletal complications of malignancy. Cancer 1997;80:1588-94.
[62] Lipton A, Theriault RL, Hortobagyi GN, et al. Pamidronate prevents skeletal complications and is effective palliative treatment in women with breast carcinoma and osteolytic bone metastases: long term follow-up of two randomized, placebo-controlled trials. Cancer 2000;88:1082-90.
[63] Lipton A, Small E, Saad F, et al. The new bisphosphonate, Zometa (zoledronic acid), decreases skeletal complications in both osteolytic and osteoblastic lesions: a comparison to pamidronate. Cancer investigation 2002;20 Suppl 2:45-54.
[64] Kohno N, Aogi K, Minami H, et al. Zoledronic acid significantly reduces skeletal complications compared with placebo in Japanese women with bone metastases from breast cancer: a randomized, placebo-controlled trial. Journal of clinical oncology : official journal of the American Society of Clinical Oncology 2005;23:3314-21.
[65] Rosen LS, Gordon D, Kaminski M, et al. Long-term efficacy and safety of zoledronic acid compared with pamidronate disodium in the treatment of skeletal complications in patients with advanced multiple myeloma or breast carcinoma: a randomized, double-blind, multicenter, comparative trial. Cancer 2003;98:1735-44.
[66] Wardley A, Davidson N, Barrett-Lee P, et al. Zoledronic acid significantly improves pain scores and quality of life in breast cancer patients with bone metastases: a randomised, crossover study of community vs hospital bisphosphonate administration. British journal of cancer 2005;92:1869-76.
[67] Barrett-Lee P, Casbard A, Abraham J, et al. Oral ibandronic acid versus intravenous zoledronic acid in treatment of bone metastases from breast cancer: a randomised, open label, non-inferiority phase 3 trial. The lancet oncology 2014;15:114-22.
[68] Wong MH, Stockler MR, Pavlakis N. Bisphosphonates and other bone agents for breast cancer. The Cochrane database of systematic reviews 2012;2:CD003474.
[69] Shapiro CL, Halabi S, Hars V, et al. Zoledronic acid preserves bone mineral density in premenopausal women who develop ovarian failure due to adjuvant chemotherapy: final results from CALGB trial 79809. European journal of cancer 2011;47:683-9.
[70] Gnant MF, Mlineritsch B, Luschin-Ebengreuth G, et al. Zoledronic acid prevents cancer treatment-induced bone loss in premenopausal women receiving adjuvant endocrine therapy for hormone-responsive breast cancer: a report from the Austrian Breast and Colorectal Cancer Study Group. Journal of clinical oncology : official journal of the American Society of Clinical Oncology 2007;25:820-8.
[71] Amadori D, Aglietta M, Alessi B, et al. Efficacy and safety of 12-weekly versus 4-weekly zoledronic acid for prolonged treatment of patients with bone metastases from breast cancer (ZOOM): a phase 3, open-label, randomised, non-inferiority trial. The lancet oncology 2013;14:663-70.
[72] Van Poznak CH, Temin S, Yee GC, et al. American Society of Clinical Oncology executive summary of the clinical practice guideline update on the role of bone-modifying agents in metastatic breast cancer. Journal of clinical oncology : official journal of the American Society of Clinical Oncology 2011;29:1221-7.

[73] Mortimer JE, Schulman K, Kohles JD. Patterns of bisphosphonate use in the United States in the treatment of metastatic bone disease. Clinical breast cancer 2007;7:682-9.
[74] Clemons MJ, Dranitsaris G, Ooi WS, et al. Phase II trial evaluating the palliative benefit of second-line zoledronic acid in breast cancer patients with either a skeletal-related event or progressive bone metastases despite first-line bisphosphonate therapy. Journal of clinical oncology : official journal of the American Society of Clinical Oncology 2006;24:4895-900.
[75] Rosen LS, Gordon D, Tchekmedyian S, et al. Zoledronic acid versus placebo in the treatment of skeletal metastases in patients with lung cancer and other solid tumors: a phase III, double-blind, randomized trial--the Zoledronic Acid Lung Cancer and Other Solid Tumors Study Group. Journal of clinical oncology : official journal of the American Society of Clinical Oncology 2003;21:3150-7.
[76] Rosen LS, Gordon D, Tchekmedyian NS, et al. Long-term efficacy and safety of zoledronic acid in the treatment of skeletal metastases in patients with nonsmall cell lung carcinoma and other solid tumors: a randomized, Phase III, double-blind, placebo-controlled trial. Cancer 2004;100:2613-21.
[77] Hatoum HT, Lin SJ, Smith MR, Barghout V, Lipton A. Zoledronic acid and skeletal complications in patients with solid tumors and bone metastases: analysis of a national medical claims database. Cancer 2008;113:1438-45.
[78] Saad F, Gleason DM, Murray R, et al. A randomized, placebo-controlled trial of zoledronic acid in patients with hormone-refractory metastatic prostate carcinoma. Journal of the National Cancer Institute 2002;94:1458-68.
[79] Saad F, Gleason DM, Murray R, et al. Long-term efficacy of zoledronic acid for the prevention of skeletal complications in patients with metastatic hormone-refractory prostate cancer. Journal of the National Cancer Institute 2004;96:879-82.
[80] Small EJ, Smith MR, Seaman JJ, Petrone S, Kowalski MO. Combined analysis of two multicenter, randomized, placebo-controlled studies of pamidronate disodium for the palliation of bone pain in men with metastatic prostate cancer. Journal of clinical oncology : official journal of the American Society of Clinical Oncology 2003;21:4277-84.
[81] Wirth M, Tammela T, Cicalese V, et al. Prevention of Bone Metastases in Patients with High-risk Non-metastatic Prostate Cancer Treated with Zoledronic Acid: Efficacy and Safety Results of the Zometa European Study (ZEUS). European urology 2014 (in press)
[82] Smith MR, Eastham J, Gleason DM, Shasha D, Tchekmedyian S, Zinner N. Randomized controlled trial of zoledronic acid to prevent bone loss in men receiving androgen deprivation therapy for nonmetastatic prostate cancer. The Journal of urology 2003;169:2008-12.
[83] Black DM, Delmas PD, Eastell R, et al. Once-yearly zoledronic acid for treatment of postmenopausal osteoporosis. *N Engl J Med*. 2007;356(18):1809–1822.
[84] Lyles KW, Colon-Emeric CS, Magaziner JS, et al. Zoledronic acid and clinical fractures and mortality after hip fracture. *N Engl J Med*.2007;357:1799–1809.
[85] McClung M, Recker R, Miller P, et al. Intravenous zoledronic acid 5 mg in the treatment of postmenopausal women with low bone density previously treated with alendronate. *Bone*. 2007;41(1):122–128.

[86] Saag K, Lindsay R, Kriegman A, Beamer E, Zhou W. A single zoledronic acid infusion reduces bone resorption markers more rapidly than weekly oral alendronate in postmenopausal women with low bone mineral density. *Bone*. 2007;40(5):1238–1243.

[87] Reid DM, Devogelaer JP, Saag K, et al. Zoledronic acid and risedronate in the prevention and treatment of glucocorticoid-induced osteoporosis (HORIZON): a multicentre, double-blind, double-dummy, randomised controlled trial. *Lancet*. 2009;373(9671):1253–1263.

[88] Reid IR, Miller P, Lyles K, et al. Comparison of a single infusion of zoledronic acid with risedronate for Paget's disease. *N Engl J Med*.2005;353(9):898–908.

[89] Hosking D, Lyles K, Brown JP, et al. Long-term control of bone turnover in Paget's disease with zoledronic acid and risedronate. *J Bone Miner Res*. 2007;22(1):142–148.

[90] Boonen S, Black DM, Colón-Emeric CS, et al. Efficacy and safety of a once-yearly intravenous zoledronic acid 5 mg for fracture prevention in elderly osteoporotic postmenopausal women aged 75 years and older. *J Am Geriatr Soc*. 2010;58(2):292–299.

[91] Orwoll ES, Miller PD, Adachi JD, et al. Efficacy and safety of a once-yearly i.v. Infusion of zoledronic acid 5 mg versus a once-weekly 70-mg oral alendronate in the treatment of male osteoporosis: a randomized, multicenter, double-blind, active-controlled study. J Bone Miner Res. 2010 Oct;25(10):2239-50

INDEX

B

C

D

E

H

I

J

K

L

M

Q

R

S

T

U

V

W

X

Y

Z